Medical Contact Lens Practice
a systematic approach

Medical
Contact Lens
Practice

a systematic
approach

Ian A. Mackie MB, ChB, DO, FRCS, FCOphth

Emeritus Associate Specialist, St George's
Hospital, London, UK
Formerly Associate Specialist, External Eye
Disease Clinic, Moorfields Eye Hospital,
London, UK

BUTTERWORTH
HEINEMANN

Butterworth-Heinemann Ltd
Linacre House, Jordan Hill, Oxford OX2 8DP

A member of the Reed Elsevier group

OXFORD LONDON BOSTON
MUNICH NEW DELHI SINGAPORE SYDNEY
TOKYO TORONTO WELLINGTON

First published 1993

© Butterworth-Heinemann Ltd 1993

British Library Cataloguing in Publication Data

Mackie, Ian A.
  Medical Contact Lens Practice:
  a systematic approach
  I. Title
  617.7523

ISBN 0 7506 0939 7

Library of Congress Cataloguing in Publication Data

Mackie, Ian A.
  Medical contact lens practice: a systematic approach/Ian A. Mackie.
  p. cm.
  Includes bibliographical references and index.
  ISBN 0 7506 0939 7
  1. Contact lenses. I. Title.
  [DNLM: 1. Contact Lenses. WW 355 M158m 1993]
  RE977.C6M24   1993
  617.7'523—dc20
  DNLM/DLC
  for Library of Congress   93-3876
                                                                 CIP

Typeset by Keytec Typesetting Ltd, Bridport, Dorset

Printed and bound in Hong Kong by Dah Hua Printing Co Ltd

Contents

Acknowledgements   vi

1   Introduction   1

2   Handling of Contact Lenses by the
    Ophthalmologist   3

3   Fitting Scleral Lenses   7

4   Fitting Hard Corneal Lenses   19

5   Gas Permeable Lenses   45

6   Fitting Soft Contact Lenses   55

7   Fitting Toric Contact Lenses   59

8   Handling of Contact Lenses by the
    Patient   67

9   Care of Contact Lenses   71

10 Refraction Problems related to Contact
    Lens Wear   101

11 Adverse Reactions to Scleral
    Lenses   107

12 Adverse Reactions to Hard Corneal
    Lenses   109

13 Adverse Reactions to Soft Contact
    Lenses   124

14 Therapeutic Uses of Contact
    Lenses   164

15 Keratoconus   191

16 Corneal Grafts and Other Surgical
    Procedures   202

17 Aphakia   208

18 Presbyopia   215

Index   223

Acknowledgements

I must thank the several ophthalmologists and opticians who read parts of this book at an early stage of its preparation.

In the intermediate stage of its gestation some chapters were read by Dr Donald Korb, OD of Boston, USA. He made many valuable suggestions and drew my attention to some important references. As a close friend for many years, he has had a large influence on my thinking about contact lenses.

I must also thank those ophthalmologists, in Europe and America, who have made their published photographs and figures available to me. They are acknowledged in the text.

In its final stages, the book was critically evaluated by Professor Noel Dilly of the Anatomy and Ophthalmology Departments of St George's Medical School and Hospital in London, and by Dr Peter Heyworth, who was a Senior Hospital Medical Officer in Ophthalmology at St George's Hospital at that time. They spent a lot of time and effort and their invaluable input is greatly appreciated.

Dr Sarah Parker (née Hamilton), a former House Surgeon in Ophthalmology at St George's Hospital, was the subject of the pictures on insertion and removal of contact lenses and I am very grateful to her.

Last, but not least, I must thank George Nissel and Company Ltd, of Hemel Hempstead, Hertfordshire, for allowing me to photograph the stages in manufacture of scleral contact lenses, and No 7 Laboratory of London, W1, for letting me photograph the stages in the making of hard corneal contact lenses. David Stubbs of A.S. Optics, Cheam, Surrey, was very helpful in calculating edge lifts of hard contact lenses and I thank him also.

1

Introduction

The ophthalmologist cannot fail to be aware of the added difficulties in diagnosis and management when a patient wearing contact lenses presents before him. There is always the bother, and perhaps difficulty, of getting the lenses in and out and then there is the question of whether or not the disease is related to the contact lenses.

The author has consistently found that a patient with contact lenses presenting in a clinic is much more likely to have contact lens related problems than other ophthalmological problems.

It is not enough for the doctor to take the easy way out and tell the patient to stop wearing the lenses altogether, as is often done. This is a tragedy for many patients and the advice is likely to alienate the patient against the doctor. Furthermore, there is a large number of patients who can only see properly with the use of contact lenses. They also can suffer from contact lens related external ocular disease. Experience in dealing with the cosmetic group problems is valuable in treating those whose sight depends on contact lenses.

It is, therefore, important to know how to diagnose and treat contact lens complications, while, at the same time, maintaining the patient's status as a contact lens wearer. It may mean referral to an ophthalmologist who specializes in contact lens problems.

There are estimated to be 2 000 000 wearers of contact lenses in the UK. This compares with about 800 000 diabetics. Both conditions have their ophthalmic complications, some of which can be very serious. Great emphasis has been made in British ophthalmology on the recognition, prevention and treatment of diabetic complications, but, sadly, little attention has been paid to the understanding of contact lenses and their adverse effects. This book attempts to redress this omission.

The fitting of contact lenses is an art and a science and keeps many people happily interested, even fascinated, in full employment. Badly fitted contact lenses, just like shoes that do not fit, can be uncomfortable and produce physical signs. Some patients find that perfectly fitting lenses are uncomfortable. They may be the wrong type for that particular patient. The discomfort leads to redness of the bulbar conjuctivae and lid margins. When this is associated with a few follicles and papillae, which may be within the bounds of normality for many eyes, it can cause some ophthalmologists to become very concerned that the patient has a chronic conjunctivitis of some sort. Such problems are not resolved with lid scrubs and antibiotics.

The problems associated with the wearing of hard corneal, hard scleral and soft contact lenses are quite different and will be dealt with in separate chapters in this book.

For the past 20 years or so, since the enthusiastic reports of Kaufman in Gainsville, soft contact lenses have been used in the treatment of all sorts of external disease and this is no longer the exclusive field of the contact lens specialist. This book outlines the author's experience in this area. He has attempted a mini review of those external eye diseases in which therapeutic contact lenses may play a part in the therapy and has tried to define their role in relation to other modalities of treatment.

The author apologizes for the detailed chapters on fitting contact lenses. He has consulted many contact lens textbooks which are complete with many diagrams, mathematical formulae, chemical formulae, tables, historical reviews and such which have actually very little information on fitting. He has tried to emphasize the principles of fitting so that the non-fitting ophthalmologist can recognize good or bad fits. After all, the problems may only be in the fitting.

There is also the vexed problem of the care of contact lenses. Here the author has always tried to present information from independent published papers rather than copy the manufacturers' promotional literature. Here there are many conflicting opinions. The reader will have to make up his or her own mind from the information given as to which products are the best to use. The care regimen is intimately related to the continuing health of the eyes in a contact lens wearer.

Many of the coloured illustrations in this book are of microscopic details and should be viewed in bright daylight.

2

Handling of contact lenses by the ophthalmologist

Many ophthalmologists never become interested in contact lenses because they have never learned to handle them. They cannot insert them and they cannot remove them and in order to save embarrassment they do not try. The author takes part in a teaching course at a London teaching hospital and finds that a considerable number of ophthalmologists have great difficulty.

This chapter details a simple methodology which can be altered or abandoned as the practitioner gains more experience, but will serve to put him on the right road.

The swan hold

Even accustomed contact lens wearers are apprehensive when having someone else insert and remove contact lenses and this apprehension is considerably greater in the patient who has never

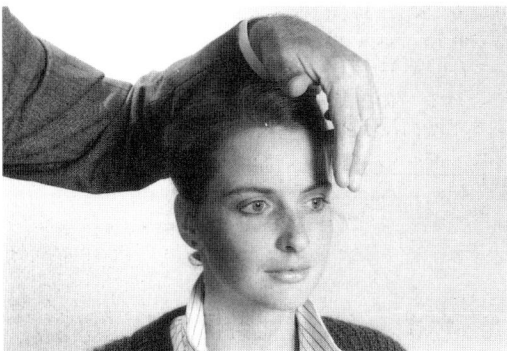

Figure 2.1 The swan hold. The left elbow is placed against the back of the patient's head and the hand drops over the patient's forehead

worn contact lenses. The instinct is to retract the head and get out of the way of the oncoming contact lens and this is where the swan hold is necessary (Figure 2.1). The ophthalmologist stands on the right hand side of the patient if he is right handed (the procedure is reversed if he is left handed). His left arm is placed in such a position that his elbow is against the back of the patient's head and his left hand, with out-stretched fingers, drops over the patient's forehead. These outstretched fingers can be used to manipulate the upper lid and, with the upper lid, the lens.

Inserting a hard corneal lens

If the lens is being inserted for the first time and for the purpose of fitting, it is convenient to instil a drop of sodium benoxinate 0.4% before applying the lens. This makes the procedure more comfortable for the patient and it also diminishes the reflex flow of tears which can interfere with the assessment of the fitting.

Do not instil amethocaine. It is epitheliotoxic. After the insertion of the lens, marked corneal epithelial staining will be found when fluorescein is introduced. This precludes the assessment of the fitting with the use of fluorescein and ultra-violet light.

The lens is washed and placed wet on the wet forefinger of the ophthalmologist's right hand. The left hand employs the swan hold and its fingers hold up the upper lid, including its lashes (Figure 2.2). The upper lid should always be kept in apposition with the eye. The right hand fore-

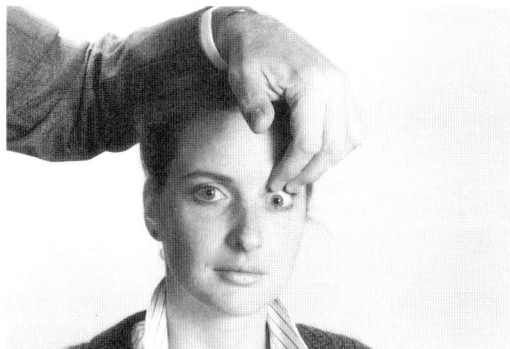

Figure 2.2 Insertion of hard corneal lens. The upper lid, including its lashes, is held up by the fingers which keep it in apposition with the eye

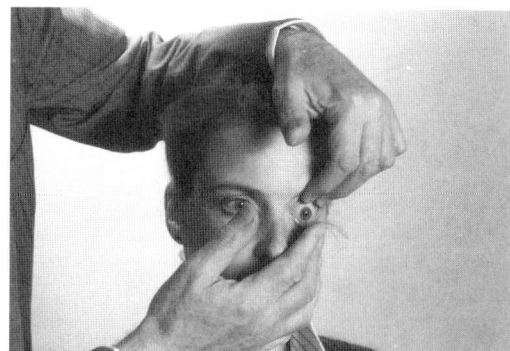

Figure 2.3 Insertion of hard corneal lens. The second finger of the right hand pulls down the lower lid and the forefinger places the lens on the cornea. This right hand is the first to be withdrawn

finger approaches the eye. The second finger of this hand pulls down the lower lid and the fore-finger places the lens on the cornea (Figure 2.3). The right hand is withdrawn first, releasing the lower lid (and this sequence is important) and then the left hand is withdrawn, releasing the upper lid.

Removing a hard corneal lens

The swan hold is employed with the left hand. The forefinger of this hand holds the upper lid in apposition with the eye above the edge of the corneal lens. The right hand forefinger holds the lower lid in apposition with the eye below the edge of the corneal lens. The two lids are then gently brought together with the forefingers so

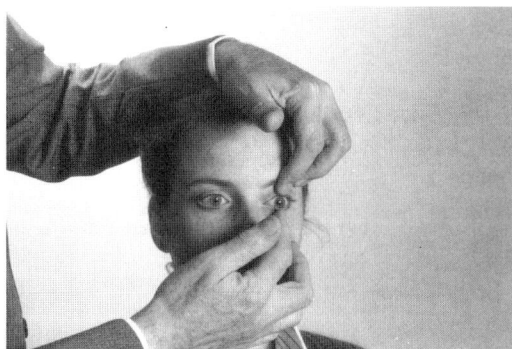

Figure 2.4 Removal of hard corneal lens. The forefinger of the left hand holds the upper lid in apposition with the eye above the edge of the lens. The right hand forefinger holds the lower lid in apposition with the eye below the corneal lens. The two fingers are gently brought together

that the corneal lens is first trapped and then ejected (Figure 2.4).

If the corneal lens is fitted according to the lens lid attachment technique, then it is frequently only necessary to touch the top lid with the left forefinger to make the hard lens lift off the eye below. It can then be grasped by the forefinger and thumb of the right hand. If the lens is displaced onto the conjunctiva on either side of the cornea the patient is instructed to look in the opposite direction to the position of the lens. This bares the conjunctiva in the area of the lens and it is removed by the forefingers acting against the lids, as above.

If the lens is displaced into the superior fornix the patient is instructed to look down and the left forefinger is used against the lid to bring it into position on the cornea, from where it can be removed as described above.

If the lens is displaced into the lower fornix the patient is instructed to look up and the lens is pushed up by the right forefinger against the lower lid onto the cornea and removed as described above. It can frequently be removed by the two forefingers acting against the lids without replacing it on the cornea.

Inserting a soft contact lens

The lens is conveniently removed from its bottle with a lens lift (Figure 2.5) (obtainable from

Lamda Polytech Ltd, 1 Lincoln Park, Borough Road, Northants NN1 3SE).

The swan hold is employed with the left hand and the forefinger holds up the lid and its lashes. The soft contact lens is placed on the right, dry forefinger with its inner side uppermost. The right hand forefinger approaches the eye. The second finger of this hand pulls down the lower lid and the forefinger places the lens on the cornea (Figure 2.6). The right hand is then withdrawn, releasing the lower lid and when the lens is seen to be settled on the cornea the left hand is withdrawn, releasing the upper lid. This sequence is important. With a tight fitting lens such as the Sauflon 85 therapeutic soft lens, it may be advisable to push it in apposition with the cornea

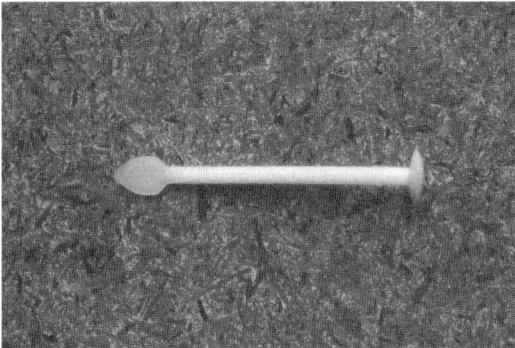

Figure 2.7 Removal of soft contact lens. The patient is instructed to look up and the second finger of the right hand pulls down the lower lid. The forefinger of this right hand brings the lens down into the lower fornix from where it is removed by gently pinching

with the right forefinger as it has a high chance of being displaced when the top lid is released, if there is a large air bubble underneath it.

Removing a soft contact lens

The head is held with the left hand. The patient is instructed to look up. The second finger of the right hand pulls down the lower lid and the forefinger is placed on the soft lens and brings it down into the inferior fornix (Figure 2.7). It is then pinched by the right forefinger and thumb and removed.

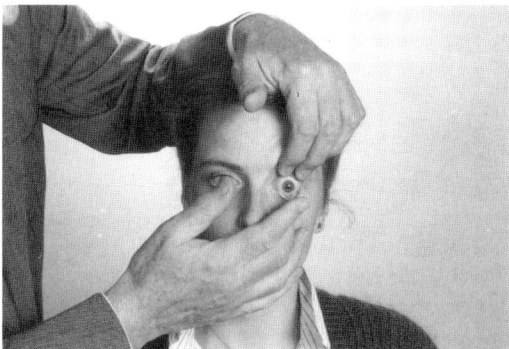

Figure 2.5 Lens lift with soft contact lens attached. This can be used for both handling and inspection of the lens with binocular operating spectacles or a slit lamp microscope

Inserting a scleral lens

The swan grip is employed by the left hand and its forefinger holds the upper lid and its lashes up and away from the globe. The scleral lens is held with the thumb and forefinger and orientated for its position on the eye with the fenestration placed temporally and any marking spot above (Figure 2.8). The forefinger of the left hand gently pulls on the upper lid and the lens is slipped under it. The forefinger of the left hand then steadies the lens while the forefinger of the right hand pulls the lower lid down and over the lower edge of the scleral lens (Figure 2.9). If the lens is not fenestrated or otherwise ventilated it must

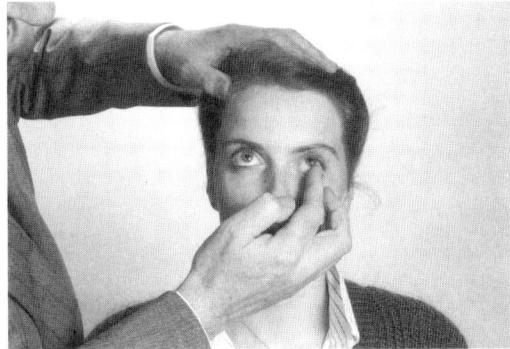

Figure 2.6 Insertion of soft contact lens. The second finger of the right hand pulls down the lower lid and the forefinger places the lens on the cornea. This right hand is the first to be withdrawn

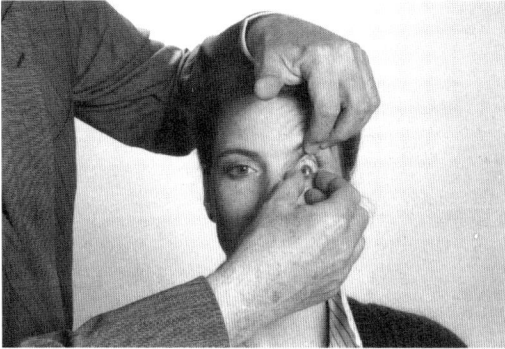

Figure 2.8 Insertion of scleral lens. The forefinger of the left hand gently pulls on the upper lid and the lens is slipped under it

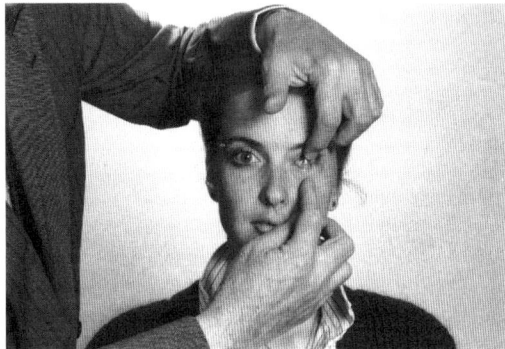

Figure 2.9 Insertion of scleral lens. The forefinger of the left hand steadies the lens while the forefinger of the right hand pulls the lower lid down over the lower edge of the lens

first be filled with saline and the patient should be instructed to bend down so that he is facing the floor before the insertion takes place.

Removing a scleral lens

The right hand is placed open under the patient's eye to catch the lens. The patient is instructed to look down. The left forefinger is placed on the upper lid which is lifted to a position above the upper edge of the lens. The lens is then lifted off the eye with the left forefinger against the lid (Figure 2.10).

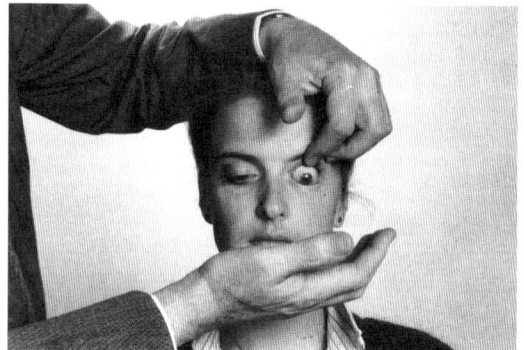

Figure 2.10 Removal of scleral lens. The left forefinger is placed on the upper lid which is lifted to a position above the upper edge of the lens. Gentle pushing will dislodge the lens from the eye

3

Fitting scleral lenses

Scleral lenses still play a part in the management of eye disorders. They were formerly called haptic lenses. They may be the only practical method of correcting the vision in many eyes in which the corneas are grossly distorted. There is a very small number of patients still wearing them having been fitted in the 1940s, 1950s and 1960s.

Scleral lenses are usually made of glass or polymethylmethacrylate. They can now be made of gas permeable materials (Ezekiel, 1983; Pullum, 1987; Pullum, Parker and Hobley, 1989; Schein, Rosenthal and Ducharme, 1990). The Pullum *et al.* lenses are 'moulded' from eye impressions. The Schein *et al.* lenses are 'preformed'. These terms will be explained later. Very few workers remain who can make the lenses in glass.

When the original scleral lenses were fitted in the late 19th and early 20th centuries tolerance was often poor, often amounting to only two or three hours due to the development of corneal oedema. However, patients varied in their susceptibility to this oedema. The practice of 'ventilation' started in the late 1940s. A 'fenestration' – a small hole 1.5–2.0 mm in diameter – was introduced into the lens just within the corneal portion on the temporal side on the horizontal axis. This procedure greatly improved the tolerance. It was found that if the bubble of air introduced behind the lens by this fenestration did not move, localized corneal drying would occur with subsequent scarring and vascularization of the cornea in the area which the bubble covered (see Figure 11.1). Accordingly, it was laid down as a principle that the bubble should rotate round the limbus as the eye moved in different directions.

Another method of ventilation was introduced at Moorfields Eye Hospital, London, in the 1950s.

This was 'channelling' (see Figure 3.3). Channels are introduced in the scleral portion of the lens, usually above. This is not such an effective method of ventilation as fenestration, but the fitting is much simpler and quicker and it may be that this is all that is required in a grossly diseased eye.

A further method of ventilation has recently been introduced. This is 'slotting' (see Figure 3.3) (Pullum, 1984; Pullum and Trodd, 1984). It had been noted that a crescentic aperture cut from the area of the superior transition in a scleral lens was often as effective in correcting ptosis as a prop which fitted to the front of the superior scleral portion. Then it was found that these slotted lenses ventilated extremely well and were easier to fit in patients without ptosis than the conventional fenestrated lens. These lenses are now used extensively in patients with keratoconus.

Two methods of fitting scleral lenses may be employed. The first is by taking an impression of the eye and moulding a lens to the shape of the impression. The second is by using preformed scleral lenses.

Experienced fitters of scleral lenses usually have their own laboratory with pressing, grinding and polishing equipment. Nowadays the demand for scleral lenses is so small that such a laboratory is only justified in large centres or when a particular contact lens practitioner has a special interest in scleral lenses.

The occasional scleral lens fitter who is remote from a specialist or a large centre can, however, fit scleral lenses by using a remote laboratory to do all the modifications and polishing and it is with this sort of person in mind that the following text has been written.

Moulded hard scleral lenses

Moulding

The patient is placed in a recumbent position with the eye fixing a target so that it is slightly convergent and is looking neither up nor down. The eye should then be covered to ensure that this fixation is maintained. If it is not, the target (as seen by the other eye) should be moved until the desired position is obtained.

The eye is then anaesthetized with sodium benoxinate 0.4% (Smith and Nephew Ltd). This anaesthetic has a minimal toxic effect on corneal epithelium, unlike amethocaine, which is toxic and rapidly produces a very friable epithelium. The moulding material is then prepared (see Appendix 3.I).

An impression shell (Figure 3.1) is then inserted into the eye so that the horizontal marker is in line with the fornices. The shell should be as large as the eye can accommodate. The moulding material is then inserted into a 10 ml syringe and injected into the impression shell while pulling the shell slightly away from the eye and moving it from side to side so that it is completely filled. The impression shell is then maintained in its original position until the moulding material has gelled.

The impression shell is then carefully removed from the eye, first from the lower fornix and then from the upper fornix by gently manipulating the lids and then it is placed in a holder with its concave surface uppermost.

Preparation of the cast

A positive cast is then made of the mould with plaster or dental stone (see Appendix 3.II). The mould should be fully filled so that its edges are overlapped with casting material. Pouring the casting material down one side of the mould and not directly into it will help to avoid the entrapment of air bubbles.

There is a conventional way of marking and identifying the cast (Figure 3.2). The horizontal line is marked on the posterior surface of the cast to be continuous on either side with the horizontal line on the impression shell. The nasal side of the cast is marked above the line with an 'N' and the temporal side is marked with a 'T'. Between these two letters is put an 'R' or 'L', according to whether it is a cast of the right or the left eye. The patient's name, with, perhaps, the date is written under the horizontal line.

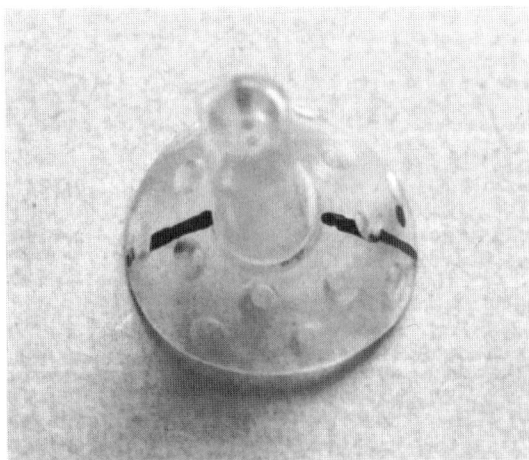

Figure 3.1 An impression shell with perforations of the scleral portion, a funnel for the introduction of moulding material and marked horizontal line

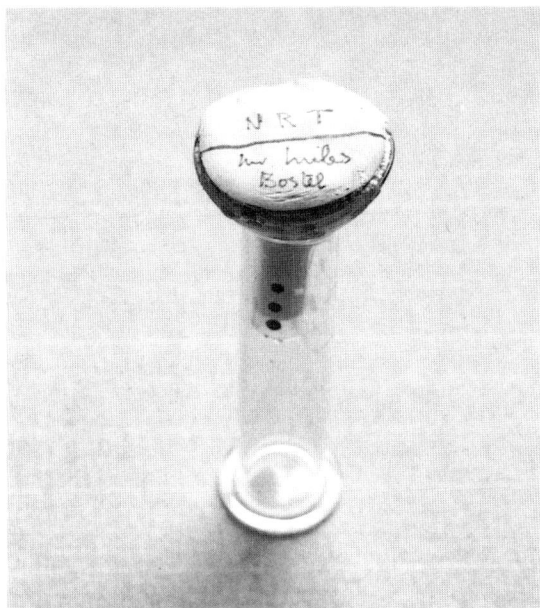

Figure 3.2 The cast is prepared by filling the mould (still in contact with the moulding shell) with casting material. The horizontal line is marked, together with the nasal and temporal orientation and the patient's name

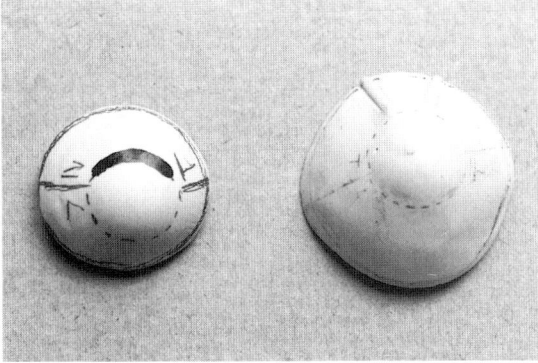

Figure 3.3 Casts for slotted and channelled scleral lenses. The cast on the left hand side has been marked with a horizontal line and with the area where a slot is to be introduced. The cast on the right hand side has had the impressions for channelling applied by the laboratory

If it is to be a channelled scleral lens, the positions of the channels are marked on the lens and the laboratory technician will modify the cast appropriately in these positions. If it is to be a slotted scleral lens, the position of the slot is marked on the cast (Figure 3.3).

Preparation of the shell

The usual direction to the laboratory is to 'prepare a shell to the full dimensions of the cast'.

The laboratory technician will take a plastic sheet of polymethylmethacrylate, 2.25 inches square (54 mm) and 2.5 mm or 3.0 mm thick, insert it in a press and, with the aid of heat, mould it over the cast (Figure 3.4).

He will then trim the shell to the dimensions of the cast (Figure 3.5). Twelve millimetre diameter 'formers' are then inserted against the inside of the corneal portion of the plastic shell to see which fits best. These formers are usually in steps of 0.25 mm radius (Figure 3.6). Conformity is assessed by noting the pattern of Newton's rings. A grinding tool, 12 mm in diameter and 0.2 mm or 0.3 mm flatter than the radius determined by the former, is then used to fashion an optical surface on the back of the corneal portion of the shell (Figure 3.7). Grinding is stopped when the grinding tool reaches the centre of the corneal portion.

The thickness of the corneal portion is then measured (Figure 3.8). The usual direction to the laboratory is to 'give 0.1 mm corneal clearance', that is, grind out from the inside of the corneal portion with a tool of the same radius as previously used, 0.1 mm in thickness. (Some fitters

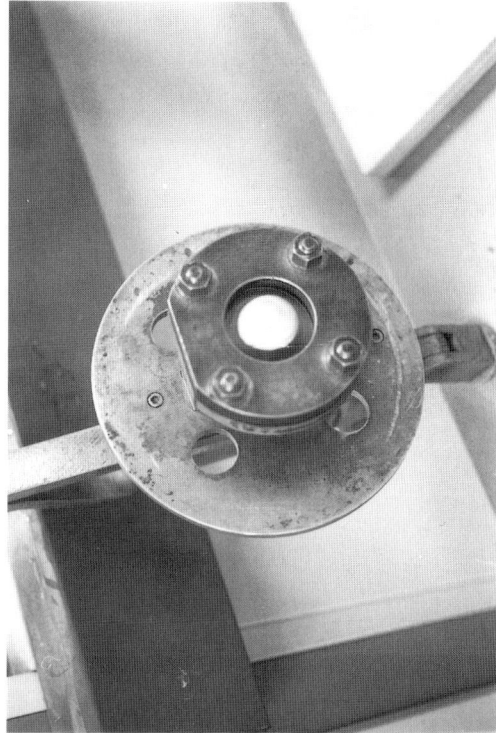

Figure 3.4 The plastic sheet is inserted in a press and, with the aid of heat from an infrared bulb below, is moulded over the cast

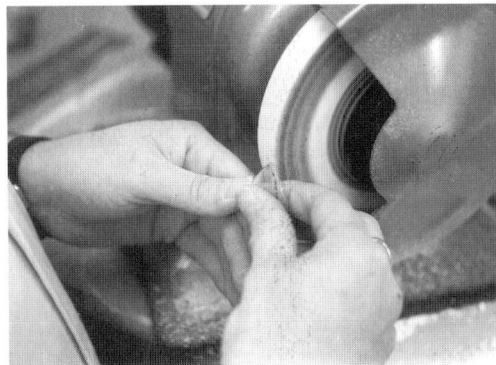

Figure 3.5 The shell is trimmed to the dimensions of the cast

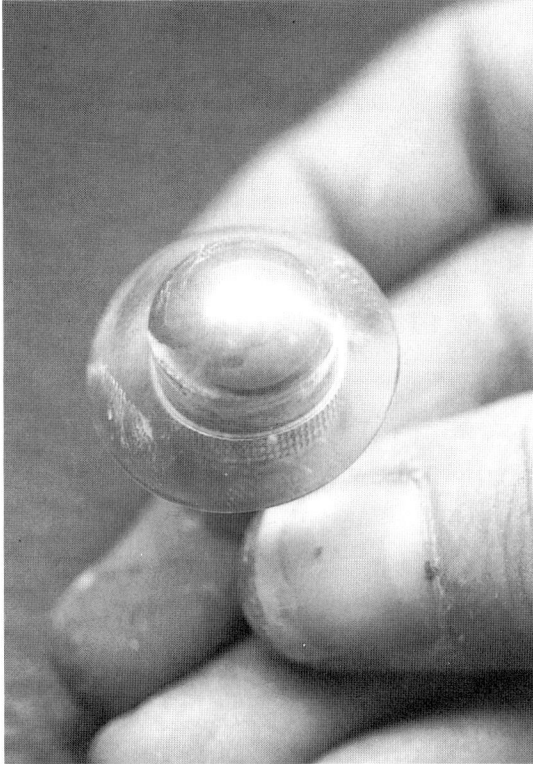

Figure 3.6 Twelve millimetre formers are inserted against the inside of the corneal portion of the plastic shell to ascertain which fits best

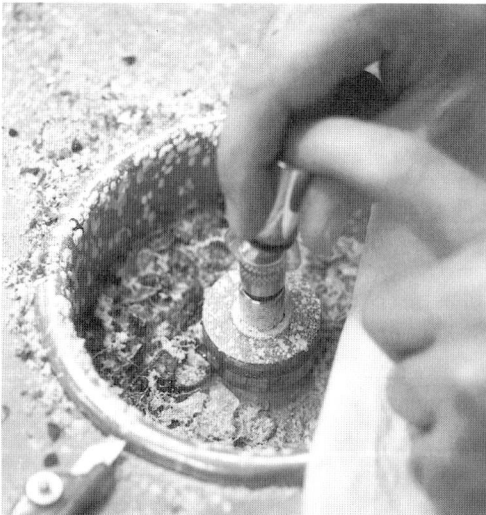

Figure 3.7 A 12 mm grinding tool, 0.2 mm or 0.3 mm flatter in radius than that determined by the former, is used to fashion an optical surface on the back of the corneal portion of the shell

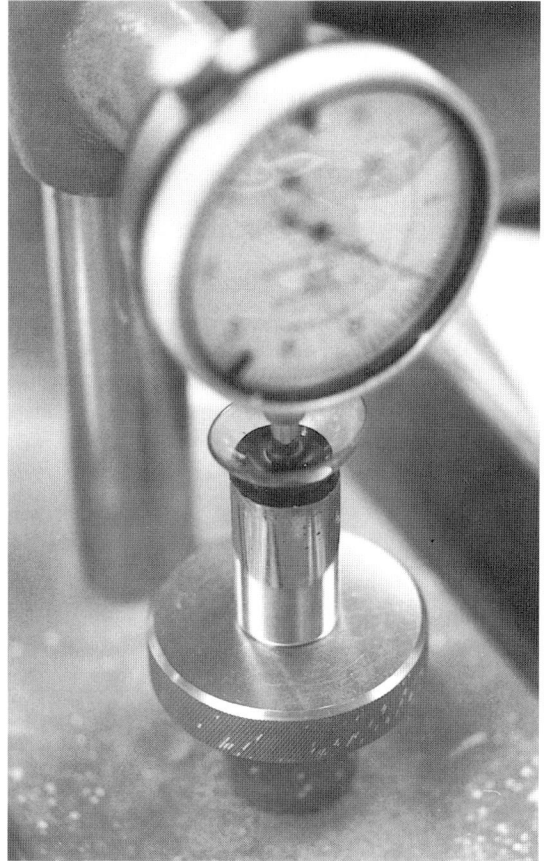

Figure 3.8 The thickness of the corneal portion is measured. After this has been done, 0.1 mm is usually ground out from the back surface of this corneal portion

order 0.2 or 0.25 mm corneal clearance, but it is best for a start to proceed slowly because excessive corneal clearance can only be remedied by extensive grinding inside the scleral portion.) Alternatively, mean keratometer readings may be taken and the direction given that 'the posterior corneal portion should be ground to a radius 0.2 to 0.3 mm flatter than the specified mean keratometer readings'. Again 0.1 mm corneal clearance should be ordered.

The laboratory technician then takes an 18 mm diameter grinding tool, usually 1.0 mm flatter than the back corneal curve which has been chosen, and generates the transition zone which is usually 1.5–2.0 mm wide on either side. This is done by moving the shell by hand over the grinding tool in a circular fashion to follow the existing

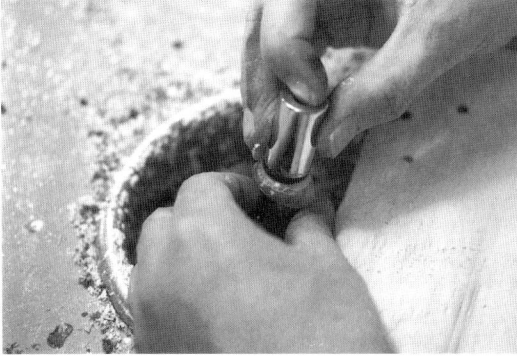

Figure 3.9 An 18 mm diameter grinding tool, usually 1.0 mm flatter than the back corneal curve, grinds out the transition zone between the corneal and scleral portions

surface and blend with curves on the corneal and scleral portions of the shell (Figure 3.9).

Preparation of the scleral lens

The shell and the cast will be returned by the laboratory. The shell should be fitted on the cast and a horizontal line marked with a waterproof pen to coincide with the horizontal line marked on the cast. The shell is filled with saline and inserted in the eye. This is done in the usual manner as described in Chapter 2, but the patient should be bent forwards so that the shell filled with saline can be held in a horizontal position. It is not necessary to fill a slotted, or fenestrated, lens with saline.

After some 15 minutes it should be ascertained whether the shell is fitting so that the horizontal line is in the correct position. Rotation is usually caused by two tight areas on the scleral portion which are opposite one another and this can usually be remedied later. If indicated, the shell should be marked for fenestration. This is usually done temporally and *within* the corneal portion, at its periphery, on the horizontal line.

The shell is removed from the eye and fenestration is performed with a drill, 1.5–2.0 mm in diameter (Figure 3.10). The hole should then be polished with a boxwood stick (obtainable from a jeweller's merchant) and Silvo polish (Reckitt and Sons Ltd, Hull).

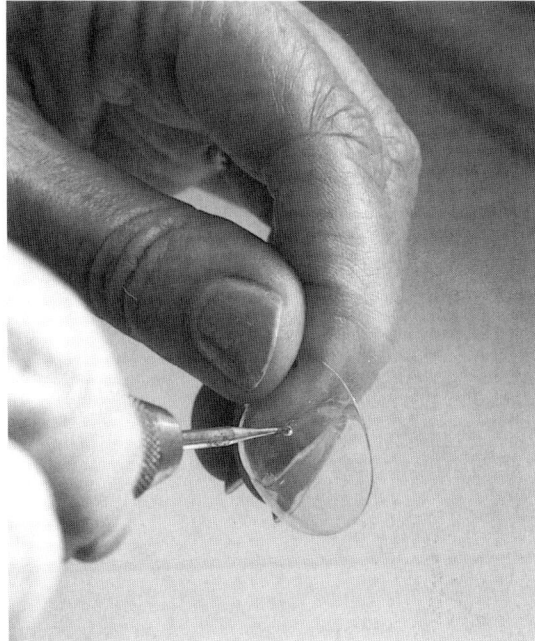

Figure 3.10 The shell is 'fenestrated' with a drill 1.5 mm to 2.0 mm in diameter. The hole is then polished with a boxwood stick and Silvo polish

The shell is reinserted. After 15 minutes, when the shell has settled back, a drop of fluorescein is introduced at the fenestration hole and the shell is examined for fit under ultraviolet black light (a Burton lamp).

The principles of fitting were laid down many years ago. The scleral portion of the shell must fit the white of the eye as evenly as possible. Unevenness of the scleral fit can be assessed by noting any areas of conjunctival vessel blanching or standoff of the edge of the shell from the conjunctiva (Figure 3.11). An uneven scleral fit will be uncomfortable, but is seldom associated with a pathological ocular reaction.

Blanched areas are marked with a waterproof pen and the shell is sent to the laboratory technician with the direction to give 0.1 mm clearance. This can be increased at a subsequent adjustment. Any edge standoff is marked for the attention of the laboratory technician, who may be able to heat the plastic and adjust the edge. This situation may, however, require a further impression of the eye being taken.

When the scleral fit is even, the fit of the corneal and transition portions of the shell can be

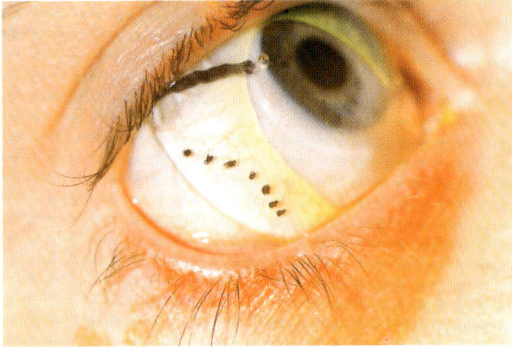

Figure 3.11 The area where the shell causes conjunctival blanching is marked with a pen so that the laboratory can grind it out to give more clearance

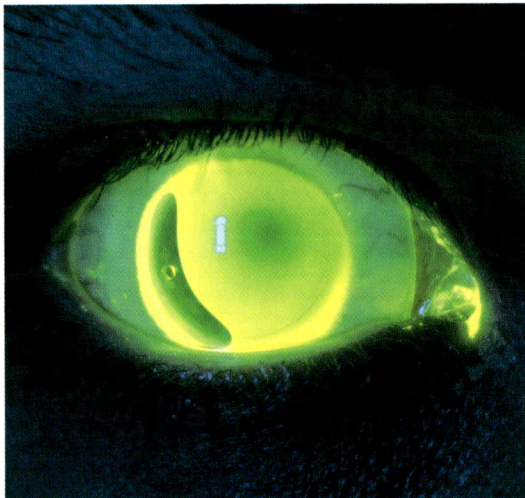

Figure 3.12 The ideal fit of a scleral lens, as viewed with fluorescein instilled and an ultraviolet black light. There is an even scleral fit, adequate limbal clearance, adequate corneal clearance and a bubble of the correct size which rotates on the versions of the eye

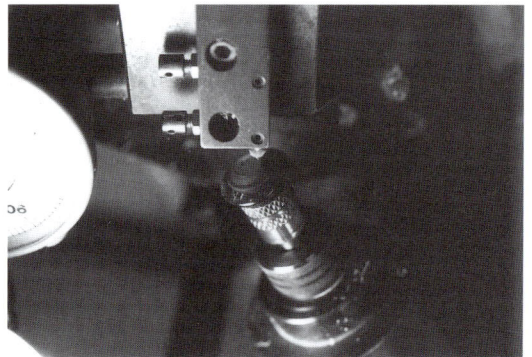

Figure 3.13 The front optical portion of the scleral lens is ground to the indicated power

examined. These portions should be completely clear of the cornea and the limbus (Figure 3.12). (After a scleral lens has been worn for a few hours it may 'settle back' so that a light corneal touch occurs, which is acceptable, but limbal touch ('compression') is not.) In some eyes which are grossly distorted the fitting of the corneal portion may have to be a compromise. It is frequently not possible to clear the cornea satisfactorily in keratoconus.

If there is corneal or limbal touch the laboratory technician is instructed to 'give 0.10 mm corneal clearance' or 'give 0.10 mm clearance at the transition'. This sort of modification is continued until the desired fitting is obtained.

The bubble of air introduced by the fenestration should be sausage shaped, no more than one-quarter of the circumference of the cornea in length after the lens has 'settled back' (Figure 3.12), and should rotate around the limbus as the eye looks in different directions. Static bubbles of air should be avoided at all cost. They give rise to corneal drying, scarring and vascularization (see Chapter 11). Great enlargement of the bubble when the eye looks in one or other direction may mean that the shell is too large in overall size at the side remote from the enlarged bubble. Poor rotation of the bubble may mean that the shell is too small in overall size. The laboratory technician should be informed accordingly.

When the fitting of the corneal and transition portions is completed and the performance of the bubble is satisfactory, the position of the centre of the pupil is then marked on the front of the corneal portion and the shell is sent to the laboratory technician with instructions to grind an optical surface on the front of the corneal portion (Figure 3.13) and it is helpful at this point to indicate the patient's spectacle refraction.

The laboratory returns a scleral contact lens and appropriate modification of its power is then done. Finally, the thickness of the scleral portion is reduced uniformly to 1.0 mm.

There are, of course, variations to the procedures outlined here, but the commonest methods have been described. In this text all corneal and scleral modifications have been

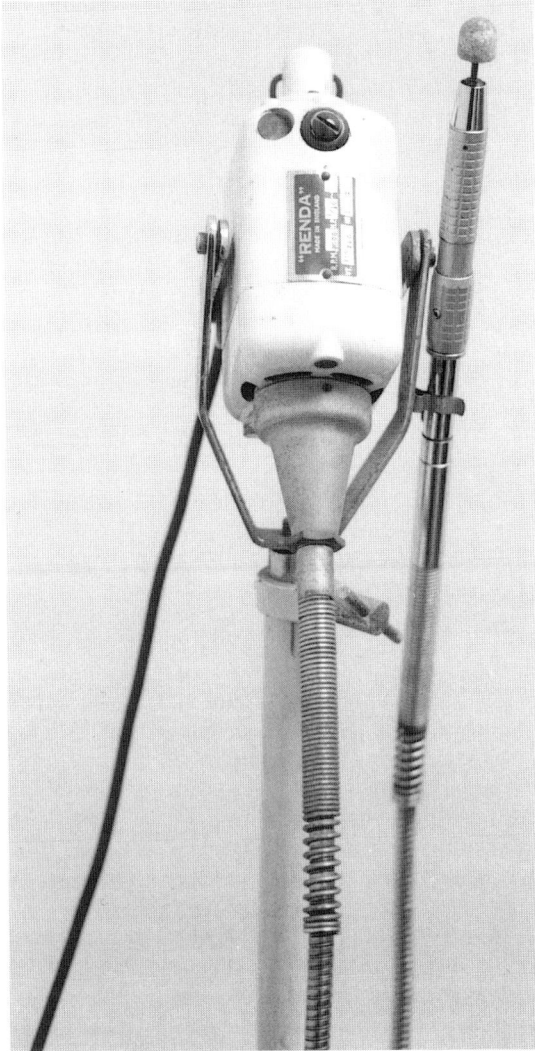

Figure 3.14 Old style dental drill used for modifying the scleral portion of the shell

ordered from the laboratory, but, of course, some scleral lens fitters do their own scleral modifications with an old style dental lathe (Figure 3.14) and grinding and polishing heads. This is a technique that needs practical training.

Flush fitting scleral lenses

Flush fitting lenses had a vogue in the 1960s and were used in pathological eyes (Ridley, 1962). The concept was to fit a therapeutic shell fashioned

from the mould, without modification, on the cornea and sclera. Ruben (1967) pointed out that, to achieve overall corneal contact of the shell, settling back of the lens by grinding and polishing the back surface of the scleral flange was often necessary.

Preformed hard scleral lenses

Preformed lenses are easier to fit and avoid the discomfort and problems of moulding. Where there are problems of fixation and steadiness of an eye, for example, with nystagmus, these may be the only hard scleral lenses which it is possible to fit. The method is not suitable for grossly toroidal or distorted eyes.

Preformed hard scleral lenses are fitted in two ways. The first uses a single lens to assess both the scleral and the optic fitting. The second uses separate lenses to assess the scleral and the optic fittings.

Single lenses

An example of these is the Wide Angle Fitting Set associated with the name of G. Nissel (obtainable from G. Nissel & Co. Ltd, Maxted Close, Hemel Hempstead, Herts., England). This usually comprises about 24 lenses with back scleral radii and back optic radii in 0.25 mm steps. The set is arranged so that steeper (more curved) scleral radii are associated with steeper back central optic radii and flatter (less curved) scleral radii are associated with flatter back optic radii. There is a cone-shaped transitional area from the optic to the scleral portion.

The lens must be inserted when filled with saline, as already described in this chapter, and fluorescein and ultraviolet black light are used to determine the corneal and limbal clearance.

The objective in fitting is to get an even scleral fit, as determined by the absence of conjunctival vessel blanching, and corneal and limbal clearance which is not excessive. The back vertex power required is ascertained by over-refraction.

The lens is ordered from the laboratory by specifying:

1. The back optic radius.

2. The back scleral radius.
3. The back scleral size.
4. The displacement of the optic.
5. The back vertex power.

Since no lens in the trial set may give the proper fit it may be required to instruct the laboratory to increase, or decrease, the corneal clearance and this is usually done in steps of 0.10 mm.

Separate lenses

An example of these is the Offset Fitting Set associated with the name of A.J. Forknall, used together with the FLOM Fitting Set associated with the name of N. Bier.

Offset fitting set

This consists of a number of lenses with back scleral radii in 0.25 mm steps, each designated by a code letter. A second code letter is added to designate the back scleral size and the displacement of the optic in millimetres.

A trial lens is chosen using the keratometry as a guide, if possible. A steep cornea will usually have a steep sclera and a flatter cornea a flatter sclera. The lens is inserted when filled with saline, as already described.

There are only two considerations – the radius of the lens and the diameter of the lens.

The lens is too large in diameter if it passes over the caruncle or the lateral check ligament, but it should be large enough so that its edges do not show in the palpebral aperture. Blanching of the scleral vessels at the periphery of the lens will indicate too steep a scleral fit. Blanching near the limbus and standoff at the edges will indicate too flat a scleral fit. A lens should be chosen which dose not show either of these features.

A drop of fluorescein is then introduced behind the lens. When viewed with ultraviolet black light this will indicate whether there is a large pool behind the optic portion, in which case the lens is too steep, or whether there is a small pool, in which case it is too flat. The ideal is a central pool which extends evenly just beyond the central portion. During this assessment of the scleral fit it is only the width of the central fluorescein pool that is of interest.

Displacement of the optic is assessed by putting lenses of known optic displacement on the eye.

Transcurve fitting set

This is a further example of the use of separate lenses and consists of at least eight lenses (it was originally 24) with variable optic and scleral radii with an intermediate transcurve radius which is the mean of the optic and scleral radii. Again, a trial lens is chosen according to the keratometry findings.

The lens is made 23.00 mm round with 1.00 mm nasal displacement of the optic, or oval 22.00 mm vertical by 24.00 mm horizontal, again with 1.00 mm nasal displacement of the optic. It is available in steps of 0.25 mm radius of curvature.

It is used to fit the scleral portion and can be used to fit the corneal portion or FLOM lenses can be used for this latter purpose.

FLOM lenses

FLOM stands for fenestrated lens for optic measurement and the lens is used to determine the optic fit.

The lens consists of an optic portion from 13 mm to 14.75 mm in diameter with a narrow scleral rim beyond this, approximately 2.0 mm in width so that the overall size is approximately 17.0 mm to 18.75 mm. The scleral portion has a radius of approximately 13.0 mm so that it is flat and stands off the sclera at its edge (Figure 3.15).

The FLOM fitting set has back optic radii ranging from 8.00 mm to 9.50 mm in 0.25 mm steps. These lenses were designed by Norman Bier and detailed consideration of their use is found in his original textbook (Bier, 1957).

The patient's eye is anaesthetized with topical sodium benoxinate 0.4% (Smith and Nephew Ltd) before these lenses are used.

A FLOM lens is chosen 0.50–0.70 mm flatter in back optic radius than the mean keratometry and in the middle of the diameter range. There are, again, only two considerations – the radius of the optic portion and the primary diameter of the optic portion. Decreasing the radius of the optic portion and increasing the primary diameter of the optic portion will both, on their own, increase the clearance of the lens from the cornea and vice

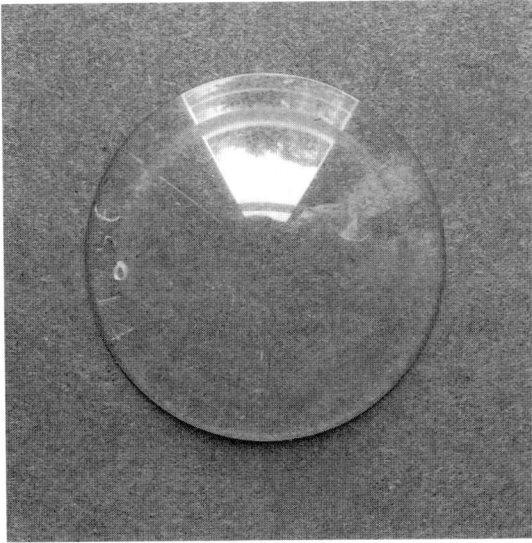

Figure 3.15 A FLOM lens (fenestrated lens for optic measurement)

versa, as is explained in the case of corneal lenses in Chapter 4.

After five minutes it is ascertained whether the lens fills with tear fluid and what shape the bubble of air is, which has been let in by the fenestration.

If the radius is too steep, the bubble tends to cross the pupil. If the radius is too flat, a ring bubble extends a considerable way around the limbus region. The correct fit is when a small sausage-shaped bubble forms with its concave surface inwards (see Figure 3.12).

Fluorescein and ultraviolet light are used to determine the corneal fit. If there is corneal touch the back optic radius should be decreased while maintaining the same primary back optic diameter.

If there is corneal touch and limbal touch the primary back optic diameter should be increased while maintaining the same back optic radius.

If there is corneal clearance, but limbal touch, then the primary back optic diameter should be increased while making a compensatory increase in the back optic radius.

An increase of 1.00 mm in primary back optic diameter will have to be accompanied by an increase of 0.50 mm in back optic radius to maintain the corneal clearance (and vice versa).

Throughout this description reference has been made to the *primary* back optic diameter. This is because, on occasions, it is necessary to introduce a centrally placed secondary back optic diameter of increased radius, to achieve satisfactory corneal and limbal clearance. Refraction is carried out over a FLOM lens of the same back optic radius as ordered and known back vertex power.

The scleral lens ordered from the laboratory will undoubtedly 'settle back' with wear and this should be anticipated. It is usual to order a primary optic diameter with an 0.25 mm addition to that used in the trial lens. This gives more corneal clearance.

The lens is ordered from the laboratory by specifying:

1. The back optic radius
2. The primary optic diameter
3. The first letter on the fitting set lens (that is the equivalent back scleral radius)
4. The size letter
5. The back vertex power

When the lens is received from the laboratory the horizontal line (between the canthi) should be marked on it with a waterproof pen and a check made to make sure that it remains in this position. The lens should then be fenestrated in the manner described for moulded lenses.

Fitting problems

Rotation

Here the horizontal line marked from the cast does not assume a horizontal position. It is usually caused by tight (pressure) areas in the haptic on opposite sides of the eye. These need to be marked and ground out. It is usually advisable to fenestrate the lens temporally at a point along the marked horizontal line and at the periphery of the corneal portion, before the grind out is delineated.

Overall lens size disparity

When the lens is obviously undersize and the moulding procedure has been used there is no other recourse but to explain to the patient that the moulding will have to be done again. This is not always welcomed. If the lens is oversized it should be marked for grinding down before the fenestration is done.

Clicking

This is a problem sometimes experienced with fenestrated scleral lenses. Every time the patient blinks a clicking noise is heard and this may be socially embarrassing. It is often due to excessive corneal clearance and too large a fenestration hole.

Frothing

In this condition, which occurs more frequently in fenestrated lenses, the large bubble fragments into froth and the visual and cosmetic result is undesirable. It may be relieved by a larger fenestration hole or by more corneal clearance.

Mucus under the lens

In this condition floating plaques of mucus appear behind the corneal portion of the lens and often interfere with vision. This condition is very difficult to remedy and some relief may be obtained by the use of Gutt. acetylcysteine 10%, three times daily. It is usually seen where there is conjunctival pathology.

References

BIER, N. (1957) *Contact Lens Routine and Practice*. Butterworths Scientific Publications. London

EZEKIEL, D. (1983) Gas permeable haptic lenses. *Journal of the British Contact Lens Association*, **6**, 158

PULLUM, K.W. (1984) Development of slotted scleral lenses. *Journal of the British Contact Lens Association*, **7**, 92–95

PULLUM, K.W. (1987) Feasibility study for the production of gas permeable scleral lenses using ocular impression techniques. *Transactions of the British Contact Lens Association Conference*, pp. 35–39. British Contact Lens Association, London

PULLUM, K.W. and TRODD, T.C. (1984) Development of slotted scleral lenses. *Journal of the British Contact Lens Association*, **7**, 28–38

PULLUM, K.W., PARKER, J.H. and HOBLEY, A.J. (1989) The Joseph Dallos Award Lecture, 1989. Development of gas permeable scleral lenses produced from impressions of the eye. *Transactions of the British Contact Lens Association Conference*, 1989. British Contact Lens Association, London

RIDLEY, F. (1962) Therapeutic uses of scleral contact lenses. *International Ophthalmological Clinics* (Diseases of the Cornea), **3**, 687–716

RUBEN, M. (1967) Types of haptic lenses in current use. *Transactions of the Ophthalmological Society of the UK*, **LXXXVII**, 643–659

SCHEIN, O.D., ROSENTHAL, P. and DUCHARME, C. (1990) A gas permeable scleral contact lens for visual rehabilitation. *American Journal of Ophthalmology*, **109**, 318–322

Appendix 3.I

Moulding materials

Kromopan

This dental alginate is distributed by F.H. Wright Dental Co. Ltd. It changes colour twice during manipulation. Initially, the mixture is violet in colour. This changes to pink, indicating the end of the spatulation period when the syringe should be loaded and, in ophthalmic work, the injection should be commenced. It turns white just before, or at the end of the injection, and gels about 30 seconds after this. The impression is removed after two minutes on the eye.

Ophthalmic Zelex

This is distributed by the Amalgamated Dental Co. Ltd. It produces very good impressions because it can be spatulated into a very smooth, free flowing cream, which gels gradually. The setting time is long – about three minutes.

Tissutex

This dental material is distributed by Dental Manufacturing Co. Ltd. It makes excellent impressions. It has a long free flow period. Spatulation time must not exceed one minute. For ophthalmic work it should be ordered free from peppermint flavouring.

Spatulation of moulding materials

Spatulation is the means of ensuring a smooth, well mixed moulding material without lumps for insertion into the syringe and then into the impression shell.

It is done in a rubber or soft plastic bowl with a spatula one inch (2.54 cm) or slightly less in width. The moulding material is mixed with water according to the directions. Warm water will speed the gelling. Cold water will retard it.

The spatula is used with a stropping motion against the side of the bowl, always smoothing the resultant paste, and a figure of eight motion helps the process.

Appendix 3.II

Casting materials

Calestone

This dental material is distributed by Amalgamated Dental Co. Ltd. It is a hard material which does not shrink. It must be mixed with water and spatulated in the same manner as moulding material.

KD plaster (Kaffir D plaster)

This dental material is distributed by Wright Dental Products Ltd. It is a plaster with limited shrinkage.

Axial edge thickness

Back optic zone diameter

Axial edge lift

Back peripheral radius

Back optic zone radius

Front optic zone diameter

Carrier

Central thickness

Front peripheral radius

Carrier thickness

Total diameter

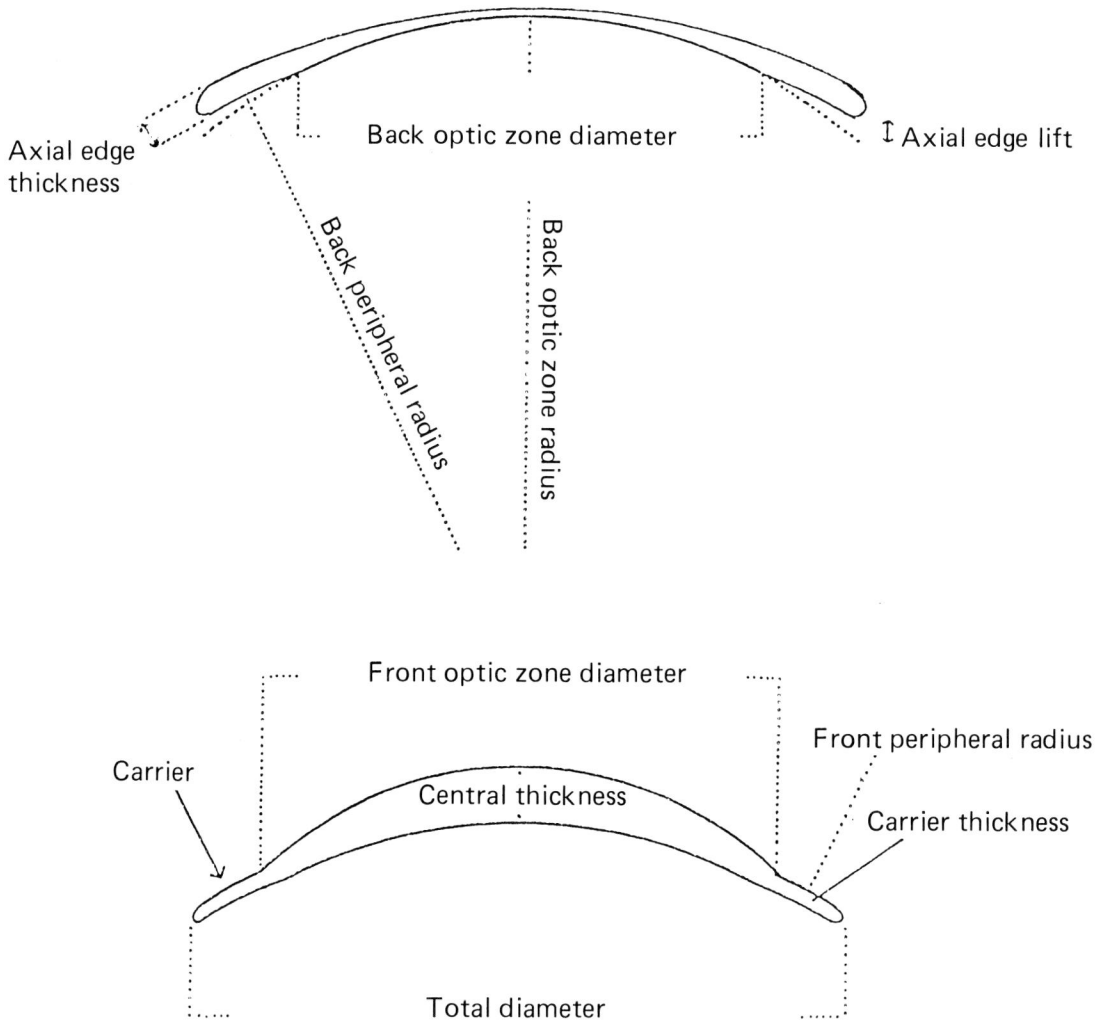

Figure 4.1 Nomenclature of hard corneal lenses

4

Fitting hard corneal lenses

Introduction

Hard corneal lenses (Figure 4.1) can be moulded to shape or manufactured on a lathe. Moulding equipment is expensive to set up and each power and design requires a separate mould. The method is only suitable for the production of lenses in large quantities and the range of designs is necessarily limited. The usual course is to manufacture the contact lens from a 'button' of plastic.

In modern manufacture this button is fixed to a lathe. The specified back peripheral curve, or curves, are then cut out on the lathe with a sharp edged tool and this is followed by the cutting out of the back central curve (Figure 4.2). (Cutting produces a smoother surface than grinding out.) A modern lathe can then reduce the diameter of the button, leaving sufficient material for edge polishing (Figure 4.3), and can perform these three steps without the necessity of resetting.

The back peripheral curves are then blended by polishing (Figure 4.4) and then the back central curve is polished (Figure 4.5).

The next step is the remounting of the lens on the lathe so that its front surface can be cut out. Devices are used to ensure that it is properly

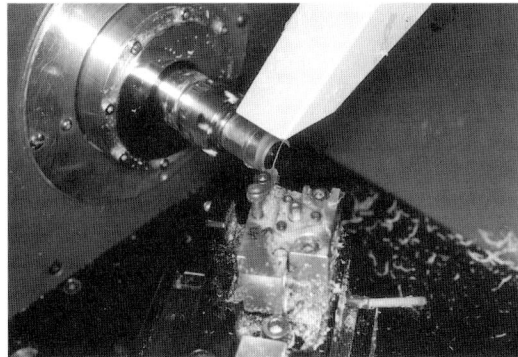

Figure 4.3 The diameter of the button is reduced, leaving sufficient material for edge polishing

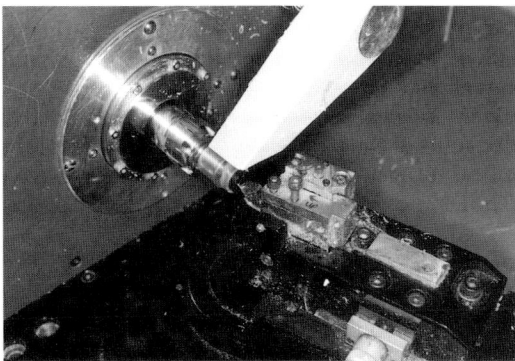

Figure 4.2 The specified back peripheral curve or curves are cut out on the lathe with a sharp edged diamond tool and this is followed by the cutting out of the back central curve

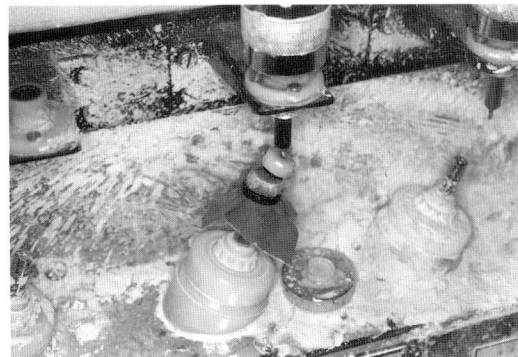

Figure 4.4 The back peripheral curves are blended by polishing

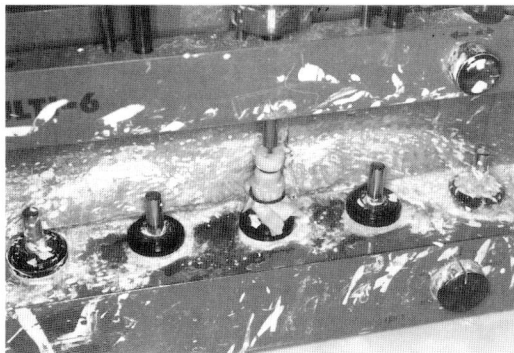

Figure 4.5 The back central curve is polished

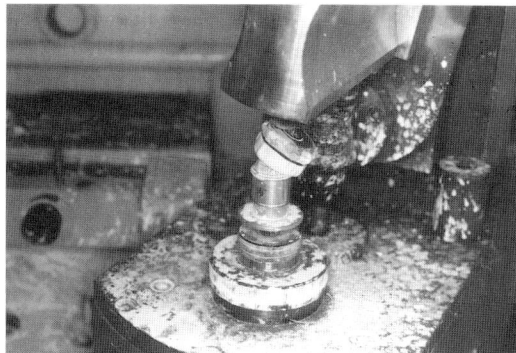

Figure 4.7 After removal from the lathe the front surface of the lens is polished

aligned, otherwise a prism would be introduced. The front peripheral curve (if ordered) is then cut out followed by the front central curve (Figure 4.6). A modern lathe will perform these two actions without resetting and it can be set so that the ordered central thickness of the lens is obtained automatically.

The lens is then removed from the lathe and its front surface is polished (Figure 4.7). The edge is then fashioned and polished (Figure 4.8).

Lathes are available which can generate aspherical curves. Small hand calculators and desk computers are available which can rapidly calculate and even graphically represent the parameters which are desirable, or indeed, possible on these contact lenses. Trial lenses are usually employed in the fitting of hard corneal lenses and sets of these lenses can be ordered using the data in the Appendices of this chapter. An alternative method is to order according to nomograms

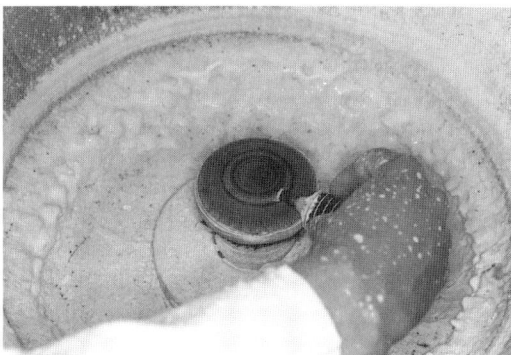

Figure 4.8 Finally, the edge of the lens is fashioned and polished

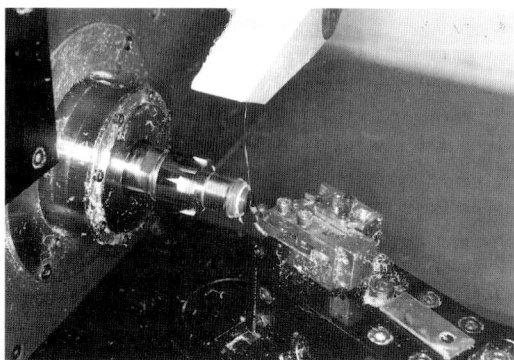

Figure 4.6 After remounting of the button, the front peripheral curve, if ordered, is cut out followed by the front central curve

worked out according to the spectacle refraction, keratometry and corneal diameter, but this is an unsatisfactory method as it does not take into account the action of the eyelids in a particular patient and it is only applicable in low minus corrections.

Hard corneal lenses are usually fitted so that the radius of the back surface is near to that of the central corneal radius. Contact lens fitters vary as to how much more curved (steep or apex clear) or less curved (flat or apex touch) they make the lens.

Lenses which have a back surface which is less curved than that of the cornea may tend to be ejected more easily because their edges will be more elevated above the corneal surface. They will have, because of a minus tear fluid lens behind them, a relatively lesser minus power, compared with the spectacle power, and thus less bulk increase at their periphery. Bulk increase at the periphery is responsible for many corneal lenses being grasped by the upper lid and controlled by it. Without it the lens may drop to rest on the lower part of the cornea.

Lenses which have a back surface which is more curved than that of the cornea will be less likely to be ejected and will require, because of a plus tear fluid behind them, a relatively greater minus power to compensate (compared with the spectacle power). They will, thus, have greater bulk increase at the periphery and they will be more likely to be grasped by the upper lid.

If the back surface of the corneal lens is too curved, tiny bubbles of gas (froth) may become visible under the lens (Figure 4.9). These bubbles may consist of carbon dioxide coming off the surface of the cornea. Alternatively, they may be bubbles of entrapped air coming from the area of the tear wedges which occur between the cornea and the lid margins. The bubbles interfere with the patient's vision while the lens is in situ. When the lens is removed, small dimples can be seen on the corneal surface, which stain with fluorescein. These, again, interfere with the patient's vision (in spectacles), but they disappear rapidly. Plus hard corneal lenses do not, of course, have bulk increase at their periphery and so have the tendency to drop to the lower part of the cornea, unless they are constrained by corneal centration forces. This tendency to drop can be overcome by putting a bevel on the front periphery of the lens (see Figure 4.27). This allows the centre thickness of the lens to be reduced and so also its mass. It also allows the top lid to grasp and control the lens (see Figure 4.28).

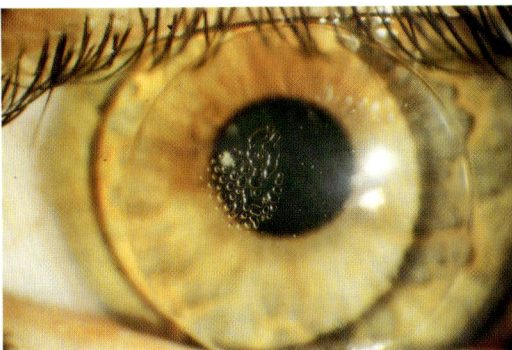

Most corneal lenses have a back peripheral curve or curves, that is, a back bevel or bevels. The less curved (that is, flatter) and more extensive these are the more the lens will be able to slide over the cornea and possibly the corneo-scleral junction and the more the interchange of tear fluid from the eye to the undersurface of the lens will be facilitated. If the back peripheral bevels are too wide and stand off too much (that is, are too flat), the lens may easily be ejected on coming in contact with a lid margin.

A back peripheral curve or curves dictate increased thickness in minus and plus lenses. The wider and more standing off the back peripheral curves are the thicker the lens must be in its centre (Figure 4.10). Central thickness is the most important factor governing lens mass. The more the lens mass, the more the tendency will be for the lens to drop to the lower part of the cornea.

Corneal lenses of different diameters are used by different fitters and under different situations. The greater the diameter of a minus corneal lens the greater the bulk of the peripheral substance will be (Figure 4.11). In manufacturing the front edge substance can be pared off, but only to a limited extent, in order to conserve the optical

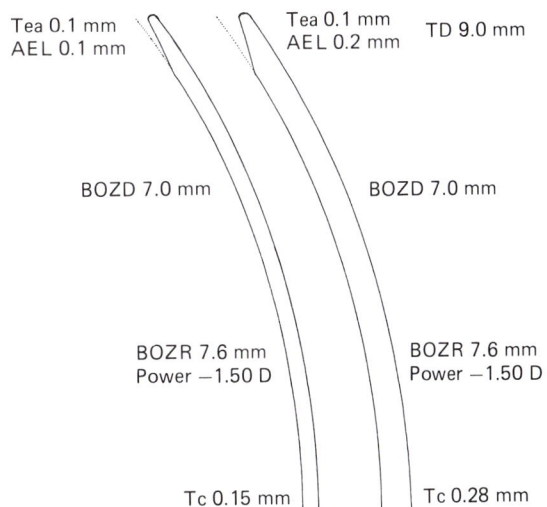

Tea 0.1 mm
AEL 0.1 mm

Tea 0.1 mm
AEL 0.2 mm
TD 9.0 mm

BOZD 7.0 mm

BOZD 7.0 mm

BOZR 7.6 mm
Power −1.50 D

BOZR 7.6 mm
Power −1.50 D

Tc 0.15 mm

Tc 0.28 mm

Figure 4.10 The wider and more stand off the back peripheral curves are the thicker the lens must be in its centre. The left hand lens has an axial edge lift of 0.10 mm and a minimum thickness of 0.15 mm. The right hand lens has an axial edge lift of 0.20 mm and a minimum thickness of 0.28 mm. Only half of each lens is shown

Figure 4.9 Small bubbles ('frothing') under a steeply fitted hard corneal lens

Tea at 10.0 mm = 0.32 mm

Tea at 10.0 mm = 0.58 mm

Tea at 8.0 mm = 0.22 mm

Tea at 8.0 mm = 0.37 mm

BOZR = 7.60 mm
Power = −5.0 D

BOZR = 7.60 mm
Power = 5.0 mm

Tc = 0.10 mm

Tc = 0.10 mm

TD = 10.0 mm AEL = 0.15 mm Te = 0.10 mm

FOZD = 8.0 mm

TD = 8.0 mm AEL = 0.15 mm Te = 0.10 mm

FOZD = 6.0 mm

BOZR = 7.60 mm
Power = +5.0 D

BOZR = 7.60 mm
Power = +5.0 D

Tc = 0.30 mm

Tc = 0.40 mm

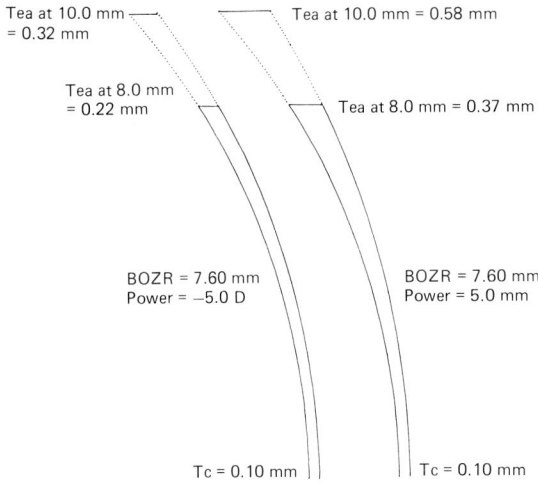

Figure 4.11 The greater the diameter of a minus corneal lens the greater the bulk of the peripheral substance will be. Only half of each lens is shown. Note that the right hand, higher minus power lens, has a disproportionately larger increase in edge thickness as its diameter is increased from 8.0 mm to 10.0 mm, compared with the left hand lens

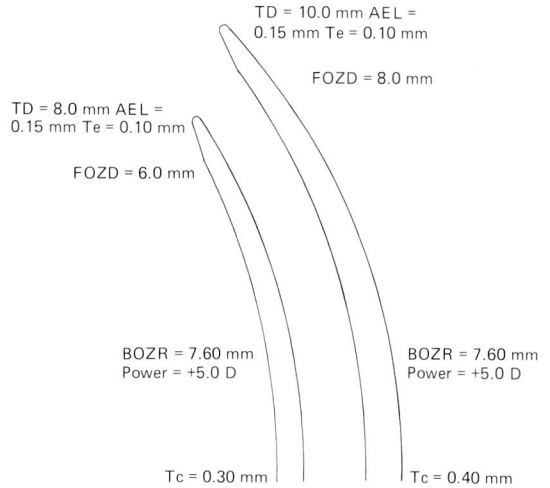

Figure 4.12 The greater the diameter of a plus corneal lens the greater its central thickness will need to be. A front peripheral curve can be created to result in a lens of lesser central thickness. Only half of each lens is shown.

efficiency of the lens. The front peripheral bevel thus created will influence the fitting of the lens in its relation to the lids.

The greater the diameter of a plus corneal lens the greater its central thickness will need to be (Figure 4.12). As already stated, a front peripheral curve or bevel can be created, resulting in a lens which can have a lesser central thickness (see Figure 4.34).

The greater the diameter of the corneal lens, the greater will be the area of cornea potentially excluded from an oxygen supply. The area is calculated by the formula πr^2. Thus, small increases in diameter can mean large increases in corneal coverage (Figure 4.13).

Corneal lenses may be seen to centre on the cornea when the lids are pulled apart. This is due to corneal centration forces related to the formation of a meniscus around the entire lens and its resistance to deformation (Mackie, Mason and Perry, 1970) (Figure 4.14). The deformation of this meniscus is created by the lift given to the lens by the protuberant central area of the cornea as the lens passes over the cornea. The centration force can be very powerful so that it exceeds the forces exerted by the lids. Without this centration force the lens can drop to the lower part of the cornea.

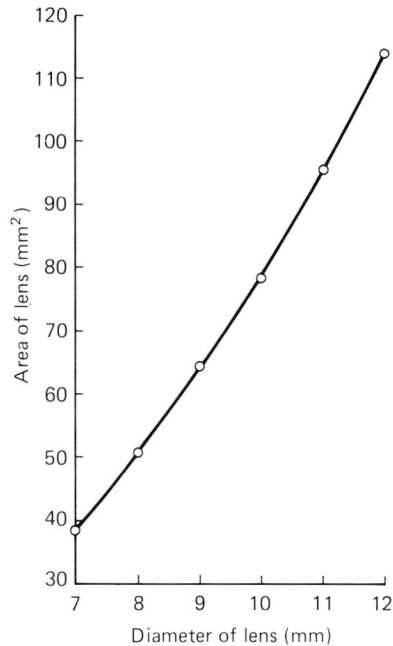

Figure 4.13 A graph to show the relationship between contact lens diameter in millimetres and area of coverage in square millimetres

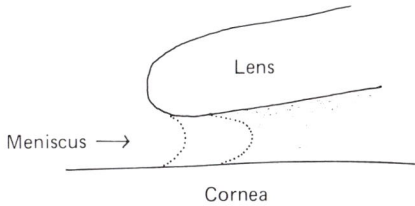

Figure 4.14 A meniscus is formed around the entire lens which resists deformation

Under conditions already stated, the lens may be grasped and controlled by the upper lid.

This latter 'lens lid attachment' (Korb and Korb, 1970) is the preferred physiological position for a lens (Figure 4.15a), being responsible for the best movement of the lens and the least interference with normal blinking mechanisms.

Next to this in physiological performance is the centralizing lens (Figure 4.15b). This may interfere with normal blinking as clarity of vision may be dependent on its central position not being disturbed by the sweep of an upper lid. This, in turn, can give rise to problems related to exposure and drying of the ocular surface in the interpalpebral areas not covered by the lens.

The worst situation is the dropping lens (Figure 4.15c), which does not move on the cornea because the lower lid has insignificant movement in a vertical direction, except when in spasm. This leads to stagnation of tears under such a lens and the certain development of corneal oedema. It also leads to grossly abnormal blinking in such a patient since the tendency will be for the upper lid, on blinking, to come down only as far as the top edge of the lens.

A so-called 'temporal ride' (Figure 4.15d), whereby the lens dislodges to the temporal side of the cornea, is a feature of thick front optic reduced aphakic corneal contact lenses (lenticular design) when fitted to certain eyes. These lenses seldom drop. The position on the cornea is dictated by the corneal toricity, the thickness of the lens and the lid cornea relationship. Little can be done to remedy the position. It does not usually give tolerance problems. It may give problems with the visual acuity and the usual course of action then is to make the lens larger and so obtain more corneal coverage.

Many cases of intolerance of hard corneal lenses can be related to the development of corneal oedema as a result of coverage of the cornea

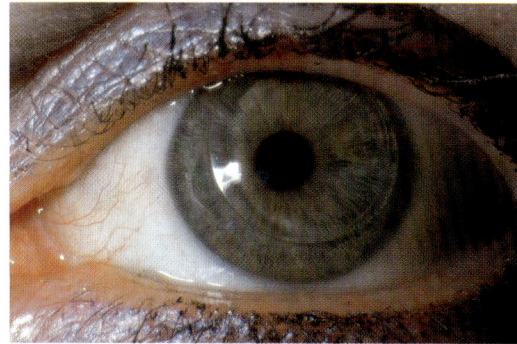

(a)

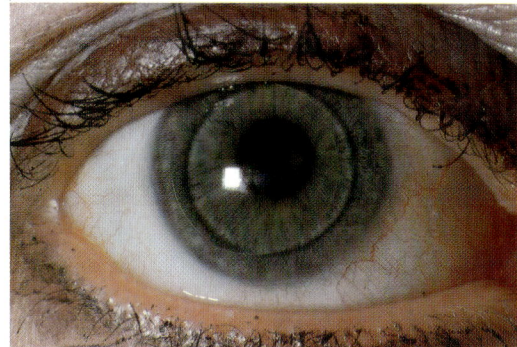

(b)

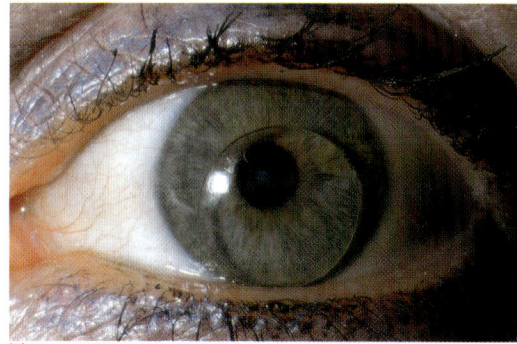

(c)

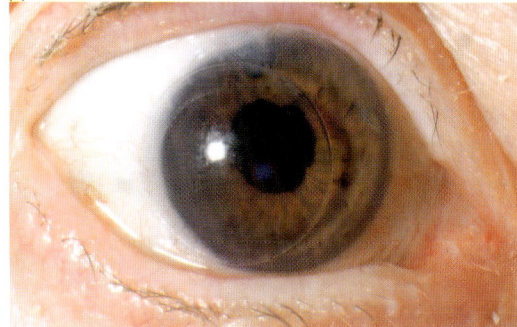

(d)

Figure 4.15 (a) Lens lid attachment; (b) centralizing lens; (c) dropping lens; (d) temporal ride of aphakic lens

and the inhibition of aerobic glycolysis (Smelser and Chen, 1955), and/or to the development of abnormal blinking mechanisms.

Objectives in fitting hard corneal lenses

The objectives in fitting hard corneal lenses can be listed as follows:

1. The lens should be stable after a blink.
2. The lens should move with the blink.
3. The lens should produce no abnormality in the pattern of blinking.
4. The lens should produce satisfactory vision.
5. The lens should produce no visible corneal oedema.

Positioning of lenses

Centring lenses

Corneal lenses may be seen to centre on the cornea when the lids are pulled apart. If the upper lid is then gently pushed so that it in turn pushes the lens downwards and if this lid is then quickly retracted it can often be seen that the contact lens will rise on the cornea and return to a central position independent of any action by the lids.

This centration has been thought to be due to the presence of a central corneal 'cap' of regular curvature which is surrounded by peripheral cornea of lesser curvature. This cap was described by Wolff (1954). Girard (1964) evolved a method of measuring its diameter by the use of a topogometer. This was an instrument designed to be attached to a Bausch and Lomb keratometer to take peripheral keratometry readings at a known distance from the optical centre of the cornea. It had a moveable fixation device which was fitted in front of the keratometer. The patient's eye followed the fixation point as it moved in different directions and when there was a difference in reading, equivalent to a change in keratometry of 0.10 mm, this was noted to be the limit of the cap. Girard found that in 90% of cases the cap measured 5–7 mm in diameter (Figure 4.16) and

advocated the adoption of the formula LD + 2 for calculating the total diameter of corneal lenses so that optimum centration was obtained. LD represented the longest diameter of the corneal cap and the expression was in millimetres. Mackie, Mason and Perry (1970) worked out the factors influencing corneal lens centration based on the existence of this corneal cap.

The existence of this cap has been disputed by Dingeldein and Klyce (1989). Using computer assisted photokeratographic analysis they did not confirm the existence of a definable apical or corneal cap. They stated that 'it appears that it is arbitrary and anatomically incorrect to divide the cornea into zones, even though the concept may be useful for the practice of fitting contact lenses'. They agree with Mandell (1981) who stated, 'It must be understood that significant variation in corneal curvature occurs in the central cornea . . . The two zone concept is an arbitrary division for convenience'.

Dingeldein and Klyce (1989) found that all the corneas they examined were steeper centrally and flattened progressively towards the limbus. The degree of peripheral flattening was asymmetric in the majority of the eyes in their study and flattening began closer to the visual axis on the nasal side in most cases. In all of the eyes they studied the cornea flattened more rapidly nasally than temporally.

The most striking finding in their study was the high degree of mirror image symmetry often found between the right and left eyes of many individuals. They compared this to the mirror image symmetry of thumbprints. In their paper, Dingeldein and Klyce show videokeratographs of corneas in which the area of highest dioptric power is, in one case, inferior to the visual axis and in the other supratemporal to the line of sight and represented in a brown colour (Figure 4.17). Both corneas were normal with 20/20 vision.

Bogan *et al.* (1990) have put forward a classification of normal corneal topography. They found five types of picture – round (22.6%), oval (20.8%), symmetric bowtie (17.5%), asymmetric bowtie (32.1%) and irregular (7.1%) (Figure 4.18). They suggest that the five patterns in colour coded maps of normal eyes probably form a continuum (Figure 4.19).

Since the paper by Dingeldein and Klyce was published, another corneal mapping device has appeared, which is commercially available and

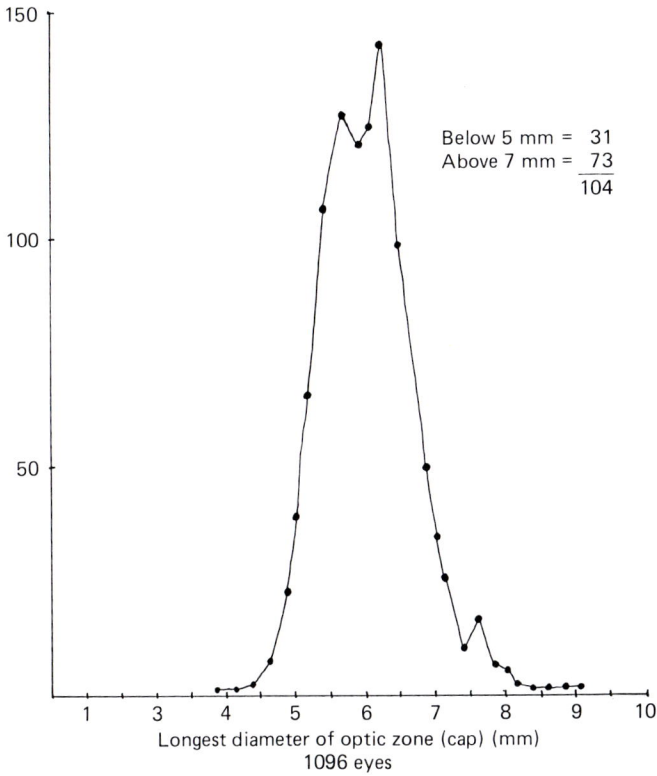

Figure 4.16 Graph of distribution of cap diameters as described by Girard (1964)

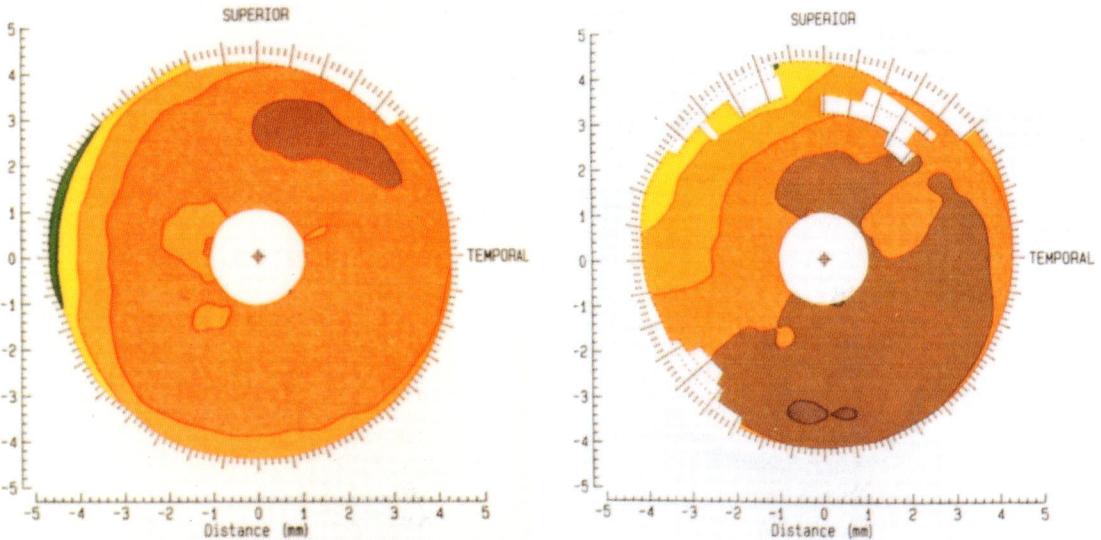

Figure 4.17 Videokeratographs of corneas in which the area of highest dioptric power is represented by the brown colour. On the right hand side videokeratograph the area of highest dioptric power is inferior to the visual axis. On the left hand side videokeratograph the area of highest dioptric power is supratemporal to the line of sight. Both corneas were normal with 20/20 vision. (Reproduced from Dingeldein, S.A. and Klyce, S.D. (1989) *Archives of Ophthalmology*, **107**, 512–517, by kind permission of Dr S.D. Klyce and the Editor of *Archives of Ophthalmology*; copyright 1989, American Medical Association)

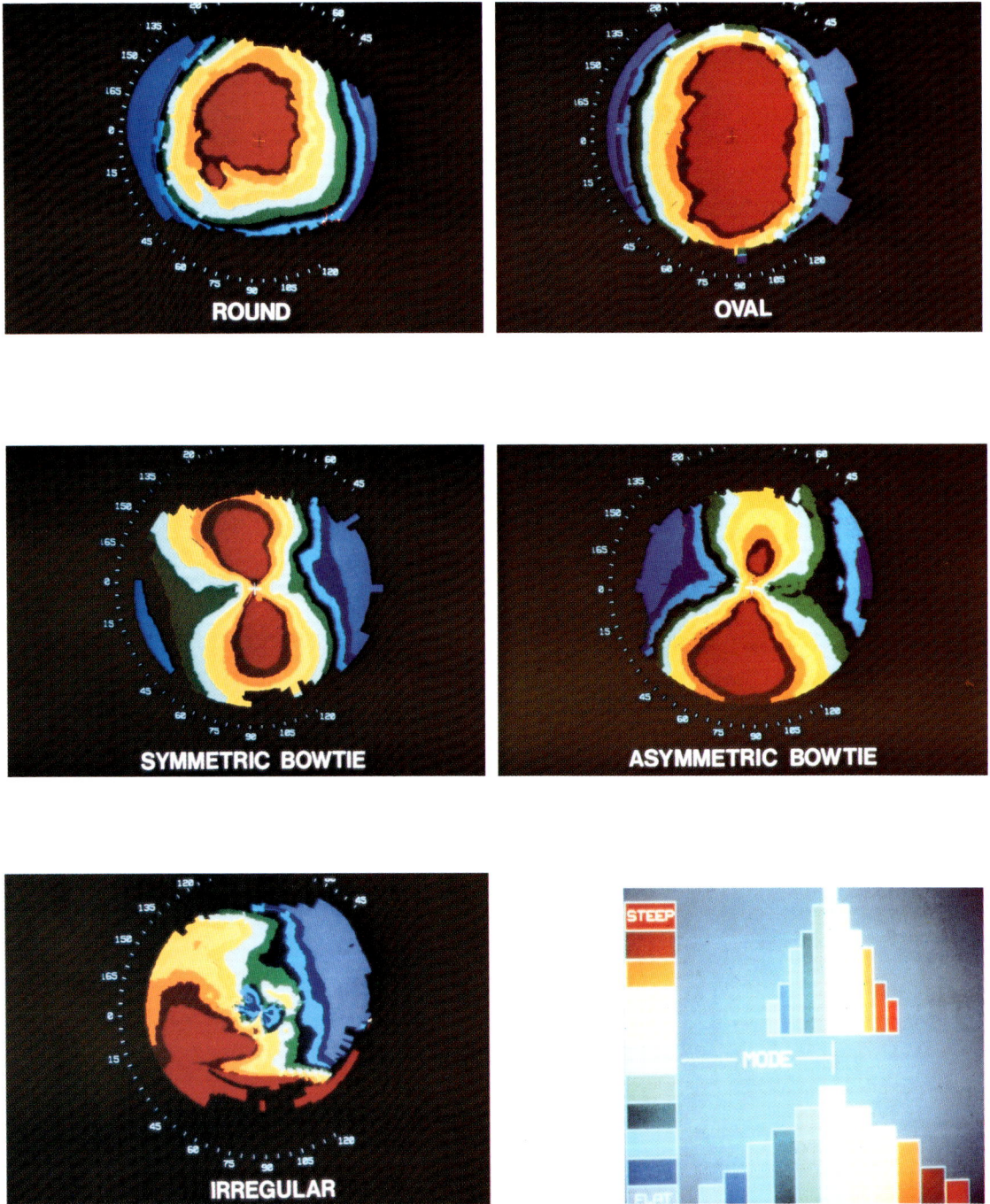

Figure 4.18 Classification of normal topography. Five qualitative patterns of corneal topography based on computer assisted videokeratography. Bottom right – in the normalized scale the range of dioptric power represented by each colour varies among eyes, depending upon the degree of corneal asphericity. (Reproduced from Bogan *et al*. (1990) *Archives of Ophthalmology*, **108**, 945–949, by kind permission of Dr G.O. Waring III and the Editor of *Archives of Ophthalmology*; copyright 1990, American Medical Association)

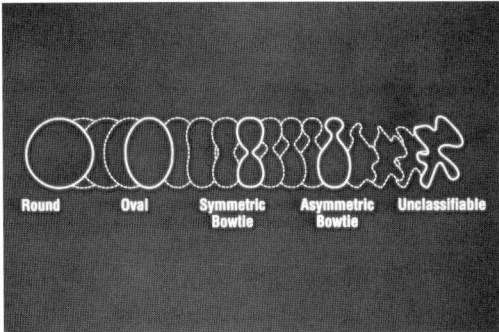

Figure 4.19 The five patterns in colour coded maps of normal eyes probably form a continuum. (Reproduced from Bogan *et al*. (1990) *Archives of Ophthalmology*, **108**, 945–949, by kind permission of Dr G.O. Waring III and the Editor of *Archives of Ophthalmology*; copyright 1990, American Medical Association)

which has been developed by Computed Anatomy Inc., New York, New York. This machine is claimed to be more sensitive and to define the central cornea in greater detail. The flattening from the centre to the periphery, as observed with this device, is very gradual and most corneas show a horizontal ellipsoid shape with nasal flattening. The superior and inferior flattening is usually greater than the temporal flattening, but less than the nasal flattening. The machine has shown up imperfections in the curvature of the central 3 mm of cornea which have not been shown before and either have been merely averaged or entirely omitted. This machine has not been able to detect any area of sharp transition from the central zone to the peripheral zone.

The corneal cap then is perhaps conceptual, rather than real. It helps us to explain the interrelationship of the back surface of the contact lens and the front surface of the cornea. The corneal lens is not sealed to the eye and such space as exists between the lens and the cornea will be filled with tear fluid. This tear fluid will be free to move into and out of this space. In the adapted eye there is usually only a minimum of tear fluid available and a meniscus is formed around the periphery of the lens (see Figure 4.14). The force holding the lens to the eye is purely the surface tension of this meniscus.

It can be shown (Figure 4.20) that as a spherical segment (the corneal lens) moves from a first

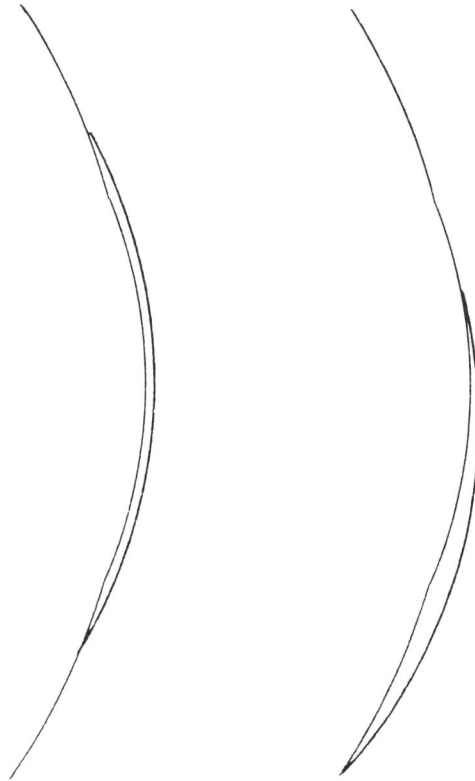

Figure 4.20 A spherical segment (the corneal lens) moves from a first surface of one radius of curvature (the corneal 'cap') to a second surface of a greater radius of curvature (the corneal periphery). The volume (of tears) enclosed between the segment and the surfaces increases. The drawing is of a cornea 12 mm in diameter with a 'cap' radius of 7.8 mm and 'cap' diameter of 6.0 mm. The flattening of the peripheral cornea has been exaggerated at 11.8 mm for illustrative purposes. A drawing of the back surface of a single cut lens of 8.0 mm diameter and 8.0 mm radius is shown mounted on the corneal profile. The increase in volume of the enclosed space would also occur if the flattening of the corneal profile towards the periphery was gradually progressive

surface of one radius of curvature to a second surface of a greater radius of curvature the volume enclosed between the segment and the surfaces increases. Although for the purposes of diagrammatic illustration, two distinct radii of curvature have been used in the surface representing the cornea, an increase in volume would occur if the increase in radius of curvature from centre to periphery were gradual.

In practice, the weight of the lens (plus its entrapped fluid) will cause the lens to move downwards. As it does this, the space between the lens and the cornea increases and since there is little extra fluid available in the adapted eye the meniscus will be deformed. This deformation will produce a resultant radial force which may oppose the motion of the lens. The meniscus can only move into those positions at which its allowed contact angle is maintained. The meniscus may be deformed in two different ways:

1. The 'overhang' meniscus is associated with corneal lenses which do not vault the cornea ('flat' or 'apex touch' lenses) (Figure 4.21). A meniscus is formed below because the central area of the cornea lifts the inferior edge of the contact lens as it moves downwards. The formation of this meniscus may be resisted by the surface tension forces resulting in centration.
2. The 'collar stud' meniscus is associated with corneal lenses which vault the cornea ('steep' or 'apex clear' lenses) (Figure 4.22). The movement downwards of the corneal lens will result

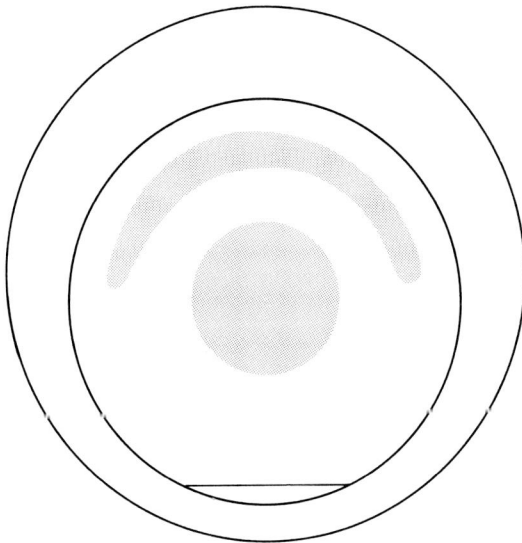

Figure 4.22 Collar stud meniscus. The menisci are below and to the sides. The shaded areas represent corneal touch in a tight fitting (that is apex clear) lens. The menisci are formed as the contact lens moves downwards because, then, a potentially greater volume of fluid can be accommodated under the central area of the lens. This is due to the fact that the superior peripheral area of the contact lens is lifted as it mounts the central protuberant area of the cornea. The formation of the menisci is resisted by surface tension forces

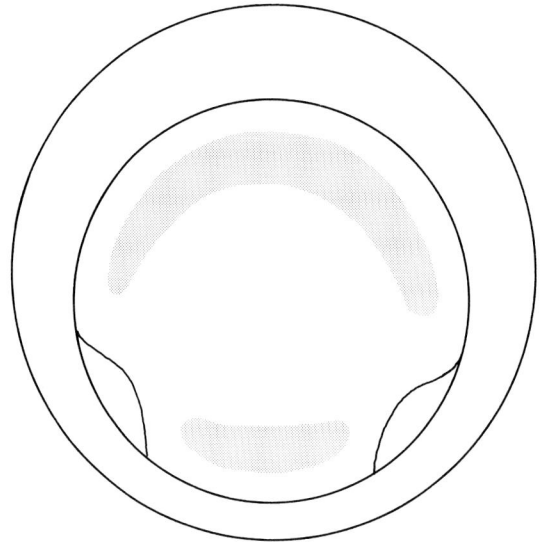

Figure 4.21 Overhang meniscus. The meniscus is below. The shaded areas represent corneal touch in a flat fitting (that is apex touch) lens. The meniscus is formed because the protuberant central area of the cornea causes a lifting of the inferior edge of the lens, as it moves downwards. The formation of the meniscus is resisted by surface tension forces

in the superior or trailing edge of the lens riding up towards the centre of the cornea before the inferior edge reaches the corneoscleral junction. This will result in the lower lateral edges of the lens being lifted from the surface of the cornea. The potential volume of fluid between the cornea and the lens will increase. The meniscus will be deformed at these areas and this may be resisted by the surface tension forces resulting in centration.

Corneal centration forces can be very strong and result in good stability of a corneal lens after a blink.

Certain factors militate against centration of a corneal lens (see Mackie, Mason and Perry, 1970):

1. *The corneal topography is such that no lift of the inferior edge of the lens is produced when a flat fitting lens moves downward over the cornea. Little can be done to remedy this situation. The*

contact lens will adopt another position on the cornea.

2. *The corneal topography is such that movement downwards of a steep fitting lens does not result in a potentially greater volume of fluid under the contact lens.* Alteration of the total diameter of the contact lens may remedy this situation and centration may be obtained. If not, the contact lens will adopt another position on the cornea.

3. *The mass of the lens is so great that it cannot be overcome by the surface tension forces resisting the deformation of the meniscus.* Central thickness of the corneal lens is the most important factor governing lens mass (Augsberger and Hill, 1971). It must, however, be remembered that to this mass of the lens must be added the mass of the entrapped fluid behind it and thus, decreasing the back radius of curvature of the lens (steepening) will increase this mass. The lens may drop to the lower part of the cornea. Here it will be stable after the blink but all our other fitting objectives will not be met.

4. *The upper lid may grasp the edge of the contact lens.* In this case the lens will be decentred upwards.

5. *There may be too much fluid in the eye.* In this case, a meniscus will not be formed at the edge of the lens. The lens will float freely and if not grasped by the upper lid will sink to the lower part of the cornea. This is often the case in the unadapted eye and is a cogent reason for using a non-epitheliotoxic local anaesthetic (sodium benoxinate 0.4% is preferred by the author) in the initial evaluation of the fitting.

It is probably true to say that 'centring lenses' are the goal of most contact lens fitters, especially on the American continent, but often these lenses which are seen to be in the centre of the cornea are maintained there by an attachment to the upper lid rather than purely centration forces.

When this is not the case, despite good centration forces, these lenses often cause problems. They are usually small diameter lenses and in conditions of dim light and dilated pupils can give rise to visual problems, especially in young adults. The teenager is less critical. These lenses can also interfere with normal blinking mechanisms and lead to suppression of the blink in the interest of stable vision, together with localized drying in the interpalpebral zones of the cornea and conjunctiva.

Lens lid attachment

It has already been stated that a lens may be decentred if the upper lid grasps it and lifts it upwards. This usually happens when the lens has bulk increase at its periphery as is the case in minus lenses. The more minus the lens the more this bulk increase will be. Borish (1961) advocated a prism base up design (Figure 4.23) for the edge of lenses with no inherent bulk increase at their periphery.

Often lenses with bulk increase at their periphery will not only be grasped by the upper lid but pressed against the eye so that a sulcus is formed in the sclera above the superior limbus. The upper edge of the lens will lodge in this sulcus so that the lens will become immobile and will not move with the blink. This is a most undesirable feature and modifications must be made to the back central and peripheral curves and also the front peripheral curves in an attempt to avoid it.

The concept of lens lid attachment was introduced as a method of fitting by Korb and Korb (1970). Kessing (1967) (Figure 4.24) showed that

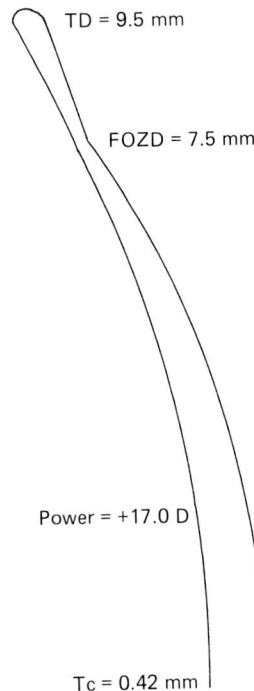

TD = 9.5 mm

FOZD = 7.5 mm

Power = +17.0 D

Tc = 0.42 mm

Figure 4.23 Prism base up edge design advocated by Borish (1961). Only half the lens is shown

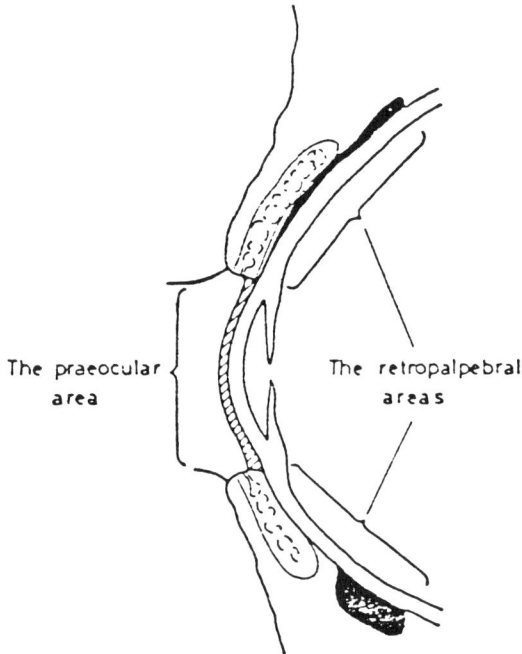

Figure 4.24 Schematic presentation of the retropalpebral space by Kessing (1967) (Reproduced from Kessing (1967) *Acta Ophthalmologica*, **45**, 680–683, by kind permission of the Editor of *Acta Ophthalmologica* (Kbn))

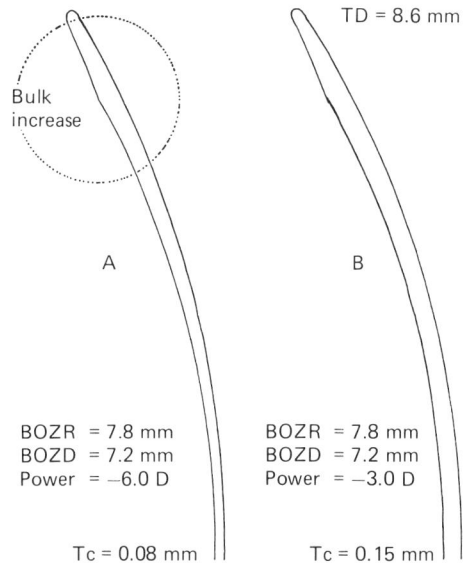

Figure 4.25 Bulk increase of −6.00 D lens compared with −3.00 D lens

only the marginal area of the upper lid is in close contact with the eye. The upper lid can thus act as a sling if there is something for it to hold on to. The bulk increase, or if you will, the prism base out at the periphery of a minus lens of over, say three dioptres, is usually enough for the lid to grasp (Figure 4.25) and the larger the lens is in diameter the more the peripheral bulk increase will be (see Figure 4.11). It may be, however, that the lens required will be of low minus or even plus power. In this case Korb and Korb advocate a lens in which there is a front peripheral zone (a front peripheral bevel) the radius of which parallels that of the back peripheral curve or curves (Figure 4.26). A back peripheral curve in a corneal lens dictates increased centre thickness. The thinner the lens the less its mass will be. The Korb and Korb design lens lid attachment lens can be thought of as a lens without a back peripheral curve or curves, but with an ideological joint which can be 'bent' forwards to achieve a hooked device (Figure 4.27). Such a lens tends to induce normal blinking (Figure 4.28). It is always in contact with the upper lid. The lens is always in the

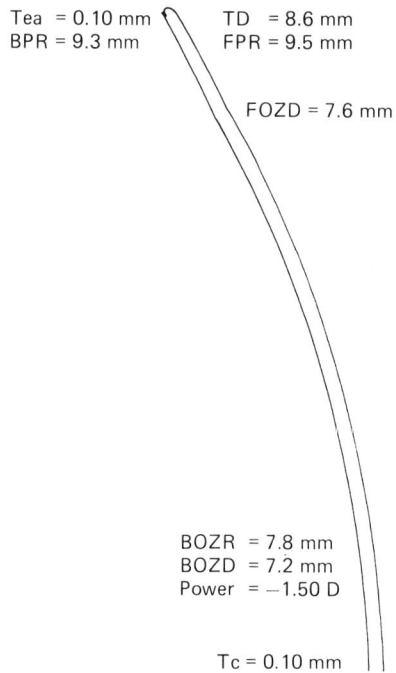

Figure 4.26 Korb technique (KT) lens −1.50 D power. Only half the lens is shown

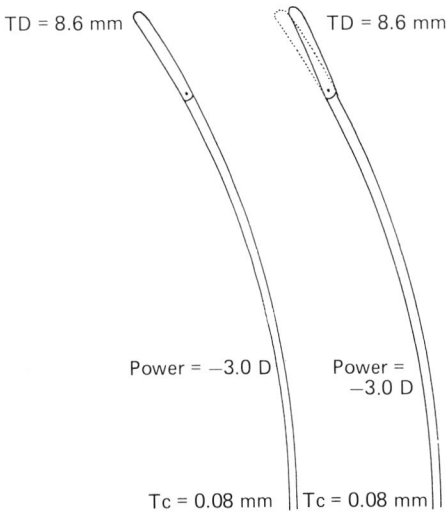

Figure 4.27 The 'ideological' joint in a Korb technique (KT) lens. Only half of each lens is shown

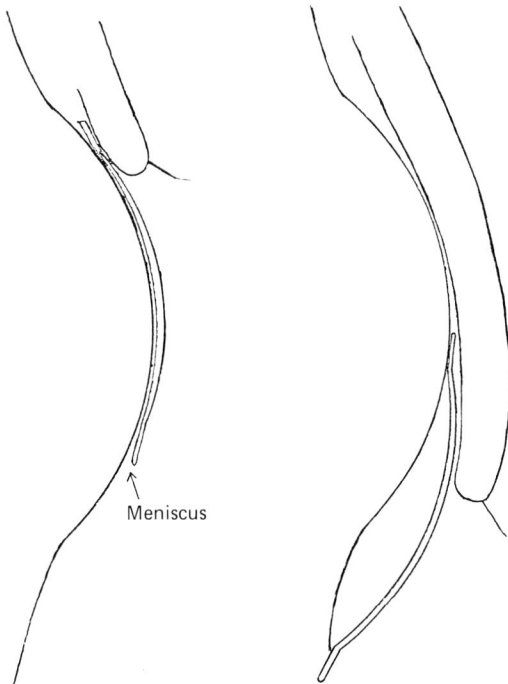

Figure 4.28 Diagrams of the Korb technique lens as it moves on the eye

correct position for vision after a blink. Since the upper lid is re-surfacing it with fresh mucus after every blink the mucus does not dry on it to blur the vision.

Some words of warning need to be inserted here regarding the patient who has worn centring or dropping lenses for many years. Sometimes refitting with lens lid attachment lenses can, in some subtle way, play havoc with the visual acuity so that the patient complains bitterly. What the precise reason for this is, is beyond the author's knowledge, but at any rate, a warning should be given to the patient before refitting.

Choosing the back optic zone radius of the lens (BOZ)

It has already been stated that hard corneal lenses are usually fitted so that the curvature of the back surface of the lens is near to that of the corneal curvature. If the curves are very near to one another it is known as an 'alignment' fit. Between the two surfaces there will be a plano tear fluid lens.

A 'steep' fit implies that the back of the lens is more curved than the cornea. In this case between the two surfaces there will be a plus powered tear fluid lens.

A 'flat' fit implies that the back of the lens is less curved than the cornea. In this case between the two surfaces there will be a minus powered tear fluid lens.

It is important to realize that, contrary to statements often found elsewhere, this relationship is not critical to the development of corneal oedema.

There are four ways of assessing whether a lens is in alignment, steep or flat:

1. A comparison of the keratometer readings with the radius reading of the back optic zone of the lens.
2. A comparison of a photokeratometer calculation for the radii of the cornea and the radius of the back optic zone of the lens.
3. The calculation of the power of the tear fluid lens.
4. The introduction of fluorescein into the tear fluid so that the pattern of its fluorescence can be studied under ultraviolet black light.

These approaches are subject to reservations.

Comparison of keratometry readings and the back central radius of the lens

Many corneas are toroidal in shape and all corneas are not uniformly curved. The keratometer measures the radius of the central cornea as it is defined by two points some 3 or 4 mm apart about the centre of the cornea. The periphery of the cornea is parabolic in shape, flattens more nasally than temporally (Wolff, 1954) and has a variable flattening factor which Brungardt (1965) found was on the average 0.13 mm in radius. The largest flattening he observed was 0.45 mm. Thus two corneas with identical keratometry readings may require entirely different corneal lens fittings.

The fit of the corneal lens depends on its sagittal height more than on its back central radius.

The sagittal height of the corneal lens depends on:

(a) the back optic zone radius
(b) the back optic zone diameter
(c) to a lesser extent, the back peripheral curve or curves.

In practice, if the back optic zone radius is the same as the average keratometry reading and the back optic zone diameter is 7–7.5 mm in diameter an alignment fit will result.

A larger back optic zone diameter will result in a more apex clear (steeper) fitting. A smaller back optic zone diameter will result in a less apex clear (flatter) fitting, or even a fitting which is manifestly flat.

In practice, increasing the back optic zone diameter by 0.5 mm is equivalent to steepening the lens by 0.05 mm in radius of curvature in terms of sagittal height. The converse applies. Although the influence is slight, wider and flatter back peripheral curves will lessen the sagittal height and therefore tend to 'flatten' the lens.

Comparison of the photokeratometer calculation for the radii of the cornea and the back optic zone radius of the lens

The photokeratometer is an instrument which photographs a series of concentric rings which it projects onto the cornea. When the photograph of the rings is enlarged by projection the radii of the cornea can be calculated from their distance apart. The diameter of the cornea can be calculated at the same time.

The calculation of the power of the fluid lens

The power of the corneal lens required can be assessed by spectacle over-refraction with a corneal lens of known power and back central optic radius in situ. However, if the spectacle lens used is over five dioptres in power then a compensation will have to be made for its vertex distance. A plano fluid lens indicates an alignment fitting.

In practice, if the back optic zone radius of the corneal lens is the same as the mean keratometry (irrespective of the diameter of the lens), then the power of the lens required will be the same as the spectacle lens power, ignoring a minus cylinder. This does not apply when the lenses are over five dioptres in power, when the spectacle cylindrical refractive error is over two dioptres in power or when there is a plus spectacle refraction.

An increase of 0.05 mm of steepness to the back optic zone radius of the lens in relation to the mean keratometry will add plus 0.25 D of power to the fluid lens and thus the total refracting power at the front of the eye. The required corneal lens will thus have to be altered by 0.25 D. The converse applies when the lens is flatter than the mean keratometry.

Fluorescein patterns

A small amount of fluorescein is instilled near the superior limbus while the lens is in situ and an ultraviolet black light is used to view the eye (Figure 4.29). Where the lens is clear of the cornea the fluorescein will fluoresce brightly. Where the lens is close to the cornea there will be blackness without fluorescence. An alignment fit is characterized by an even pattern of fluorescence over the area of the back optic zone. Bronstein (1959) and Orsborn *et al.* (1989) have drawn attention to the inaccuracies of this assessment, even in experienced hands. Nevertheless, in some cases, for example, young children, or patients with nystagmus, this may be the only practicable method.

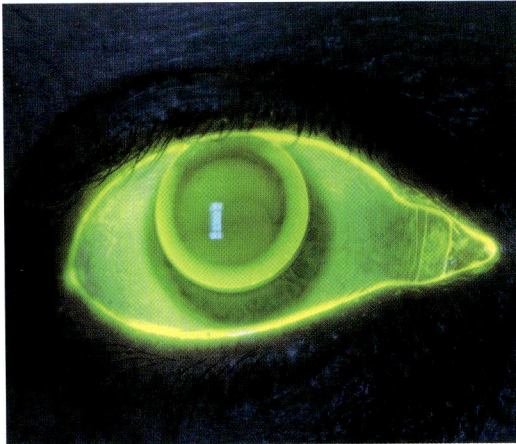

(a)

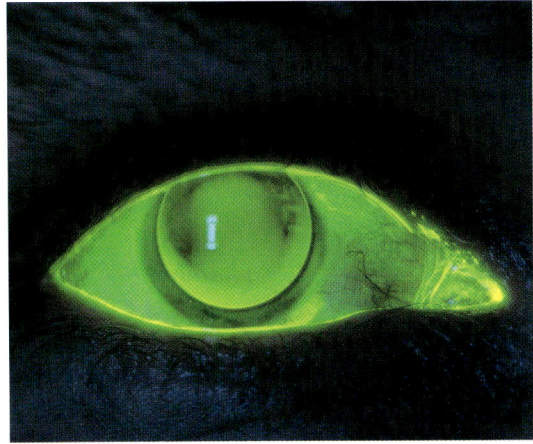

(b)

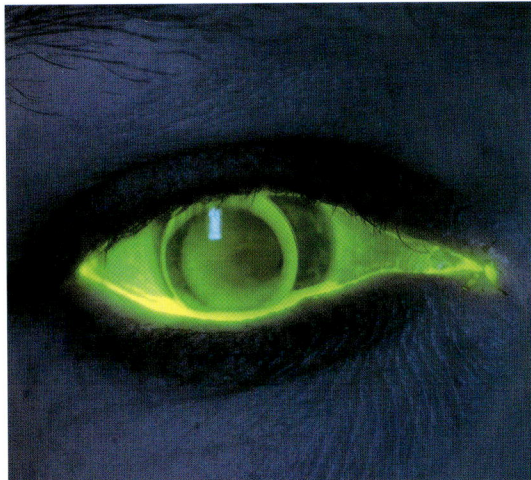

(c)

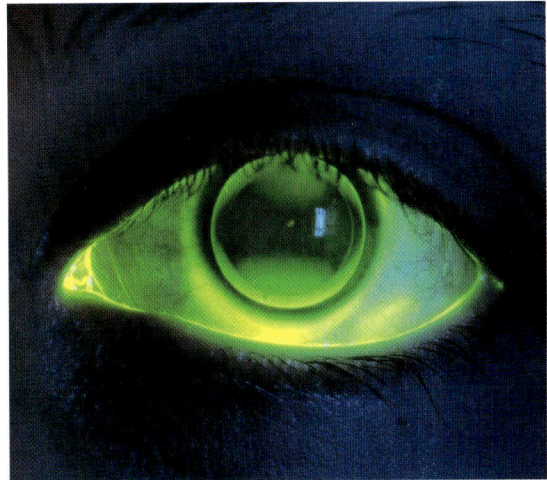

(d)

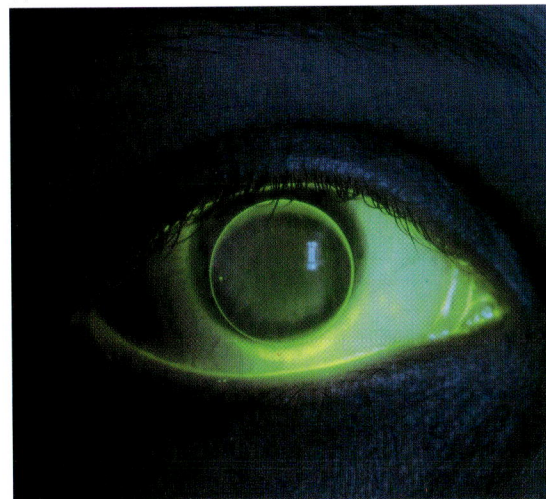

(e)

Figure 4.29 Fluorescein patterns. (a) Apex clear (note the wide flat back peripheral curve); (b) apex clear astigmatic; (c) flat fitting (the lens is decentred down and out); (d) flat astigmatic (note the moderate width back peripheral curve); (e) alignment (note the narrow back peripheral curve)

Choosing the total diameter of the lens

This was like choosing between the devil and the deep blue sea before the advent of gas-permeable hard corneal lenses in the late 1970s and most fitters before that time had experience of starting at one time with small lenses and at another time with large lenses.

By and large, a small cornea demands a small lens and vice versa, but there are other considerations.

The small lens (7.0 to 8.5 mm total diameter)

1. This may give inferior visual performance. This is often the case when lighting is low (such as in the cinema) and the pupil is large. This would appear to be much more noticeable to the mature adult than the teenager and the reasons for this visual failure are hard to understand. One can see a person with a small 8.0 mm lens perched up on the cornea so that its inferior edge almost bisects the pupil and yet there are no complaints about the vision. In another person, the lens may be centred perfectly on the cornea in an eye with a small pupil, adequately covered by the lens, and yet the patient will complain bitterly.
2. It covers a smaller area of cornea. It thus, potentially, gives rise to less corneal oedema. This was the most pertinent reason for using the small lens in the days before gas-permeable lenses.
3. It tends to centre on the cornea. It is often clear of the upper lid and it is lighter than a larger lens. Centration forces tend to be optimal with a small lens.
4. It has less bulk increase at its periphery if it is a minus lens. This may be a desirable feature in a high minus lens. It is undesirable in a low minus lens because there is not adequate substance for the upper lid to grasp to give lens lid attachment.
5. It tends to create problems of drying of the cornea and conjunctiva in the interpalpebral zones. This is because it tends to centre on the cornea and may, because of this, interfere with

the normal patterns of blinking. The patient may tend to avoid contact between the upper lid and the upper edge of the lens.

The large lens (9.0 to 10.0 mm total diameter)

1. It tends to give superior visual performance. This is due to larger coverage of the pupil and more stability in position. However, there may still be visual problems if the patient has been used to a centring or dropping lens.
2. It covers a larger area of cornea. It thus potentially gives rise to more corneal oedema. This was the main reason for the swing to smaller diameter lenses in the middle of the 1960s. Corneal oedema had just started to be acknowledged and detected then. Its presence was probably the main cause of the intolerance which had been experienced with hard corneal lenses. This problem has largely been removed with the advent of gas-permeable lenses.
3. It tends to give lens lid attachment if it is a minus lens. This is due to the increase in bulk at the periphery of the lens as the diameter increases. The lens is more likely to be grasped by the upper lid and this is a desirable feature.
4. It has more bulk increase at its periphery if it is a minus lens. This is an undesirable feature if it is a high minus lens as the peripheral substance may be excessive. It is a desirable feature tending to give a greater possibility of lens lid attachment in a low minus lens.
5. It tends to drop on the cornea if it is a plus lens. This is because of the greater mass. A dropping lens may lead to vascularization of the cornea below. It may also lead to problems of drying of the cornea and conjunctiva in the interpalpebral zones because of the interference with normal blinking patterns. Contact between the upper lid and the upper edge of the lens may be avoided.

Corneas do not vary much in diameter, but small variations can make a large difference in terms of area. It is very difficult to measure the corneal diameter, either by estimating it visually or by special instruments. One of the problems is the ill-defined boundary zone of the limbus which, of course, is on both sides of the measuring instrument. The curvature and steadiness of the eye are other problems. The best way of assessing the diameter is by putting on a corneal lens of known diameter and comparing.

In practice and especially with the advent of gas-permeable lenses, think in terms of two common total diameters, say, 8.6 mm and 9.6 mm with excursions below, between and above in special cases. This standardization helps the stocking of trial lenses in a practice committed to the lens lid attachment technique. If centralization is being aimed at, a diameter of 8.0 mm is often necessary. An important consideration in the choice is that of the corneal diameter of the eye being fitted, as too small a lens may not give satisfactory performance on a large cornea.

Choosing the back optic zone diameter (BOZD)

This amounts to choosing how wide the back peripheral curves should be. A small back optic zone diameter may give problems with the visual acuity, especially if the lens rides high and the junction of the back central curve and the back peripheral curve is within the pupillary area. However, many patients are unaware of the encroachment of this junction within their pupil. On the other hand, a smaller back central optic diameter will cover less cornea, with benefit so far as corneal oxygenation is concerned, and thus compensate, in part, for a larger diameter lens.

Choosing the back peripheral curve or curves

Here there are two principal considerations:

- The diameter of these curves (BPD)
- The radii of these curves (BPR)

On these two factors depends the standoff or 'edge lift' of the lens.

The *radial edge lift* (Figure 4.30) is measured along a line from the centre of curvature of the back central optic radius of the lens. It is the distance between the edge of the back peripheral curve or curves and the projection of the back

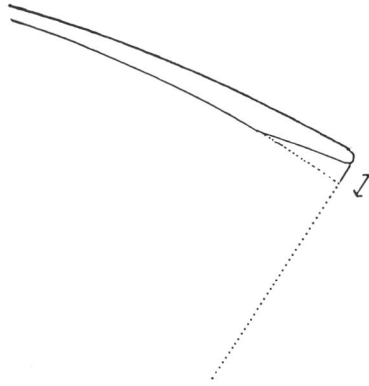

(Not drawn to scale)

Figure 4.30 Radial edge lift. This is measured along a line from the centre of curvature of the back central optic radius of the lens. It is the distance between the edge of the back peripheral curve, or curves, and the projection of the back central optic curve

optic zone curve. The radial edge lift gives a clear picture to the contact lens fitter of how much the edge of the lens is lifting or standing off. Unfortunately, laboratories use the axial edge lift as their guide because it is easier for them to calculate and to measure.

The *axial edge lift* (Figure 4.31) is measured along a line parallel to the optical axis of the lens and is the distance between the edge of the lens and the projection of the back central curve. The axial edge lift is always a little greater in length than the radial edge lift.

Flatter peripheral curves:

- facilitate the passage of fresh tears under the corneal lens;
- facilitate the passage of the corneal lens over the flattening corneal periphery and perhaps

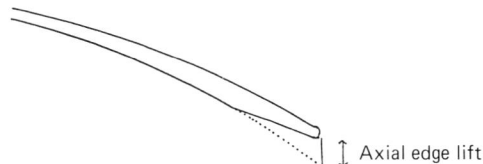

(Not drawn to scale)

Figure 4.31 Axial edge lift. This is measured along a line parallel to the optical axis of the lens and is the distance between the edge of the lens and the projection of the back central curve

on to the sclera during blinking movements (see Figure 4.28)

but,

- give a lens which is more easily ejected or displaced in coming into contact with a lid;
- give a lens which may be more uncomfortable because the patient can feel the edge.

In practice the axial edge lift is usually from 0.10 mm to 0.20 mm in lenses ranging in diameter from 8.6 mm to 10.0 mm. The diameter of the peripheral curve or curves is usually 1.0 mm to 2.0 mm (overall) in lenses ranging from 8.6 mm to 10 mm in overall diameter. More than one back curve is often used to get a smoother transition to the edge lift.

There was a fashion for 'offset' or 'parabolic' back peripheral curves in the early 1970s. The idea was that the transition from spherical back optic zone to the parabolic back peripheral optic zone would be very smooth and special lathes were produced to manufacture these lenses. Since there was no such thing as gas-permeability in those days the parabolic curves were wide and the edge lifts large. In the event, with mass manufacture, these lenses often had a very sharp transition between the spherical and parabolic areas which produced concentric corneal abrasions when the lenses were worn (see Figure 12.20). These abrasions can also be caused by sharp transition in multicurve lenses. Sharp transitions can be detected by inspecting the lens against a light source using a linen measuring device (Figure 4.32), but the curved nature of the abrasion and its position in the intermediate corneal zone between edge and centre should alert the ophthalmologist to the problem. These lesions are usually asymptomatic, or only mildly symptomatic. The laboratory can be instructed to blend the curves. A light, medium or heavy blend can be specified and these terms really relate to the width of the blended area. The laboratory will choose a polishing tool midway in radius of curvature between the two adjacent curves and will do this at the polishing stage after the posterior curves have been ground on the lathe. For accuracy, the back peripheral curves should be ground on a corneal lens as a preliminary procedure while the lens is in the 'button' stage before the front surface is worked. Cutting the posterior curves after the front surface has been

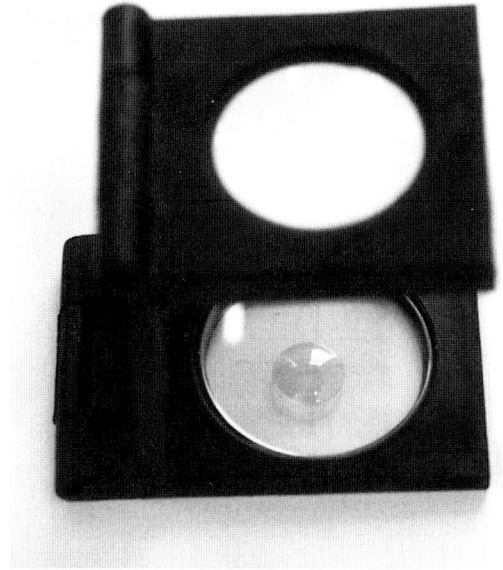

Figure 4.32 Linen measuring device

fashioned leads to inaccuracy due to the flexing of thin lenses.

The British Standards Institution has adopted the International Standards Organisation (ISO 8320–1986) for describing the parameters of a corneal lens (BS 3521 Part 3, 1988). This nomenclature is used in this book.

Figure 4.33 (which is drawn to scale) can be used to explain the system.

The back surface is described in the following way:

C3   7.80 / 7.10 / 8.60 / 8.50 / 10.50 / 9.50

No. of BOZR BOZD BP1R BP1D BP2R   TD
curves

Appendix 4.I gives typical back profiles for 8.0 mm, 8.6 mm, 9.0 mm and 9.6 mm total diameter tricurve lenses with axial edge lifts varying from 0.09 to 0.17 mm.

Appendix 4.II gives typical back profiles for two 9.5 mm total diameter tricurve lenses in which an attempt has been made to keep the edge lifts as constant as possible throughout the range of back optic zone radii. One profile is for a smaller BOZD of 7.10 mm with axial edge lifts varying

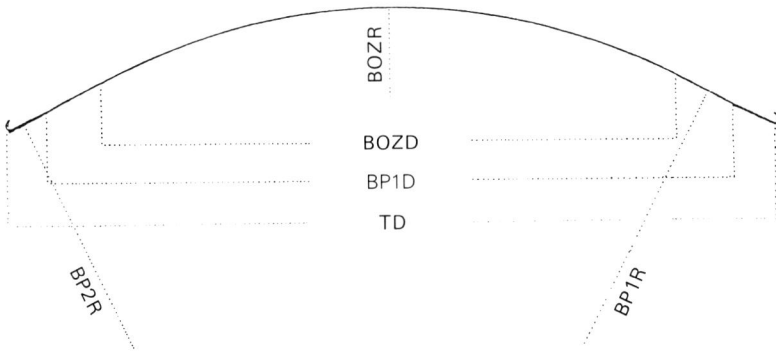

Figure 4.33 Diagram of the back of a corneal lens. BOZR: back optic zone radius; BOZD: back optic zone diameter; BP1R: first back peripheral radius; BP1D: first back peripheral diameter; BP2R: second back peripheral radius; TD: total diameter

from 0.13 to 0.20. The other is for a larger BOZD of 7.80 mm with axial edge lifts varying from 0.09 to 0.15 mm.

Appendix 4.III gives typical back profiles for 9.5 mm total diameter bicurve lenses with small axial edge lifts varying from 0.11 mm at 7.20 mm back optic zone radius to 0.07 mm at 8.40 mm back optic zone radius. The axial edge lift at 7.80 mm back optic zone radius is still only 0.80 mm.

Choosing the front optic zone diameter (FOZD)

This amounts to choosing how large the optically worked, window area (Figure 4.34) of the lens will be. A small, front central optic diameter may give problems with the visual acuity, especially if the lens rides high and the junction of the front central curve and the front peripheral curve are within the pupillary area. However, many patients are unaware of the encroachment of this junction within their pupil. On the other hand, in a plus lens, a smaller front central optic diameter will result in a potentially thinner and, thus, lighter lens, and lens lid attachment will be facilitated. In a minus lens a smaller front central optic diameter will mean an overall thinner and, thus, lighter lens, and will facilitate lens lid attachment.

Appendix 4.V gives figures for reduced optic construction lenses to give lens lid attachment.

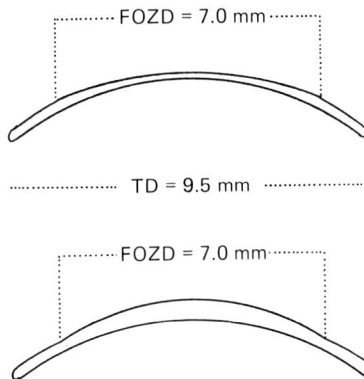

Figure 4.34 Diagram to show front optic reduction in both a minus and a plus lens

Choosing the geometrical centre thickness (Tc)

The factors influencing minimum centre thickness are:

1. The power of the lens
2. The total diameter of the lens if it is of plus power
3. The axial edge lift
4. Reduced front optic zone construction.

The power of the lens

The power of a minus lens can influence the minimum central thickness if that lens has a back peripheral optic curve or curves.

In practice, 0.05 is the lower limit for central thickness, but low powered minus lenses cannot be made so thin because the back peripheral curves would result in little or no edge thickness (Figure 4.35). Plus lenses must have enough centre thickness to allow a satisfactory edge thickness and the incorporation of a back peripheral curve or curves (Figure 4.36).

The total diameter of the lens

The larger the total diameter of a minus lens the greater will be the thickness of its periphery (edge substance), and the more substance there will be for the incorporation of back peripheral curves. A large total diameter, low minus lens with back peripheral curves can thus be thinner than a smaller one with the same back peripheral curves.

The larger the total diameter of a plus lens the greater the central thickness will need to be.

The axial edge lift

A larger edge lift may demand a greater geometric central thickness.

Reduced front optic zone construction

Reduced front optic zone construction allows smaller central thicknesses in both plus and some minus lenses of low power.

Advantages of minimum geometric centre thickness

1. In a gas-permeable lens it gives maximum oxygen transmission for the material used.
2. It minimizes the mass of the lens. Central thickness is the most important factor governing lens mass (Augsberger and Hill, 1971).

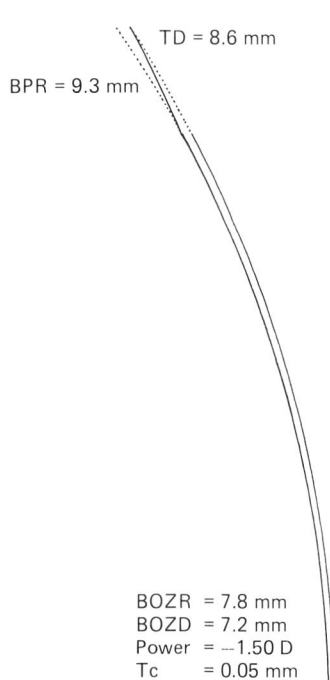

TD = 8.6 mm
BPR = 9.3 mm

BOZR = 7.8 mm
BOZD = 7.2 mm
Power = −1.50 D
Tc = 0.05 mm

Figure 4.35 Low powered lens (−1.50) at 0.05 mm central thickness – there is no substance for the edge if there is a back peripheral curve

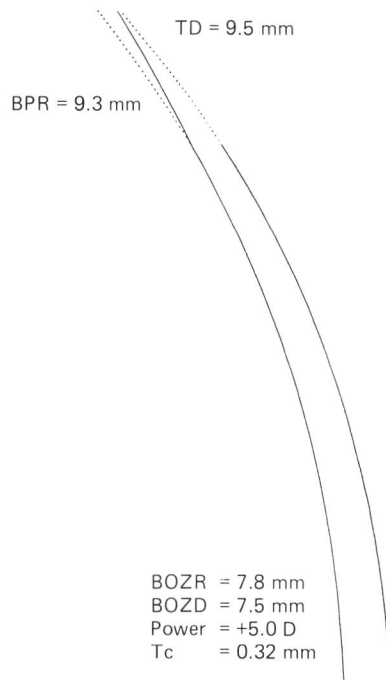

TD = 9.5 mm
BPR = 9.3 mm

BOZR = 7.8 mm
BOZD = 7.5 mm
Power = +5.0 D
Tc = 0.32 mm

Figure 4.36 Plus lens without sufficient centre thickness to allow the incorporation of back peripheral curves. Only half the lens is shown

3. It minimizes the amount of edge substance in both minus and plus lenses.

Disadvantages of minimum geometric centre thickness

1. The lens is more fragile.
2. The lens is more flexible and the effects of this are often seen in the case of more flexible gas-permeable material. The gas-permeable lens tends to conform to any corneal toricity and poor and variable vision may result. A central thickness not less than 0.13 mm may be more appropriate for such lenses.
3. The lens is more difficult to manufacture. Any lack of parallelism of the front and back curves results in no edge at one part of the circumference and this is why manufacturers' stated minimal thicknesses are usually much in excess of the possible minimal thickness.

Appendix 4.IV gives minimum centre thicknesses in the types of lenses for which back profiles have been given.

Choosing the edge thickness (Tea)

According to the British Standards Institution BS 3521 Part 3, 1988, it is now necessary to measure this thickness parallel to the primary axis of the lens and not radially as before.

If the edge is too thick the lids will have difficulty in passing over the lens and they will tend to retract rather than pass over. This will result in abnormal patterns of blinking. Excessive edge thickness will also increase the tendency for the lens to be ejected when the lid comes in contact with it. These are grossly undesirable features. On the other hand, excessively thin edges tend to shatter in use and this is especially the case in gas-permeable material.

Much has been written about edge form, but when an edge is as thin as recommended in this text there is little room for shapes. The edge should be rounded and not sharp at any point. Special edges have been advocated for the control of giant papillary conjunctivitis (see Chapter 12).

In practice an edge thickness of 0.08 to 0.10 should be used, bearing in mind that when a lens is easily ejected the thinner edge will be better and that 0.08 can be too thin for a more fragile gas-permeable lens.

Choosing the front peripheral curve or curves

A front peripheral curve (or curves) is necessary in many high minus lenses and the radius and diameter can be calculated as described in the following text. Front peripheral curves are also frequently found in hard corneal lenses used in aphakia. In this case, it is often enough to specify their diameter and leave the calculation of the radius to the laboratory, merely specifying that the front peripheral zone should be 'plano', that is parallel to the back peripheral zone or zones. The normal diameter of the front peripheral zone in a 9.5 mm aphakic lens is 2 mm, leaving a front central optic diameter of 7.5 mm. A front peripheral zone curve is used in a low minus lens to achieve lens lid attachment and a reduced centre thickness. The calculation of the radius and diameter of this curve can be made as detailed in the following text, or by the more convenient use of the table given in Appendix 4.V.

Calculating the parameters of a hard corneal lens

When lenses are designed or when it is necessary to know, for example, how thin a lens can be, or what its front peripheral radius should be, the calculations can be done mathematically, on a computer, or on a drawing board.

Prescribing by these methods leaves nothing to the judgment, or whim, of the laboratory technician.

These methods aid:

1. Precise specification.
2. The determination of what is possible.
3. Precise reproducibility.

Mathematical calculation

Mathematical calculation has the disadvantage that it is very tedious and, in the end, gives no idea of the appearance the lens will have.

Computerization

A small hand computer can be obtained with a program for calculating the parameters of hard corneal lenses (and soft lenses in both their dry and hydrated states). It will give axial edge lifts, geometric central thicknesses, front optic zone curves, etc. (G. Nissel & Co. Ltd, Hemel Hempstead, Herts., England, supply such an instrument.) Pye, Lin and Nhieu (1986) have discussed the problems of visualizing contact lens designs. They have developed computer-aided design software that greatly improves visualization. There are options of displaying magnified cross-sections of any part of the lens, making detailed measurements of these cross-sections and displaying colour-coded, three-dimensional views of the lens surfaces.

A large computer is available. It is programmed in a similar manner to the hand held instrument, but the lens can be visualized on a video screen. Such a computer can be obtained from Contek Ltd, Cambridge, England.

Drawing contact lenses

Provided that the equipment is laid out, this can be done in a few minutes.

Some contact lens designers draw at a scale of 100 to one on graph paper one metre wide. This makes the calculation very easy, but this magnitude is impracticable for most contact lens fitters and a scale of 40 to one is used.

The following materials are required:

1. Sectional pads. These are pads ruled in millimetre squares. Most lenses can be drawn on a pad measuring 40×25 cm but in the case of minus lenses, over 10 D in power, a chart measuring 50×40 cm will be required.
2. Beam compass. This is an alternative to the conventional compass and is used when parts

of large circles are required. The beam should measure at least 50 cm in length.
3. Nissel slide ride (obtainable from G. Nissel and Co. Ltd, Hemel Hempstead, Herts., England). This instrument, designed by A.G. Bennett (1963), gives the surface power of the back optic radius and also gives the outer optic radius according to the nominal front surface power and the centre thickness. The centre thickness influences the final front surface power.

The lenses are drawn to a magnification of $\times 40$. This makes the mathematics easy. Converting the contact lens parameters, which are given in millimetres to centimetres, and multiplying by four simplifies the procedure in the chart.

The method is as follows:

- Draw only half the lens, as if it had been divided along a diameter.
- The back central curve is the first to be drawn.
- The axial edge lift is then determined, together with the diameter of the back peripheral curve, which, of course, has to be divided by two. The radius necessary to join these two points together while maintaining the centre of the compass on the base line can then be determined.
- A trial central thickness can then be taken. A Nissel rule is then used to calculate the front optic zone radius according to the power of the lens and the centre thickness chosen. Alterations can be made to the centre thickness as necessary, so that the lens has sufficient edge thickness.
- A front peripheral curve can be drawn in by joining two points between a chosen axial edge thickness and the limitation of the front optic zone curve. For lens lid attachment, the front optic radius should parallel the back peripheral curve, or curves.

The main reasons for drawing a contact lens are to determine central thickness and the front peripheral curve.

The drawings of contact lenses in this book were done by this method. Appendix 4.V, as an alternative to drawing, gives a set of figures which can be used for designing low minus and plus lenses with a front peripheral curve so as to obtain lens lid attachment.

References

AUGSBERGER, A.R. and HILL, R.M. (1971) Contact lens mass: the most elusive design feature. *Journal of the American Optometric Association* **42**, 78–82

BENNETT, A.G. (1963) *Optics of Contact Lenses*. Association of Dispensing Opticians, London

BOGAN, S.J., WARING, G.O., IBRAHIM, O., DREWS, C. and CURTIS, L. (1990) Classification of normal corneal topography based on computer-assisted videokeratography. *Archives of Ophthalmology*, **108**, 945–949

BORISH, I.M. (1961) *Bulletin No. 7*. Indiana Contact Lens Co., Marion, Indiana

BRONSTEIN, L. (1959) The accuracy of fluorescein for determining corneal curvature. *Contacto*, **3**, 170–171

BRUNGARDT, T.F. (1965) Sagittal height of the cornea. *American Journal of Optometry*, **42**, 525–533

DINGELDEIN, S.A. and KLYCE, S.D. (1989) The topography of normal corneas. *Archives of Ophthalmology*, **107**, 512–517

GIRARD, L.J. (ed.) (1964) *Corneal Contact Lenses*. C.V. Mosby Co., St Louis

KESSING, S.V. (1967) A new division of the conjunctiva on the basis of X-ray examination. *Acta Ophthalmologica*, **45**, 680–683

KORB, D.R. and KORB, J.E. (1970) A new concept in contact lens design. Parts 1 & 2. *Journal of the American Optometric Association*, **41**, 12, 1023–1032

MACKIE, I.A., MASON, D. and PERRY, B.J. (1970) Factors influencing corneal lens centration. *British Journal of Physiological Optics*, **25**, 2, 87–103

MANDELL, R.B. (1981) *Contact Lens Practice*, 3rd edn. Charles C. Thomas, Springfield, Illinois

ORSBORN, G.N., ZANTOS, S.G., GODIO, L.B., JONES, W.F. and BARR, J.T. (1989) Aspheric rigid gas permeable contact lenses: practitioner discrimination of base curve increments using fluorescein pattern evaluation. *Optometry and Visual Science*, **66**, 4, 209–213

PYE, D.C., LIN, G.C.I. and NHIEU, T. (1986) Computer-aided design of hydrophilic contact lenses. *Clinical and Experimental Optometry*, **69**, 3, 93–97

SMELSER, G.K. and CHEN, D.K. (1955) Physiological changes in cornea induced by contact lenses. *Archives of Ophthalmology*, **53**, 676–679

WOLFF, E. (1954) *The Anatomy of the Eye and Orbit*, H.K. Lewis, London

Appendix 4.1

Back profiles of tricurve 8.00 mm total diameter lenses with axial edge lifts varying from 0.13 mm at 7.20 mm radius to 0.09 mm at 8.40 mm radius (after Korb).

BOZR	according to the choice made
BOZD	6.70 mm
BP1R	2.4 mm flatter than the BOZR
BP1D	7.8 mm
BP2R	12.00 mm
TD	8.0 mm

For example:

C3	7.20/6.70/ 9.60/7.80/12.00/8.00	AEL 0.13 mm
C3	7.80/6.70/10.20/7.80/12.00/8.00	AEL 0.10 mm
C3	8.40/6.70/10.80/7.80/12.00/8.00	AEL 0.09 mm

Back profiles of tricurve 8.6 mm total diameter lenses with axial edge lifts varying from 0.14 mm at 7.20 mm radius to 0.09 mm at 8.40 mm radius (after Korb).

BOZR	according to the choice made
BOZD	7.2 mm
BP1R	1.5 mm flatter than the BOZR
BP1D	8.2 mm
BP2R	12.00 mm
TD	8.6 mm

For example:

C3	7.20/7.20/8.70/8.20/12.00/8.60	AEL 0.14 mm
C3	7.80/7.20/9.30/8.20/12.00/8.60	AEL 0.11 mm
C3	8.40/7.20/9.90/8.20/12.00/8.60	AEL 0.09 mm

Back profiles of tricurve 9.00 mm total diameter lenses with axial edge lifts varying from 0.17 mm at 7.20 mm radius to 0.10 mm at 8.40 mm radius (after Korb).

BOZR	according to the choice made
BOZD	7.50 mm
BP1R	1.40 mm flatter than the BOZR
BP1D	8.4 mm
BP2R	12.00 mm
TD	9.00 mm

For example:

C3	7.20/7.50/8.60/8.40/12.00/9.00	AEL 0.17 mm
C3	7.80/7.50/9.20/8.40/12.00/9.00	AEL 0.14 mm
C3	8.40/7.70/9.80/8.40/12.00/9.00	AEL 0.10 mm

Back profiles of tricurve 9.60 mm total diameter lenses with axial edge lifts varying from 0.27 mm at 7.20 mm radius to 0.16 mm at 8.40 mm radius (after Korb).

BOZR	according to the choice made

BOZD   8.00 mm
BP1R   1.4 mm flatter than the BOZR
BP1D   8.8 mm
BP2R   12.00 mm
TD   9.6 mm

For example:

C3   7.20/8.00/8.60/8.40/12.00/9.60   AEL 0.27 mm
C3   7.80/8.00/9.20/8.80/12.00/9.60   AEL 0.18 mm
C3   8.40/8.00/9.80/8.40/12.00/9.60   AEL 0.16 mm

Appendix 4.II

Back profiles of tricurve 9.5 mm total diameter lenses in which there has been an attempt to keep the axial edge lift as constant as possible throughout the range of back central optic radii so that all lenses are likely to have similar peripheral clearances on the eyes to which they are fitted. This is in contrast to lenses in which there is a standard flattening of the back peripheral radii, in which case the flatter lenses with larger back optic zone radii have a much smaller edge lift than the steeper lenses with smaller back optic zone radii.

(a) With small back optic zone diameters

C3   7.20/7.10/7.90/8.50/10.00/9.50   AEL 0.20 mm
     7.25/7.10/7.95/8.50/10.00/9.50
     7.30/7.10/8.00/8.50/10.00/9.50   AEL 0.19 mm
     7.35/7.10/8.05/8.50/10.00/9.50
     7.40/7.10/8.10/8.50/10.25/9.50   AEL 0.19 mm
     7.45/7.10/8.15/8.50/10.25/9.50
     7.50/7.10/8.20/8.50/10.25/9.50   AEL 0.18 mm
     7.55/7.10/8.25/8.50/10.25/9.50
     7.60/7.10/8.30/8.50/10.25/9.50   AEL 0.17 mm
     7.65/7.10/8.35/8.50/10.25/9.50
     7.70/7.10/8.40/8.50/10.50/9.50   AEL 0.17 mm
     7.75/7.10/8.45/8.50/10.50/9.50
     7.80/7.10/8.60/8.50/10.50/9.50   AEL 0.16 mm
     7.85/7.10/8.65/8.50/10.50/9.50
     7.90/7.10/8.70/8.50/10.50/9.50   AEL 0.16 mm
     7.95/7.10/8.75/8.50/10.50/9.50
     8.00/7.10/8.80/8.50/10.50/9.50   AEL 0.15 mm
     8.05/7.10/8.85/8.50/10.75/9.50
     8.10/7.10/8.90/8.50/10.75/9.50   AEL 0.15 mm
     8.15/7.10/8.95/8.50/10.75/9.50
     8.20/7.10/9.00/8.50/10.75/9.50   AEL 0.14 mm
     8.25/7.10/9.05/8.50/10.75/9.50
     8.30/7.10/9.10/8.50/10.75/9.50   AEL 0.13 mm
     8.35/7.10/9.15/8.50/10.75/9.50
     8.40/7.10/9.20/8.50/10.75/9.50   AEL 0.13 mm
     8.45/7.10/9.25/8.50/11.00/9.50
     8.50/7.10/9.30/8.50/11.00/9.50   AEL 0.13 mm

(b) With large back optic zone diameters

C3   7.20/7.80/7.90/8.70/ 9.75/9.50   AEL 0.15 mm
     7.25/7.80/7.95/8.70/ 9.75/9.50
     7.30/7.80/8.00/8.70/10.00/9.50   AEL 0.15 mm
     7.35/7.80/8.05/8.70/10.00/9.50
     7.40/7.80/8.10/8.70/10.00/9.50   AEL 0.14 mm
     7.45/7.80/8.15/8.70/10.00/9.50
     7.50/7.80/8.20/8.70/10.25/9.50   AEL 0.14 mm
     7.55/7.80/8.25/8.70/10.25/9.50
     7.60/7.80/8.30/8.70/10.25/9.50   AEL 0.13 mm
     7.65/7.80/8.35/8.70/10.25/9.50
     7.70/7.80/8.40/8.70/10.50/9.50   AEL 0.13 mm
     7.75/7.80/8.45/8.70/10.50/9.50
     7.80/7.80/8.60/8.70/10.50/9.50   AEL 0.13 mm
     7.85/7.80/8.65/8.70/10.50/9.50
     7.90/7.80/8.70/8.70/10.50/9.50   AEL 0.12 mm
     7.95/7.80/8.75/8.70/10.50/9.50
     8.00/7.80/8.80/8.70/10.50/9.50   AEL 0.12 mm
     8.05/7.80/8.85/8.70/10.50/9.50
     8.10/7.80/8.90/8.70/10.75/9.50   AEL 0.12 mm
     8.15/7.80/8.95/8.70/10.75/9.50
     8.20/7.80/9.00/8.70/10.75/9.50   AEL 0.11 mm
     8.25/7.80/9.05/8.70/10.75/9.50
     8.30/7.80/9.10/8.70/10.75/9.50   AEL 0.10 mm
     8.35/7.80/9.15/8.70/10.75/9.50
     8.40/7.80/9.20/8.70/10.75/9.50   AEL 0.10 mm
     8.45/7.80/9.25/8.70/10.75/9.50
     8.50/7.80/9.30/8.70/10.80/9.50   AEL 0.09 mm

For lenses of larger or smaller overall size the back optic zone diameter, the first peripheral diameter and the total diameter can be adjusted proportionately.

For example:

C3   7.80/7.60/8.60/9.00/10.50/10.00
                    (smaller BOZD) AEL 0.19 mm

and

C3   7.80/7.30/8.60/8.20/10.50/ 9.00
                    (larger BOZD) AEL 0.12 mm

Appendix 4.III

Back profiles of bicurve lenses of 9.5 mm in total diameter, giving an axial edge lift varying from 0.11 mm at 7.20 mm radius of curvature to 0.07 mm at 8.40 mm radius of curvature. These are small axial edge lifts.

BOZR   according to the choice made
BOZD   7.50 mm
BPR   0.80 mm flatter than the BCOR
TD   9.50 mm

Specify a light blend on the transition.
  For example:

C2   7.20/7.50/8.00/9.50   AEL 0.11 mm
C2   7.80/7.50/8.60/9.50   AEL 0.08 mm
C2   8.40/7.50/9.20/9.50   AEL 0.07 mm

  For lenses of larger or smaller total diameter the back central optic diameter and the overall size can be adjusted proportionately.

Appendix 4.IV

Minimal geometric centre thicknesses of minus lenses described in Appendix 4.I

(a) Without a front peripheral curve

	Total diameter			
	8.0	8.6	9.0	9.6
Plano	0.13	0.13	0.14	0.16
−1.00	0.12	0.13	0.14	0.16
−1.75	0.11	0.11	0.12	0.13
−2.50	0.10	0.10	0.11	0.12
−3.00	0.09	0.09	0.10	0.11
−4.00	0.08	0.08	0.09	0.10
−5.00	0.07	0.07	0.08	0.09
−6.00	0.07	0.07	0.08	0.08
−7.00	0.05	0.05	0.05	0.05

(b) With a front peripheral radius for lens lid attachment (see Appendix 4.V)

Plano	0.12	0.12	0.13	0.13
−1.00	0.11	0.11	0.12	0.12
−1.75	0.11	0.11	0.11	0.11
−2.50	0.10	0.10	0.10	0.11
−3.00	0.09	0.09	0.10	0.10
−4.00	0.08	0.08	0.08	0.09
−5.00	0.07	0.07	0.07	0.07

(c) Minimal geometric central thicknesses of minus lenses described in Appendix 4.II

−1.00	0.15	0.15	0.15	0.15
−2.00	0.14	0.14	0.14	0.14
−3.00	0.13	0.13	0.13	0.13
−4.00	0.12	0.12	0.12	0.12
−5.00	0.10	0.10	0.10	0.10
−6.00	0.08	0.08	0.08	0.08
−7.00	0.05	0.05	0.05	0.05

Minimal centre thicknesses of low plus lenses

In this instance the front optic zone diameter should be taken as a reference rather than the total diameter if the front optic is reduced.

	Front optic zone diameter or total diameter				
	7.00	7.5	8.00	8.5	9.00
+1.00	0.17	0.19	0.20	0.22	0.23
+3.00	0.20	0.22	0.24	0.26	0.28
+4.00	0.22	0.24	0.26	0.28	0.31
+5.00	0.24	0.26	0.28	0.30	0.33
+6.00	0.25	0.28	0.30	0.33	0.36
+7.00	0.27	0.30	0.32	0.35	0.39

Appendix 4.V

Front optic zone diameters and front peripheral radii for lens lid attachment

Minus and plus lenses

Overall size	Power	FOZD	FPD
8.00	Plano to −2.50	7.00	2.00*
	−2.75 to −6.00	7.20	1.70*
	+0.25 to +4.00	7.00	2.00*
	+4.25 to +7.00	6.90	2.00*
8.60	Plano to −2.50	7.60	1.70*
	−2.75 to −6.00	7.60	1.50*
	+0.25 to +4.00	7.40	1.80*
	+4.25 to +7.00	7.30	2.00*

The upper-right continuation:

−4.00	0.08	0.08	0.08	0.09
−5.00	0.07	0.07	0.07	0.07

9.00	Plano to −2.50	7.80	1.70*
	−2.75 to −6.00	8.00	1.50*
	+0.25 to +4.00	7.60	1.80*
	+4.25 to +7.00	7.50	1.80*
9.60	Plano to −2.50	8.20	1.50*
	−2.75 to −6.00	8.40	1.50*
	+0.25 to +4.00	8.20	2.00*
	+4.25 to +7.00	8.20	2.00*

*Flatter than the back optic zone radius

Ordering hard corneal lenses

From the foregoing a typical lens may be ordered from the laboratory as follows:

C3   7.80/7.20/9.30/8.20/12.00/8.60

BVP −1.50   Tint light grey (912)
Tc 0.11   Tea 0.10
FOZD 7.6
FPR 9.5

Where C3 denotes that there are three back curves
    912 is a specific tint in CQ (controlled quality ICI) polymethylmethacrylate plastic
    BVP is the back vertex power
    Tc is the geometric centre thickness
    Tea is the edge thickness
    FOZD is the front optic zone diameter
    FPR is the front perpheral radius

Modifying rigid corneal lenses

There is equipment readily available for in practice, do it yourself, modification of rigid corneal lenses.

Powers can be adjusted, edges reworked, total diameters reduced and even new back peripheral curves introduced. The lenses can also be polished.

It has not been the author's practice to indulge in this activity, but rather to re-order a lens if the parameters have to be changed. He then carefully labels and stores the first lens as a trial lens. The only exception has been the light polishing of lenses and a convenient instrument is available for this from Specialist Optical, 57 Dukes Wood Drive, Gerrards Cross, Bucks. SL9 7L7, England.

Changing the parameters of a contact lens by in practice modification introduces the problem of reproducibility in the future and attempting to change the power, which is usually done by polishing the front surface on a fabric drum impregnated with polish, often leads to a lens which has a different power in its centre to that of the periphery. This has dire consequences in a lens lid attachment design. It can also be seen that reducing the total diameter of a plus lens will result in a lens which is much thicker than it need be and which will have excessive edge substance.

5

Gas permeable lenses

Introduction

The avascular cornea has an affinity for atmospheric oxygen for the maintenance of normal aerobic metabolism (Smelser and Ozanics, 1952). One of the difficulties encountered with the fitting of contact lenses is the interruption of the supply of this oxygen to the cornea, because the lens, to a greater or lesser extent, covers the cornea. When a gas impermeable lens is fitted, the cornea has to rely on tear bulk flow exchange under the lens for its oxygenation. This exchange is related to blink frequency (Cuklanz and Hill, 1969; Fatt and Hill, 1970; Efron and Ang, 1990).

The term, gas permeable lens, is commonly used by patients and fitters to denote a contact lens which is permeable to gases such as oxygen, which the cornea derives from surrounding air, and carbon dioxide which comes off the surface of the cornea. The term usually implies a hard corneal lens, but it must be realized that all soft lenses are gas permeable. The words 'rigid' or 'hard' should always be used to define precisely what is meant.

There is an important physical difference between the terms gas permeability and gas transmissibility.

Gas permeability – the Dk value – is a property of the particular material at a given temperature, where D is the diffusion coefficient for oxygen in the sample and k is the solubility of oxygen in the sample. It is usually given for a fixed temperature – nowadays 35 °C.

Gas transmissibility – the Dk/L value – is a property of the sample of material where L is the sample thickness. The diffusion coefficient D is a measure of how fast dissolved molecules of oxy-

gen move in the contact lens material. The term k is the number of oxygen molecules dissolved in the material. The term L is the thickness of the lens across which the oxygen must move in travelling from the front to the back surface of the lens.

The permeability, or Dk, of a contact lens material describes its intrinsic ability to carry oxygen. The transmissibility, or Dk/L, of a particular lens describes the passive ability of the lens to allow oxygen to move from the front to the back surface.

A lens with optical power has thickness that depends upon the distance from the centre of the lens. The lens will be thinner at the centre if it is minus and thicker at the centre if it is plus. De Donato (1981) has presented a technique which shows how lens mass can be used to determine the average lens thickness. This average thickness can be used to calculate the oxygen transmissibility of a contact lens of material of known oxygen permeability. Brennan, Efron and Holden (1986) have produced graphs which give a good estimate of average transmissibility. Nowadays, many soft lenses are designed to be as near plano as possible in shape by reducing the front central optic (Figure 5.1). This is frequently impracticable so far as rigid contact lenses are concerned because they often do not centre on the cornea and, in this case, the optically worked portion of the lens is not over the area of the pupil.

The food packaging industry has established standards for gas permeability. This has yet to be done for the contact lens industry. In a recent communication, Fatt (1986) has discussed the problems of assessing gas permeability.

When a gas permeable lens is in the eye, the

(a)

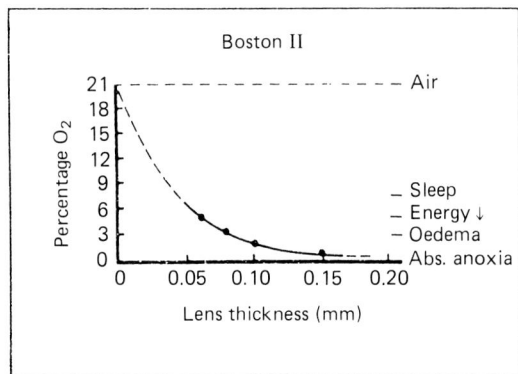

(b)

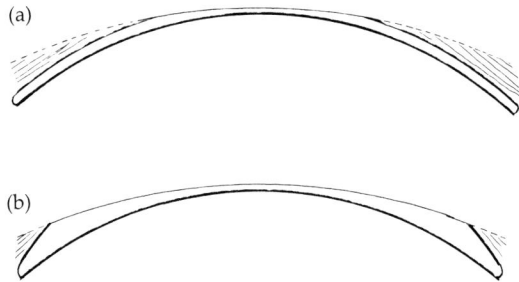

Figure 5.1 (a) A soft minus lens treated by front optic reduction to be as near as possible in shape to a plano lens. (b) The same lens without the front optic reduction

tear film between the lens and the cornea adds to the resistance encountered by oxygen, diffusing from the front surface of the lens to the cornea. This can lead to an apparent reduction in the transmissibility of the lens. The tear film under a lens varies in thickness. At the apex the reduction in transmissibility due to the tear film may be 5%. At the periphery it might be as much as 20%.

The effect of transmissibility, for any lens, is composed of three components – the lens material, boundary barriers and the tear film. Only the lens material transmissibility is well understood. The barrier and tear film effects will require much further study.

The transmissibilities of two common hard gas permeable lenses – the Boston II and the Polycon II – are shown in Figure 5.2. Note that this transmissibility varies with the centre thickness of the contact lens in a non-linear fashion.

Bonanno and Polse (1987) have shown that contact lens wear causes corneal acidosis by the production of protons from hypoxic metabolism and the accumulation of carbon dioxide behind the lens due to low carbon dioxide transmissibility.

Efron and Ang (1990) used the term hypercapnia to denote carbon dioxide accumulation and found that all the contact lenses examined in their study caused an accumulation of carbon dioxide at the anterior corneal surface under open-eye and closed-eye conditions. The physiological implications of the disruption to the normal pCO_2 cycle are unclear. The acidic shift in the cornea resulting from the interference with carbon dioxide efflux from the corneal surface may be associated with clinical and subclinical effects, such as endothelial morphological changes and stromal thinning.

Cohen *et al*. (1991) have shown that the corneal deswelling response is slower after swelling caused by a contact lens than that caused by mere deprivation of oxygen.

There was a limited availability of gas permeable hard lenses to investigators in the mid 1970s and, commercially, these lenses were available by the end of the 1970s. They represented a considerable advance. Before that time fitters were used to making modifications to lenses to try to avoid corneal oedema. Lenses were made with wide posterior peripheral curves or parabolic posterior curves. This resulted in small optic zones and, thus, less close coverage of the cornea, but this often led to visual problems, notably flare. Large edge standoffs (axial edge lifts) were used to

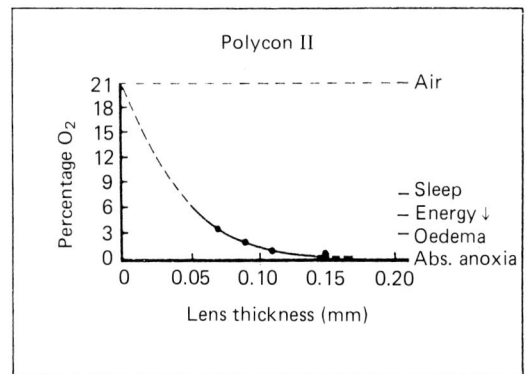

Figure 5.2 Oxygen permeability compared to lens thickness in Boston II and Polycon II rigid gas permeable contact lenses

encourage 'venting' under the lenses and these often gave rise to unstable lenses which were easily injected. In an attempt to occlude as little cornea as possible, small lenses of 8 mm or less in overall diameter were fitted to centralize on the cornea. The reduced coverage of the cornea gave less oedema, but again there was a visual problem of flare, typically in a cinema or when driving at night, when the pupils were dilated. Some lenses did not, in fact, centre on the cornea and gave marked problems, not only with vision but with tolerance.

Another effective device for relieving the oedema was the introduction of fenestrations into the lenses. These holes pass through the lens. They had to be central, or paracentral, and have a diameter of at least 0.3 mm to be effective. Again, there were visual problems in at least 30% of cases. The more numerous and the larger the diameter of the holes, the more the visual problems would increase. These problems originated from reflections from the internal surface of the holes. Blackening this surface would probably have resulted in a diminution in the annoying reflections reported. However, this was technically difficult in a hole 0.30 mm wide and 0.10 mm deep. There were, however, many people who were visually completely unaware of the holes.

Lens lid attachment (Korb and Korb, 1970) encouraged normal blinking. With this technique (see Chapter 4) the contact lens is always in contact with the upper lid. Without lens lid attachment normal blinking can be suppressed to avoid decentring a centring contact lens, or even the upper lid touching a dropping contact lens. Fink, Hill and Carney (1990) have shown that in the oxygen impermeable contact lens wearer a higher blink frequency is associated with higher corneal oxygenation.

Efron (1986) has shown that there is an inter-subject variability in the corneal swelling response to anoxia. This was always suspected by contact lens fitters in the days before gas permeable lenses. In the days before gas permeable hard lenses there were no rules as to what diameter to start with. One could start large and run into gross oedema problems, or start small and run into gross visual problems. All this has been changed by the advent of hard gas permeable lenses and it would appear that the optimum size for these is 9.5 mm in most corneas and 8.6 mm in small corneas.

Disadvantages of hard gas permeable lenses

After their introduction, gas permeable materials were soon found to have disadvantages when compared with conventional polymethylmethacrylate.

Some patients who had been long-term wearers of the latter material just did not like the feel of the new material, for no reason that they could logically explain. The new material was more flexible and it was more easily broken. Patients who had never broken a hard lens suddenly found that they broke a lens of the new material while cleaning it. (There have been reports of the new high Dk extended wear lenses breaking while in the eye.)

The lens was much more prone to attract deposit on its surface (see Figure 9.1). This deposit had been an occasional problem in certain patients with polymethylmethacrylate lenses and consisted either of magnesium and calcium carbonates or of protein. With hard gas permeable lenses it was a frequent problem, appearing a few months after the lenses started to be worn. The manufacturers quickly produced special cleaning solutions in an attempt to deal with this problem, but it still remains.

One of the first gas permeable hard materials was cellulose acetate butyrate (CAB). Stone (1978) was quick to point out the dimensional instability of this material which she found to be greatly in excess of polymethylmethacrylate. She found that changes brought about by hydration were similar in style, but much greater in magnitude than those in polymethylmethacrylate. High minus cellulose acetate butyrate lenses were very unstable. The back central optic radii of these could vary up to 0.2 mm according to the state of hydration. Low minus and low plus lenses were more stable. The alteration in back central optic radius did not, of course, affect the power of the lens itself, but it did alter the effective power when the lens was in situ on the eye due to alteration in the fluid lens and, thus, its power. A variation of 0.2 mm back central optic radius is equivalent to a variation of one dioptre in in situ contact lens power. A similar state of affairs was found with changes in temperature.

Stone (1978) also assessed the plastic memory of cellulose acetate butyrate. Squeezing a thick, or thin, or high minus lens would result in a toric lens which might take two hours to regain its spherical shape. In some cases, when this was done with thin lenses, recovery was not complete until the lens had been soaked for a day. These lenses could, thus, after a short time on the eye, drape themselves round a toric cornea so that the corneal astigmatism became uncorrected and the visual acuity was diminished. The main indication for fitting a gas permeable lens at that time was a patient who, because of significant astigmatism, could not easily be fitted with a soft lens after failing with a conventional hard lens. The flexibility of the material was a great disadvantage.

The original cellulose acetate butyrate lenses made by Danker and Wohlk had a centre thickness of 0.16 mm in a −5.75 lens. This was an excessive thickness for a lens of such power and was presumably set at that value in the interest of maintaining its shape. The increased thickness, of course, decreased lens oxygen transmissibility and increased the tendency of the lens to drop and assume a low position on the cornea.

The dimensional stability of lenses of the silicone co-polymers of methylmethacrylate (such as Polycon and Boston), which were also introduced at that time, was more acceptable, but not as high as polymethylmethacrylate.

The phenomenon of flattening in high minus lenses made from second generation, higher Dk materials was noted at an early stage in the development of routine hydration and stability trials. At about −10.0 D these lenses would flatten about 0.10 mm in a period of wear lasting from two days to three months. Lenses of −15.00 D would flatten by 0.15 mm over a period of wear lasting from one to three months.

Third generation very high Dk fluoropolymers have now arrived which have such oxygen permeability that centrally thick aphakic lenses (0.40 or more) can be used on an extended wear basis.

Cavanagh *et al.* (1989) have shown that corneal swelling responses caused by these high Dk rigid gas permeable lenses differ with extended wear in naive and adapted subjects. They contend that, at least for the lenses they tested, adaptation to contact lens wear down-regulates the overnight swelling response to levels at or near no lens wear, or daily wear values. They hypothesize that corneal neural sensitivity to lens wear lessens with time and this decreasing sensitivity down-regulates the overnight swelling response.

It is now apparent that these lenses can steepen in wear by as much as 0.50 mm, causing an unacceptably tight fit (Kerr and Dilly, 1988). Frothing, debris retention, indentation and binding (see below) would occur.

Kerr and Dilly (1988) have shown, by electron microscopy, what is happening at a molecular level. They coated the lenses with a thin layer of gold and electrically charged the material. Charging favours the regions of molecular stress and sharp polymer chain edges within the system, thus, as it were, allowing the charged polymer chains to shine, causing these regions to light up at the cut up surface of the lens. In normal, unworn 'virgin' lenses, these lines are infrequent and, where present, run directly from the front to the back surface of the lens (Figure 5.3).

In the worn, steepened lenses these charge lines are distorted, such that the anterior surface appears to have moved radially towards the perimeter of the lens, compared with the posterior surface (Figure 5.4). The steepening distortion can most easily be explained by the forces of a mass polymer flow, radially towards the border of the lens. Dimensional instability gives rise to the problem of lenses flexing during wear. Non-gas permeable and gas permeable hard lenses both exhibit this disadvantage. It appears that the higher the Dk value, the higher the flexibility.

Harris and Chu (1972) studied the effect of contact lens thickness and corneal toricity on flexure and residual astigmatism, that is, astigmatism remaining after the fitting of a hard corneal lens. They used hard corneal (PMMA) lenses.

On spherical and near spherical corneas none of the lenses flexed significantly or altered the residual astigmatism. On toric corneas, thick lenses in excess of 0.13 mm central thickness did not flex significantly. However, thin lenses of less than 0.13 mm central thickness did flex significantly and did alter residual astigmatism in a predictable manner. Lens flexure and residual astigmatism increased as centre thickness decreased. These observations should apply, but more so, to gas permeable lenses.

Harris *et al.* (1982) have studied flexure and residual astigmatism with both Polycon and PMMA lenses in toric corneas. They found that Polycon lenses undergo significantly more flexure and alter residual astigmatism more on toric corneas than PMMA lenses at all centre thicknesses

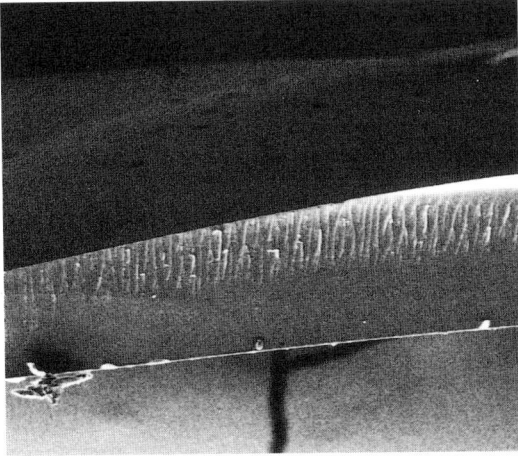

Figure 5.3 A 'virgin' high plus, fluoropolymer lens showing undistorted, vertical, charging lines. (Courtesy C. Kerr and P.N. Dilly)

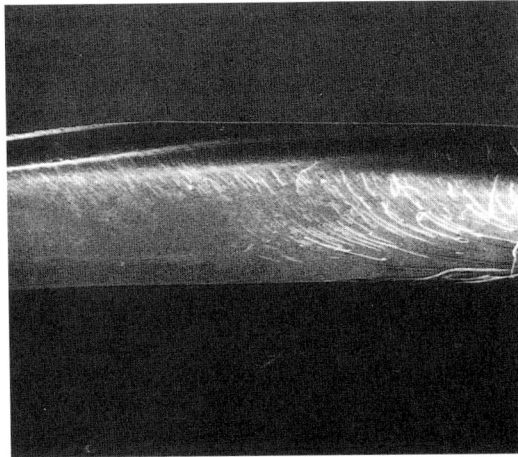

Figure 5.4 A worn, high plus, fluoropolymer lens showing curved charging lines induced by material flow in a lens steepened by wear. (Courtesy C. Kerr and P.N. Dilly)

evaluated (0.07 mm–0.16 mm). For both materials flexure and residual astigmatism increased as centre thickness decreased.

Herman (1983) has studied the flexure of rigid contact lenses on toric corneas as a function of the back optic zone radius fitting relationship. He used gas permeable lenses (Polycon at 9.5 mm diameter). He found that the amount and the direction of the flexure were determined by the relationship of the back central optic radius to the cornea. As the lenses were fitted steeper than K (the flattest keratometer reading) with the rule flexure occurred. As lenses were fitted flatter than K, against the rule (that is with the minus cylinder at 90°) flexure occurred.

He also found that if the upper lid covered the superior portion of the lens, an against the rule flexure component was usually introduced. Aphakic lenses normally have a thickness in excess of 0.40 mm. Examination of Figure 5.2 will show what a disadvantage this is in terms of oxygen transmission in the second generation of Polycon and Boston materials (siloxane methacrylates, Polycon II and Boston II). There is, in fact, little oxygen transmission.

Spurred on by the fact that there is a substantial extended wear hard contact lens market and that soft extended wear lenses can be dangerous, the manufacturers have searched for hard materials with very high oxygen permeability (Dk) values.

These enable aphakic hard contact lenses to be worn on an extended wear basis. There is now a plethora of hard materials with Dk values greatly in excess of anything obtainable in hydrophilic soft lenses. The highest Dk value for a soft hydrophilic contact lens is about 35×10^{-11} and this is a high water content lens. The highest Dk value for a hard gas permeable lens is about 85×10^{-11} according to Brennan, Efron and Holden (1986). Allergan quotes a Dk value of 100×10^{-11} for their Advent lens which contains no silicone. These high gas permeable hard materials are silicone elastomers, perfluorether-N-vinylpyrrolodine-methylmethacrylate, siloxane acrylate and methacrylate, fluorosiloxane acrylate and perfluoroalkyl-itaconate-siloxane.

The newer materials contain fluorocarbon monomers. The combination of silicon and fluorocarbon monomers has enabled very high oxygen permeability to be obtained without detriment to other properties, such as hardness, stability and wettability, that were apparent with the silicon methacrylate lenses. There appears to be synergism between the two monomers that enhances the oxygen permeability such that less of the monomer need be added which would otherwise cause a reduction of hardness, stability and wettability.

Materials for hard and soft contact lenses have recently been listed with their specifications by

Burki (1989). Since 1983, the Association of Contact Lens Manufacturers in the UK (ACLM) has developed a system of classifying contact lens materials. This system is widely used by the UK industry and it is being proposed for adoption as a Standard nomenclature to the British Standards Organisation. The Food and Drugs Administration in the USA has another system called the United States approved name (USAN). The problem there is that almost every different polymer has been given an approved name.

The classification of the ACLM divides contact lens materials into two main groups, Filcon for soft lens materials and Focon for hard lens materials (which happens to be the stem names in the USAN system). The classification is given in Appendix 5.I.

Lenses made of high gas permeable materials are now being made available for wear by myopes. It has been shown by Korb *et al.* (1980) that 10.5% of wearers of hard corneal lenses develop giant papillary conjunctivitis after a period of 5 years. It can be expected that with extended wear of hard gas permeable lenses this percentage would increase. The aphakic patient does not have a long life expectancy, but giant papillary conjunctivitis is a problem.

With young myopes the problem looms larger. Many observers feel that giant papillary conjunctivitis is a problem of trauma in susceptible wearers of contact lenses. Extended wear doubles the time that they are worn. Furthermore, the surfaces of gas permeable lenses are not as clean as those made of hard polymethylmethacrylate. There are more deposits which may become abrasive and also add to the antigen load. A major problem with the use of high Dk gas permeable rigid lenses worn on an extended basis is that of binding ('glued on syndrome' in the American literature), that is, the lens is found adherent to the cornea, on opening the eye in the morning. Typically, the lens is bound in a decentred position, often overlapping the limbus. A ring of tear debris is frequently seen trapped behind the mid periphery of the lens. At this stage, the lens is not uncomfortable, but the vision is blurred due to the tear debris and the decentred position of the lens. The most frequent position of decentration is nasally.

Spontaneous movement of the lens generally occurs within the first hour of eye opening, although the lens may remain bound for several hours. As the lens begins to move there may be a foreign body sensation. Punctate fluorescein staining of the central cornea and inferior conjunctiva can be seen once the lens is mobile, together with a complete or partial indentation ring on the cornea (Figure 5.5). A severe abrasion may ensue binding, especially if there is forceful removal of the lens.

Swarbrick and Holden (1987) found in a retrospective analysis that the incidence of binding was 22% in 279 cases of overnight wear of rigid gas permeable lenses in a variety of materials and designs.

They found that overnight lens binding occurred more frequently with lenses of:

1. Large diameter.
2. Flat back optic zone radius.
3. Minimal edge lift.
4. Lenses fitted 'on K' (that is in alignment) or flat relative to the central corneal curvature.
5. Lenses exhibiting less than optimal on-eye lens movement before closure.

Swarbrick (1988) assessed the effect of central fenestration of a lens which repeatedly bound to the eye of a young, male contact lens wearer. The fenestrated lens was worn in the right eye over a 10-day period, during which time the lens was left out for one night. Over the nine nights that

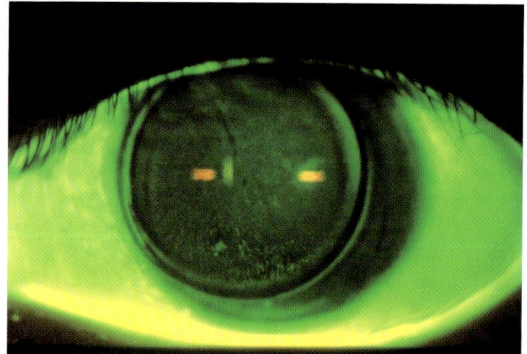

Figure 5.5 Corneal indentation ring immediately after removal of a bound rigid gas permeable lens. The indentation ring rarely stains with fluorescein. Instead, the tears either pool in the indentation, or appear to thin in this area if the indentation is shallow. Mild punctate staining of the central cornea is also apparent. The lens had been bound for nine hours. (Reproduced from Swarbrick, H.A. (1988) *International Contact Lens Clinic*, **15**, 13–19, courtesy of Dr Helen Swarbrick and the Editor, *International Contact Lens Clinic*)

the lens was worn, lens binding was noted on eight occasions.

Swarbrick and Holden (1989) suggest that lens binding is primarily a patient-dependent phenomenon.

Zabkiewicz *et al*. (1988) have also studied the problem of binding. They observed a group of patients wearing different lens designs, but all fitted to give minimum clearance fluorescein patterns, over a period of 15 months. Sixty eight per cent of patients (21 out of 31) showed signs of binding. During the first month binding was more frequent with the tricurve design, but later there was a significant increase in frequency with both aspheric and tricurve designs. They concluded that:

1. Binding is most likely to occur in subjects with a thin lipid pre-corneal layer and little corneal astigmatism.
2. Fitting lenses with mid peripheral bearing and with narrow or tight (that is less axial edge lift) edges will increase binding.
3. Binding increases with time due to the 'moulding' effect on the cornea from the lens back surface.
4. Lens movement has little influence on binding.

It appeared to them that repeated episodes of binding after one month of successful wear can result in severe corneal distortion. There can be gradual steepening of the corneal curvature and lenses can begin to ride high. That is, the BOZR can become relatively flatter.

A further problem with gas permeable lenses is wettability. The newer polymers differ from PMMA in that they include silicon and/or fluorine which are two hydrophobic substances. The addition of hydrophilic groups such as methacrylic acid and hydroxyethylmethacrylate is necessary to provide a wettable surface.

Doane, Korb and Miller (1984) studied the influence of lens design and fitting characteristics on the stability of the pre-contact lens tear film. They found that an edge that is too thick or poorly shaped can inhibit the normal blink process and result in accelerated drying of the lens surface.

Doane and Gleason (1987) studied the effect of lens position in relation to the marginal tear menisci (of the lids) and found that it had a significant effect on lens front surface drying time. Their high speed motion pictures showed that the lenses were wetted by tears from the inferior meniscus being dragged over the surface of the lens by the upper lid as the eye opens following a blink. Shortly thereafter the tear film begins to drain away from the surface, producing varying degrees of exposure depending on the individual patient and the material from which the lens is made. There is, thus, a period of time between blinks when the surface of the lens is all, or partially, dry. These authors have also photographed new dry lenses on human subjects. The lenses wet very poorly at first but as the surface becomes coated with mucin, wettability gradually increases. It is important that new polymers have a strong affinity for mucin which increases the energy of the solid surface of the contact lens, facilitating wettability.

Doane (1989) has described an instrument for in vivo tear film interferometry. This instrument allows objective evaluation of the break up characteristics of the tear film on contact lens surfaces and provides a means of examining the dynamic changes in thickness, thickness distribution and wetting properties during sequential interblink periods. The effects of contact lens material, wetting solutions and cleaning regimens can be compared objectively.

A final and major problem with gas permeable lenses, worn on an extended wear basis, has been the occurrence of three and nine o'clock staining, together with its sequelae. This would appear to be more pronounced than in daily wear lenses and may be related in part to the tendency of extended wear lenses to bind. Three and nine o'clock staining is discussed in Chapter 12.

Certain facts related to the fitting of gas permeable lenses are relevant.

1   Lid attachment

(a) This reduces the effect of flexure on a with the rule astigmatic cornea and allows a thinner lens for any material now in use.
(b) The problem of lenticular residual astigmatism, which is almost always against the rule, is exacerbated by lid attachment since this method of fitting can induce against the rule astigmatism.
(c) Drying is increased with the use of gas permeable lenses. The larger the lens the more surface evaporation. Lid attachment increases the

efficiency of blinking, giving better closure and decreasing evaporation.
(d) The tendency to three and nine o'clock staining is diminished by lid attachment which promotes increased efficiency in blinking and better closure.

2   *Lens thickness*

(a) A thicker lens will give less problem with flexure but will not be so oxygen transmissible.

3   *Back central optic curve relationship to corneal curvature*

(a) A flatter lens will give less flexure on any with the rule cornea.
(b) For extended wear the fitting should be flat, and flatter and wider back peripheral curves are desirable to avoid binding.

Gas permeable scleral lenses

Scleral lenses can now be made of gas permeable material (Ezekiel, 1983, Pullum, 1987; Pullum, Parker and Hobley, 1989; Schein, Rosenthal and Ducharme, 1990). The lenses described by Pullum and Pullum, Parker and Hobley are moulded from eye impressions. The lenses described by Schein, Rosenthal and Ducharme are preformed. The latter are fitted by using trial lenses.

The advantage of gas permeability in a large coverage scleral lens is obvious. With polymethylmethacrylate, oxygen availability to the cornea depends on fenestrations which introduce air bubbles behind the lens. These air bubbles have to be mobile, rotating round the limbus with the versions of the eye. These bubbles have to be just the right size so that they are large enough to function and yet do not interfere with vision. This often presents great fitting difficulties.

SoftPerm lenses

One gas permeable lens is available (the SoftPerm lens, Sola/Barnes Hind, USA) in which a rigid centre and a soft outer skirt are molecularly interwoven and made from a single piece of Synergicon A material (Figure 5.6).

The water content of the skirt is 25%. The rigid centre has a diameter of 8.0 mm. The optic zone is 7.0 mm in diameter and the lens has an overall diameter of 14.3 mm. It is available in powers ranging from +6.0 D to −13.0 D. The oxygen permeability of the centre is 14×10^{-11} and the skirt 5.5×10^{-11}.

SoftPerm lenses are fitted mainly from the keratometry findings, but fluorexan, the high molecular weight dimer of fluorescein, which is not absorbed by hydrophilic materials, can be used in the assessment of the fit (see Chapter 9).

SoftPerm lenses are the third generation of the hybrid lenses which were formerly called Saturn I

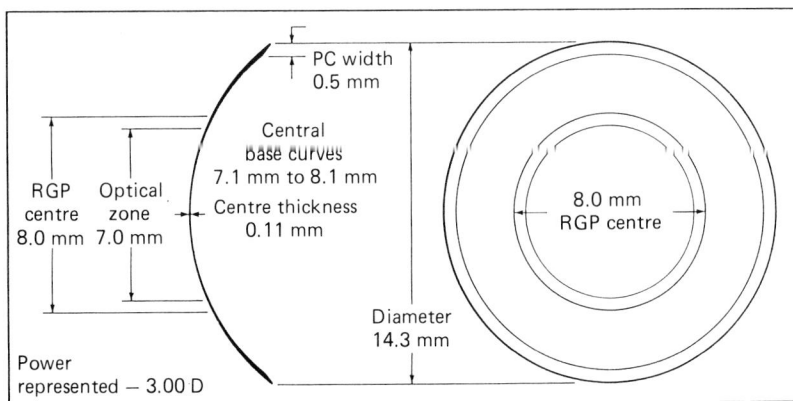

SoftPerm lens design

Figure 5.6 Diagram of a SoftPerm (Synergicon A) contact lens (Sola/Barnes Hind, USA)

and Saturn II. These lenses are useful in the management of astigmatism when a stable vision is not obtained with toric soft contact lenses. They are also useful in keratoconus, especially when there is mild disease associated with atopic conjunctivitis.

The manufactures of SoftPerm lenses advise against the use of solutions containing chlorhexidine and against the use of heat disinfection. They advise their peroxide system for disinfection.

References

BONANNO, J.A. and POLSE, K.A. (1987) Corneal acidosis during contact lens wear: effects of hypoxia and CO_2. *Investigative Ophthalmology and Visual Science,* **28**, 1514–1520

BRENNAN, N.A., EFRON, N. and HOLDEN, B.A. (1986) Oxygen permeability of hard gas permeable contact lens materials. *Clinical and Experimental Optometry,* **69**, 82–89

BURKI, E. (1989) Materials for hard and soft contact lenses. *Contactologia,* **1**, 1–4

CAVANAGH, H.D., ICHIKAWA, H., MACKEAN, D., KAZEL, A. and JESTER, J.V. (1989) Corneal swelling responses differ with extended wear in naive and adapted subjects with high DK RGP contact lenses. *Investigative Ophthalmology and Visual Science* (Suppl.), **30**, 3, abstract 13, p. 481

COHEN, S.R., POLSE, K.A., JANIC, G., BRAND, R.J. and BONANNO, J.A. (1991) Stromal acidosis reduces corneal hydration control. *Investigative Ophthalmology and Visual Science* (Suppl.), **32**, 4, 731

CUKLANZ, H.D. and HILL, R.M. (1969) Oxygen requirements of contact lens systems. *American Journal of Optometry and Archives of American Academy of Optometry,* **46**, 228–230

DE DONATO, L.M. (1981) Determination of the average thickness of a contact lens. *American Journal of Optometry and Physiological Optics,* **58**, 10, 846–847

DOANE, M.G. (1989) An instrument for in vivo tear film interferometry. *Optometry and Visual Science,* **66**, 6, 383–388

DOANE, M.G. and GLEASON, W. (1987) The marginal meniscus; a major factor in contact lens wetting. *Investigative Ophthalmology and Visual Science,* **28**, (Suppl.), 372

DOANE, M.G., KORB, D. and MILLER, D. (1984) Diagnostic high speed photography in ophthalmology. *Investigative Ophthalmology and Visual Science,* **25**, Suppl. 192

EFRON, N. (1986) Intersubject variability in corneal swelling response to anoxia. *Acta Ophthalmologica,* **64**, 302–305

EFRON, N. and ANG, J.H.B. (1990) Corneal hypoxia and hypercapnia during contact lens wear. *Optometry and Visual Science,* **67**, 7, 512–521

EZEKIEL, D. (1983) Gas permeable haptic lenses. *Journal of the British Contact Lens Association,* **6**, 158

FATT, I. (1986) Now do we need 'effective permeability'. *Contax,* July, 6–23

FATT, I. and HILL, R.M. (1970) Oxygen tension under a contact lens during blinking – a comparison of theory and experimental observations. *American Journal of Optometry and Archives of American Academy of Optometry,* **47**, 50–55

FINK, B.A., HILL, R.M. and CARNEY, L.G. (1990) Corneal oxygenation: blink frequency as a variable in rigid contact lens wear. *British Journal of Ophthalmology,* **74**, 168–171

HARRIS, M.G. and CHU, S.C. (1972) The effect of contact lens thickness and corneal toricity on flexure and residual astigmatism. *American Journal of Optometry,* **49**, 304–307

HARRIS, M.G., KADOYA, J., NOMURA, J. and WONG, V. (1982) Flexure and residual astigmatism with Polycon and polymethylmethacrylate lenses on toric corneas. *American Journal of Optometry and Physiological Optics,* **59**, 3, 263–266

HERMAN, J.P. (1983) Flexure of rigid contact lenses on toric corneas as a function of base curve fitting relationship. *Journal of the American Optometric Association,* **54** (3), 209–213

KERR, C. and DILLY, P.N. (1988) Problems of dimensional stability in rigid gas permeable lenses. *Contact Lens Monthly,* in *Optician,* Feb. 5th

KORB, D.R., ALLANSMITH, M.R., GREINER, J., HENRIQUES, A.S., RICHMOND, P. and FINNEMORE, V. (1980) Prevalence of conjunctival changes in wearers of hard contact lenses. *American Journal of Ophthalmology,* **90**, 336–341

KORB, D.R. and KORB, J.E. (1970) A new concept in contact lens design. Parts 1 and 2. *Journal of the American Optometric Association,* **41**, 12, 1023–1032

PULLUM, K.W. (1987) Feasibility study for the production of gas permeable scleral lenses using ocular impression techniques. *Transactions of the BCLA Conference,* 1987, pp. 35–39, British Contact Lens Association, London

PULLUM, K.W., PARKER, J.H. and HOBLEY, A.J. (1989) The Joseph Dallos Award Lecture, 1989. Development of gas permeable scleral lenses produced from impressions of the eye. *Transactions of the BCLA Conference,* 1989, British Contact Lens Association, London

SCHEIN, O.D., ROSENTHAL, P. and DUCHARME, C. (1990) A gas permeable scleral contact lens for visual rehabilitation. *American Journal of Ophthalmology,* **109**, 318–322

SMELSER, G.K. and OZANICS, V. (1952) Importance of atmospheric oxygen for maintenance of the optical properties of the human cornea. *Science,* **115**, 140

STONE, J. (1978) Changes in curvature of cellulose acetate

butyrate lenses during hydration and dehydration. *Journal of the British Contact Lens Association*, **1**, 1, 22–35

SWARBRICK, H.A. (1988) A possible etiology for RGP binding (adherence). *International Contact Lens Clinic*, **15**, 1, 13–19

SWARBRICK, H.A. and HOLDEN, B.A. (1987) Rigid gas permeable lens binding: significance and contributing factors. *American Journal of Optometry and Physiological Optics*, **64**, 11, 815–823

SWARBRICK, H.A. and HOLDEN, B.A. (1989) Rigid gas permeable lens adherence: a patient dependent phenomenon. *Optometry and Visual Science*, **66**, 5, 269–275

ZABKIEWICZ, K., SCHNIDER, C., HOLDEN, B.A. and TERRY, R. (1988) Poster at International Contact Lens Centenary Congress, London, 25–28th May, 1988

Appendix 5.I

Classification of contact lens materials by Association of Contact Lens Manufacturers (from Parker, J. The Classification of Contact Lens Materials. *Contact Lens Year Book*, 1990, pp. 52–54 (C. Kerr, ed.). Medical and Scientific Publishing Ltd, Hythe, Kent, UK).

The classification divides contact lens materials into two groups:

Filcon – for soft lens materials
Focon – for hard lens materials

The parameter component, in brackets, is given to distinguish performance characteristics which have great significance to the practitioner. In the case of soft lens materials it is the water content. In the case of hard lens materials it relates to the oxygen permeability.

Table 5.1 Chemical group classification – soft lens materials: Filcon

Group 1a (38)
Essentially pure 2-hydroxyethylmethacrylate, containing not more than 0.2% weight of any ionizable chemical (e.g. methacrylic acid).
Group 1b (65)
Essentially pure 2-hydroxyethylmethacrylate, containing more than 0.2% weight of any ionizable chemical

Table 5.1 (*cont.*)

Group 2a (36)
A copolymer of 2-hydroxyethylmethacrylate and/or other hydroxyalkylmethacrylates, dihydroxyalkylmethacrylates and alkyl methacrylates, but not more than 0.2% weight of any ionizable chemicals.
Group 2b
As described in Group 2a, but containing more than 0.2% weight of any ionizable chemicals.
Group 3a
A copolymer of 2-hydroxyethylmethacrylate with an N-vinyl lactam and/or an alkyl acrylamide but containing not more than 0.2% weight of any ionizable chemicals.
Group 3b (71)
As described in Group 3a, but containing more than 0.2% weight of any ionizable chemicals.
Group 4a (71)
A copolymer of alkyl methacrylate and N-vinyl lactam and/or an alkyl acrylamide, but containing not more than 0.2% weight of any ionizable chemicals.
Group 4b
As described in Group 4a, but containing more than 0.2% weight of any ionizable chemicals.
Group 5 (200)
Soft lens materials formed from polysiloxanes

Table 5.2 Chemical group classification – hard lens materials: Focon

Group 1a
Essentially pure polymethylmethacrylate (99.0%). Dk essentially zero.
Group 1b
Copolymers of PMMA with not more than 10% max. of other monomers that may alter hardness, wettability and stability. Dk essentially zero.
Group 2a (5)
Essentially pure CAB (90%). Dk range typically of 2 to 8.
Group 2b
Copolymers or mixtures of CAB and other monomers.
Group 3 (12)
Copolymers of one or more alkyl methacrylates with one or more siloxanylmethacrylates, plus other water active monomers and cross-linking agents. Typical Dk of more than 6.
Group 4
Hard lens materials formed from polysiloxanes.
Group 5 (160)
Copolymers of one or more alkyl methacrylates and/or siloxanylmethacrylates, plus other water active monomers, cross-linking agents, and at least 5% by weight of a fluoroalkyl methacrylate or other fluorine containing monomers. Typical Dk of more than 20.

CAB: cellulose acetate butyrate

6

Fitting soft contact lenses

Soft hydrophilic contact lenses are now mainly manufactured from three different materials – the original hydroxyethylmethacrylate (HEMA), vinylpyrrolidine co-polymers and glycerylmethacrylate co-polymers. They can be lathe cut or spun cast in moulds. They are then hydrated.

The fitting of soft lenses depends to a certain extent on the nature of the material with which they are made – its firmness and its water content.

Just as in the case of the hard lens, one must think not so much in terms of the back optic zone radius, but in terms of the sagittal height of the lens which is determined by its total diameter as well as its back optic zone radius. Thus, a lens of larger diameter will require a flatter, that is, less curved back optic zone radius in order to maintain the sagittal height and thus the fitting relationship with the eye (Figure 6.1).

The precision which is necessary with a hard corneal lens is not required with the soft lens. Thus, in a hard lens, one tends to work in steps of 0.05 mm of radius of curvature, whereas in soft lenses the steps are at least 0.20 mm and usually 0.30 mm.

Each variety or make of soft lens has a radius, together with a total diameter which will fit over 60% of normal eyes. There will be a second radius, perhaps 0.3 mm steeper, at the same diameter, which will fit most of the remaining eyes.

Occasionally one will have to make excursions into radii 0.2 mm or 0.3 mm flatter than the flattest radius above and 0.2 mm or 0.3 mm steeper than the steepest radius above.

So far as the diameter is concerned almost all eyes can be fitted with a lens of 13.5 to 14.00 mm in total diameter. Occasionally a lens of up to 15.50 mm in total diameter will have to be used and small cornea may be fitted with a lens of 13.0 mm in total diameter.

There is still a small cottage industry making soft lenses and here one can specify one's own radii and diameter, but most lenses are made by large manufacturers who set their own radii and diameters. One can ask them what the most popular radii and diameters are and order trial lenses accordingly.

Most soft contact lenses do not have a back peripheral curve. This dictates extra centre thickness in a soft lens, but there may be some advan-

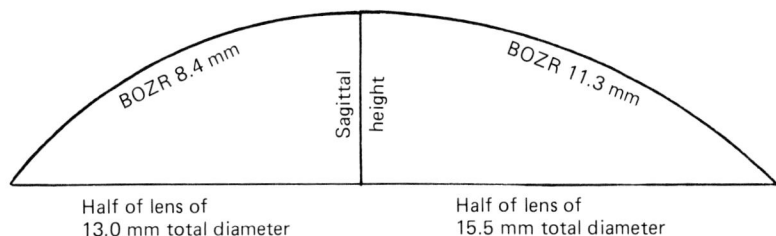

Figure 6.1 Diagrams of half of the back central optic curve of two lenses of the same sagittal height, shown adjacently. Changing the diameter requires a change in back central optic radius to maintain the sagittal height and vice versa

tage in such a curve in terms of tear fluid inter-change under the lens and the disposal of corneal epithelial debris.

Most soft lenses have a reduced front optic zone. This may only amount to a chisel edge (Figure 6.2) being put on to finish the lens. In the case of plus lenses and high minus lenses the front optic zone is usually reduced to 8.0 mm, but in the opinion of the author this is too large. There are seldom any visual problems with a 7.0 mm optic (Figure 6.3). The ideal in a minus lens is to achieve as near as possible to the profile of a plano lens by front edge reduction (Figure 6.4). Oxygen transmissibility is usually thought of in relation to the centre thickness of a soft lens, but the average overall thickness is a better guide.

A small hand computer can be obtained for calculating the parameters of soft corneal contact lenses, according to specific requirements. It will give the minimum central thicknesses for lenses of various water content, powers, curvatures and diameters and will compensate these for front optic reduction and back peripheral curves (G. Nissel & Co. Ltd , Maxted Close, Hemel Hemp-stead, Herts., UK, supplies such an instrument.)

Pye, Lin and Nhieu (1986) have developed computer-aided design software, that greatly im-proves visualization, for designing soft contact lenses.

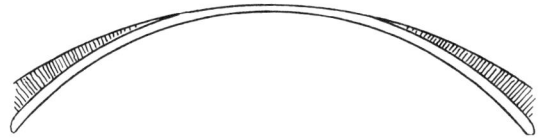

Figure 6.4 Diagram of a minus lens constructed to be as near to plano form as possible to achieve minimal overall thickness. Front peripheral substance is removed

Technique

It is best to employ some magnification in order to see the lens in the eye and this is best achieved by using times two magnification, binocular oper-ating spectacles. A slit lamp is not ideal for fitting. A good halogen ophthalmoscope producing a bright and even circle of light is ideal as an illuminator. A soft lens is inserted and it is al-lowed to settle down. The patient is asked to look up and to blink. If, on inspection, the lens hardly moves or there is a visible bubble under it, it is removed and the lens of the next flatter radius is inserted. If the lens moves excessively and does not centre on the cornea it is removed and a lens of a steeper radius is inserted. The ideal is to fit a lens which moves 1 or 1.5 mm when the patient looks up and blinks and which centralizes on the

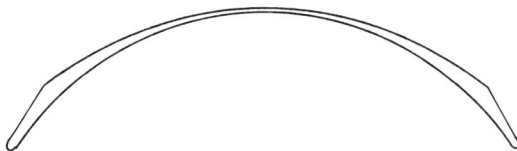

Figure 6.2 Diagram of a soft contact lens with chisel edge

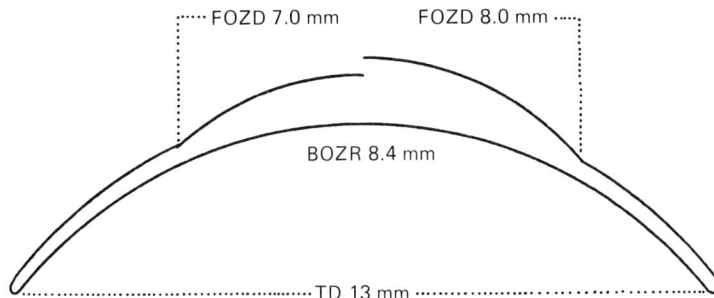

FOZD 7.0 mm   FOZD 8.0 mm

BOZR 8.4 mm

TD 13 mm

Figure 6.3 Front optic reduction to 7.0 mm and 8.0 mm. A diagram of two adjacent halves of lenses of the same plus power are shown. Compare the central thicknesses

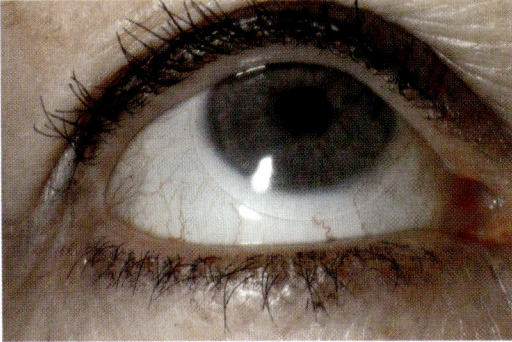

Figure 6.5 Fitting a soft contact lens. When the patient looks up and blinks the lens should move 1–1.5 mm. The lens should centralize on the cornea in this up position as well as in the primary position

cornea in this up position as well as in the primary position. In both positions no area of the cornea should be uncovered (Figure 6.5). One can only tell that the fitting is right if the lens of the next flatter radius is obviously too mobile or does not centre. Sometimes the lens will produce an indentation on the conjunctiva at its periphery. This is not necessarily an indication that the fitting is incorrect.

On the whole, smaller diameters are preferable to larger diameters in that there is less likelihood of giant papillary conjunctivitis with their use.

Choice of lens

Plastic material

Various plastic materials have different characteristics. Some are more fragile than others. Some may be less flexible than others. Thus, Sauflex 55 (Contact Lenses Manufacturing) is a very firm material, useful when there is a small degree of astigmatism to cover up or in aphakic fitting where the displacement of the thick soft lens (especially into the upper fornix) may be a problem. The Elite lens (Pilkington Barnes Hind) has a plastic specially formulated to resist protein deposition and may be useful in cases where there is rapid deposition when other soft contact lenses are worn. The CSI lens (Pilkington Barnes Hind) is conspicuous for the small pore size of the glycerylmethacrylate material and has been shown to be less liable to accumulate deposits (Levy, 1984).

Water content

Oxygen permeability is roughly proportional to the water content of the lens, but it is oxygen transmissibility that is important. Transmissibility depends not only on the permeability of the material, but also on its thickness. The relationship of permeability to thickness is not linear (see p. 46). In the case of a powered soft contact lens the thickness should be assessed as the average thickness over a diameter of 12.00 mm (the corneal diameter) and not its central thickness.

In the case of a minus lens the peripheral thickness can be pared off from the front surface to get as near to a plano lens form as possible in the finished lens (see Figure 6.4). In the case of a plus lens the optic can be reduced to, say, 7.00 mm and the surround of this optic can be of plano power and thin.

The paring off of peripheral thickness in minus lenses is more effective in reducing average central thickness than is front optic reduction in a plus lens. A minus three dioptre soft lens can have a central thickness of 0.035 mm in low water content material and still be an easy to handle lens (e.g. CSI therapeutic lens). A plus three dioptre soft lens of 55% water content with the front central optic reduced to 7.00 mm has to have a central thickness of 0.24 mm and a similar lens of 75% water content has to have a central thickness of 0.30 mm. This is because the expansion factors on hydration, which takes place after manufacture, are different, and there is a minimum central thickness to which the lens can be manufactured in the dry state.

Mobilia, Dohlman and Holly (1977) found, in a comparison of various plano soft contact lenses for therapeutic purposes, that a thin low water content one (the CSI at 0.06 central thickness, 38% water content and plano power) performed best so far as oxygen transmission was concerned. Higher water content minus lenses cannot be made very thin. Above a water content of 55% it is not possible to get down to thicknesses of 0.05 or less and 0.10 and 0.15, or even more, is the norm in many commercially available lenses.

Myopes can be fitted with a thin (0.05 mm)

58 *Medical Contact Lens Practice*

central thickness low water content (38%) contact lens or a thicker (0.15 mm) central thickness high water content (70%) contact lens and comparable oxygen transmission will be achieved.

Hypermetropes, on the other hand, have to be fitted with a higher water content lens to obtain comparable oxygen transmission to the myope, because of the central thickness of their lenses. It is, however, true that some hypermetropes will be content with a medium water content lens and some will get by with a low water content lens.

Most hypermetropes who present for contact lens fitting are middle-aged adults and they need high water content lenses to get the oxygen supply their corneas demand. The young hypermetropes who present are usually highly hypermetropic in excess of four dioptres. They may have the problem of strabismus and they cannot easily produce the accommodative effort to get consistent clear distance vision. High hypermetropia dictates increase central thickness in a soft contact lens.

Most soft contact lenses are now produced in large quantities by large companies. Their lenses usually have fixed parameters and there is an almost universal front optic reduction to 8.00 mm. Considerable saving in central thickness can be made by reducing the front central optic diameter to 7.00 mm in plus lenses, and Appendix 6.I gives minimal central thicknesses for such lenses of 38%, 55%, 61% and 75% water contents which may be ordered from some laboratories on a custom-made basis.

References

LEVY, B. (1984) Calcium deposits on glyceryl methyl methacrylate and hydroxyethyl methacrylate contact lenses. *American Journal of Optometry and Physiological Optics* **61**, 9, 605–607

MOBILIA, E.F., DOHLMAN, C.H and HOLLY, F.J. (1977) A comparison of various soft contact lenses for therapeutic purposes. *Contact and Intraocular Lens Medical Journal*, **3**, 1, 9–15.

PYE, D.C., LIN, G.C.I. and NHIEU, T. (1986) Computer-aided design of hydrophilic contact lenses. *Clinical and Experimental Optometry*, **69**, 3, 93–97.

Appendix 6.I

Minimal central thicknesses for plus lenses of 38%, 55%, 61% and 75% water content with front optic zones reduced to 7.0 mm.

Power	38% water	55% water	61% water	75% water
+1.0	0.21	0.21	0.21	0.26
+2.0	0.22	0.23	0.23	0.28
+3.0	0.24	0.24	0.24	0.30
+4.0	0.25	0.26	0.26	0.32
+5.0	0.27	0.27	0.28	0.33
+6.0	0.28	0.29	0.29	0.35
+7.0	0.30	0.31	0.31	0.37
+8.0	0.32	0.32	0.33	0.39

7

Fitting toric contact lenses

A toric surface is one that is not spherical and has two principal meridians of different regular curvature lying at right angles to each other. Such surfaces can sometimes be utilized on contact lenses to overcome fitting problems associated with the positioning of these lenses and visual problems associated with astigmatism.

Toric hard corneal lenses

A toric hard corneal lens can be a lens with a toric back peripheral radius or a toric back optic zone radius, or a combination of both. It can be a lens with a toric front optic zone radius alone or with a toric back optic zone radius in addition, in which case it is called a bi-toric lens.

A toric back optic zone radius is sometimes used to obtain a better physical fit on a highly toric cornea and, in this case, the back peripheral zone may or may not be toric. Sometimes a toric back peripheral zone only is used. Only the cornea is involved in such fitting techniques. Contact lens fitting should take into consideration the action of the lids and with the advent of lens lid attachment techniques the author has seldom found it necessary to use toric back optic zone or back peripheral curves in the interest of fitting. The main reason for fitting a toric hard lens is residual astigmatism. This is caused by lenticular astigmatism which is present at the interface of the crystalline lens and the aqueous humour and which is not neutralized by the fluid lens behind a hard corneal lens, as is corneal astigmatism.

Residual astigmatism is almost always against the rule, that is, with the minus axis at approximately 90°. It is rarely more than 1.5 dioptres in amount, except when there is a pathological condition, such as Marfan's sydrome when the crystalline lenses may be dislocated. Residual astigmatism would appear to be an autosomal dominant condition, although there has been nothing published in this respect. It is prevalent in European royalty; two kings and one prince wear toric contact lenses for visual reasons.

Fitting hard corneal toric lenses

The principle here is to fit a standard hard corneal lens and then to take measures to prevent it rotating. This stabilization can be achieved in three ways.

Truncation

This can be single or double (Figure 7.1) and is usually 0.5 mm in extent. The truncation, or truncations, are incorporated so that the lid margins will stabilize the lens as they butt against it. A conventional lens is used for preliminary fitting. An over refraction is then done and a lens with the spherical correction only, together with the truncation, or truncations, is ordered. This is inserted and the refraction is then repeated. A new lens with a trucation or truncations and the appropriate spherical and astigmatic correction incorporated on its front surface, is ordered, taking into account any deviation of the truncation or truncations from the 180° position. The cylindrical

59

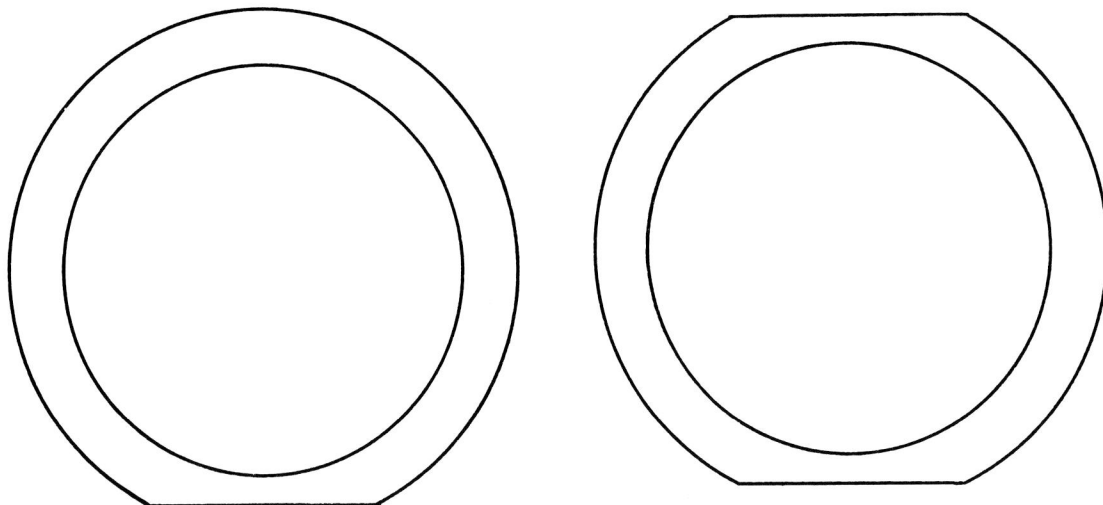

Figure 7.1 Diagrams of single and double truncated hard corneal lenses. Overall size 9.5 mm, BCOD 7.5 mm and truncation 0.5 mm

axis ordered on the contact lens must be related to this.

A single truncation can be incorporated in a lens designed for lens lid attachment and in this way a very satisfactory fit can be achieved.

Prism ballast

In this technique a two or three dioptre prism is incorporated in the lens. The axis of the prism is marked with a waterproof pen. The lens is inserted and shortly afterwards the base of the prism will be orientated downwards. An over refraction is then done and a new lens with prism ballast and the appropriate spherical and astigmatic correction incorporated on its front surface is ordered, taking into account any deviation of the axis of the prism from the 90° position on the eye. A truncation may be incorporated at the base of the prism to discourage further rotation.

This lens has the disadvantage that it tends, because of its weight, to drop and assume a low position on the cornea. This will give a very unsatisfactory fit (see Chapter 4).

Toric back optic zone

This method is sometimes used when there is a considerable degree of corneal astigmatism.

A trial lens with a toric back optic zone is inserted. The disparity in the two meridians should be about 0.6 mm. This lens will induce astigmatism into the system because the toric back optic zone portion bounds two surfaces of different refractive indices. The lens is allowed to settle and an over refraction is done. A new lens is then ordered with a toric back optic zone and the appropriate spherical and astigmatic correction incorporated on its front surface. This is a very difficult lens to manufacture.

Fitting toric soft lenses

Minor degrees of astigmatism (up to 1.0 D cyl), which are uncorrected by soft contact lenses, are sometimes worrying to patients and yet the visual impairment is not enough to warrant the use of toric soft contact lenses. Toric soft contact lenses are more difficult to wear than spherical soft contact lenses and often, themselves, give imperfect visual results.

A possible way out of this dilemma is the use of a non-spherical lens. The Nissel SV38 (G. Nissel and Co. Ltd, Hemel Hempstead, Herts., UK) has a spherical back curve. Its front curve is non-spherical, but does not fall into any standard aspheric category. In minus form, the rate of steepening of curved values, within the continuous non-spherical curve, is just sufficient to eliminate the progressive power increase that would be inherent in a conventional lens through aberration. This means that all light rays from infinity, incident on the lens surface, are taken to a common focal point. Elimination of spherical aberration limits the size of the circle of least confusion and, where there is a certain degree of astigmatism, this lens produces superior results compared with the equivalent conventional lens.

Lydon (1990) has assessed the performance of the Nissel SV38 lens. He found that cylinders up to 1.50 D were generally covered at least as effectively as they were by Optima toric soft lenses (Bausch and Lomb) and the superiority was significant where target contrast was low and in low luminance conditions. The corneal swelling response was also assessed and was not significantly different from that caused by the Hydron Z6T lens (Allergan Optical) or the Optima toric lens.

A common reason, nowadays, for fitting soft toric lenses is late intolerance of hard, or rigid, gas permeable lenses. In these late cases of intolerance there is often induced corneal astigmatism. Since ordinary soft lenses 'drape' on the cornea, the corneal astigmatism is transmitted through them with unsatisfactory visual results.

Toric soft lenses can be either back surface toric or front surface toric. In soft contact lens practice they are used not to refine the fitting, but to correct astigmatism.

Astigmatism can be either corneal or lenticular. A comparison of the amount and axis of the corneal astigmatism, as assessed by the keratometer, and the amount and axis of the spectacle astigmatism, as assessed by refraction, will show if there is residual astigmatism. It is assumed that total astigmatism equals corneal astigmatism plus lenticular astigmatism.

Thus, if there is no corneal astigmatism, as measured by the keratometer, and one and a half dioptres of astigmatism at 90° on refraction, it is obvious that this astigmatism is lenticular and therefore will not be corrected by a shperical or a back toric soft contact lens. However, in some subtle way, the visual acuity obtained with a spherical soft lens, in the presence of residual astigmatism, is often surprisingly good.

If the keratometer shows two dioptres of minus astigmatism at 90° (the reading at an axis (i.e. direction) of 180° will be more in millimetres of curvature than the reading at an axis of 90°) and the refraction shows one dioptre of minus astigmatism then there is obviously lenticular astigmatism.

Stabilization or the prevention of rotation of the soft lens can be achieved by:

1. a toric back surface
2. prism ballast
3. single or double truncation
4. dynamic stabilization (or lens thinning in defined areas).

Toric back surface lenses

This method is of most use in correcting the visual acuity if the astigmatism is corneal and not lenticular. The back toric surface essentially neutralizes the astigmatic cornea and replaces it with a front spherical refracting surface. These lenses tend to lock on to a toroidal cornea and stabilization is often assisted by the incorporation of a base down prism or a truncation.

An example of a back surface toric soft contact lens is the Hydrocurve II toric (Pilkington Barnes Hind) (Figure 7.2). This lens is manufactured from either 45% water content or 55% water content material. In the latter it is suitable for extended wear, or daily wear. It incorporates a prism ballast and has an added back peripheral curve. The prism ballast adds stability when the cornea has little toricity, but the lens is less satisfactory on a spherical cornea. When a thin toric back surface lens, such as the Hydrocurve II, is put on a spherical cornea, it will 'drape' on this surface and its toric back surface will be transmitted to the front of the lens, but some toricity is lost. However, this induced front cylinder corrects some of the corneal astigmatism. When there is lenticular astigmatism in addition to corneal astigmatism, and when these two are at different meridians, there is real difficulty in obtaining a satisfactory visual outcome.

The lens is fitted in the normal manner. Most corneas can be fitted with a lens of 8.8 mm back optic radius and 14.5 mm in total diameter. A steeper lens is available. The prism is marked by three laser induced lines or 'spokes' below, which are 20° apart, the middle and longer one being at the axis of the prism.

In fitting, the manufacturer suggests that the

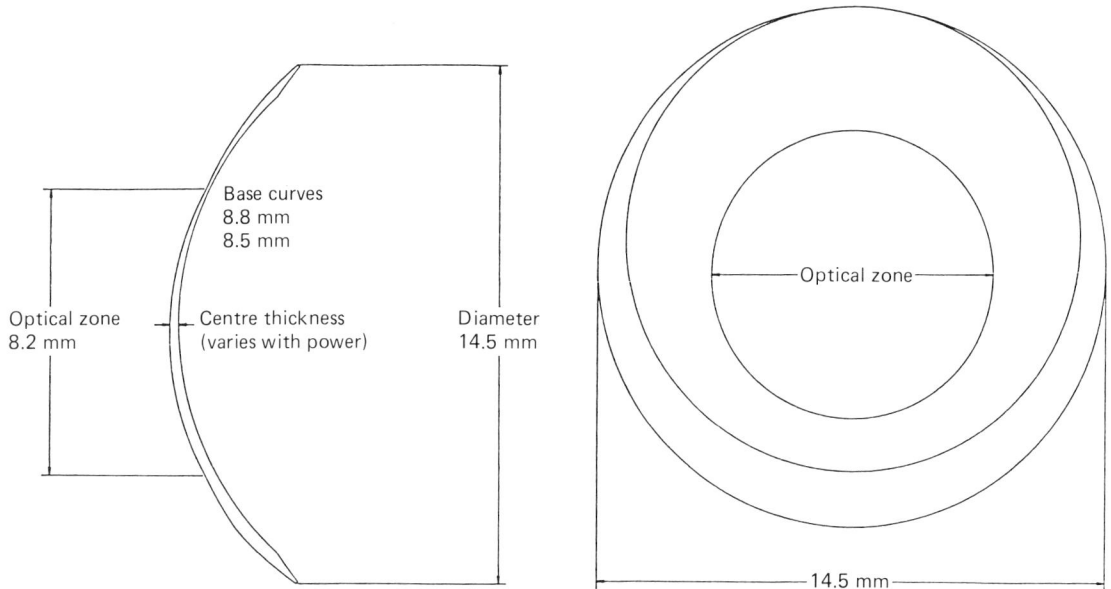

Figure 7.2 Diagrams of the Hydrocurve II toric soft contact lens

cylinder power be chosen first, according to indications from the spectacle refraction. There are three available cylindrical powers: minus 0.75 D, minus 1.25 D and minus 2.0 D. A lens is then chosen close to the spectacle refraction.

After settling, the location of the axis of the prism ballast is established, using the laser markings as a guide. The patient's lens will rotate to the same position as the trial lens. If the centre laser mark rotates to the examiner's left of the slit beam the number of degrees of rotation is added to the patient's refractive axis. If the centre laser mark rotates to the examiner's right of the slit beam the number of degrees of rotation is subtracted from the patient's refractive axis.

Further examples of toric back surface soft lenses are the Hydroflex/m-T (Wohlk) which incorporates a base down prism of 0.15 D and the Hydroflex-TS (Wohlk) which incorporates both a base down prism of 0.10 D and a truncation (Figure 7.3). In these lenses only the back optic zone is toroidal and is ellipsoidal in shape, the precise dimensions depending upon the lens power and radius. They are made of hydroxyethyl methacrylate of 38.4% water content. The lenses are engraved at the periphery with two short reference markings at exactly 90° to the base apex line of the prism and they will settle, ideally,

at the 180° axis of the eye. Compensation must be made for any deviation from this axis.

The fitting is done from a spherical trial set which incorporates other features, apart from the toric back surface, which stabilize the lenses. Alternatively, a standard spherical Wohlk soft lens can be used.

The spherical power and the cylindrical power are best ascertained by over refraction with a fully settled trial lens. The astigmatic difference to correct the cylinder is then determined using a table which equilibrates radius of curvature in millimetres with surface power in dioptres where the refractive index of the plastic (n) is 1.4448 (Appendix 7.I).

The Hydroflex/m-T is fitted as large and as flat as possible. The Hydroflex-TS has a standard overall size of 14.00 mm and an additional size of 15.00 mm for large corneas since the truncation results in a smaller vertical diameter.

An example may be quoted as follows:

Patient refraction −0.50 D sph. /−4.00 D cyl.ax.
  15
Truncation or reference markings settle at 10°
T setting (toric axis compensated for rotation of
  lens) 5

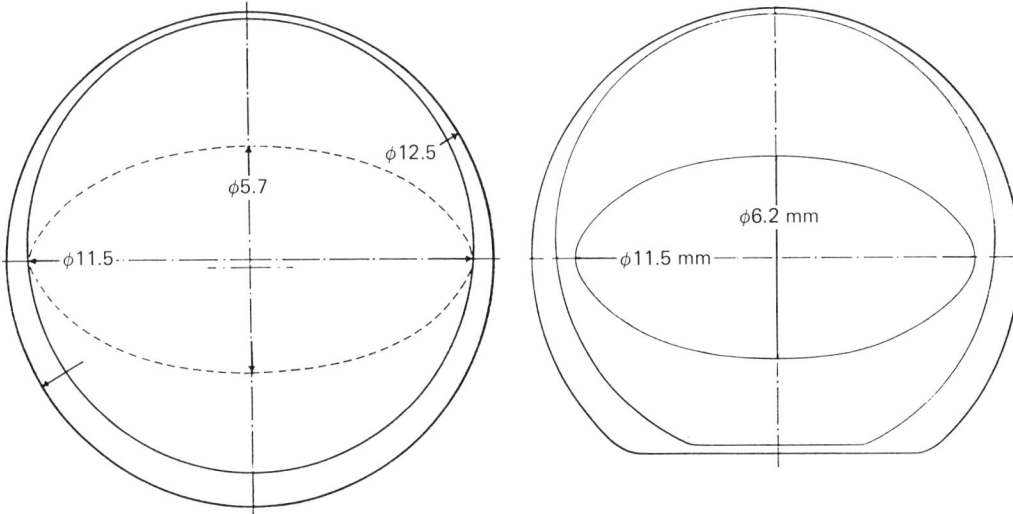

Figure 7.3 Diagrams of the Hydroflex/m-T and Hydroflex-TS toric soft lenses

Best fitting lens 9.30 mm radius at 14.00 mm diameter
Surface power of 9.30 mm radius $\quad = -47.83$ D
$\qquad\qquad\qquad$ Add $\quad \underline{-4.00\ \text{D}}$
Surface power of steeper meridian $= -51.83$ D
Nearest radius value to this is $\qquad = 8.60$ mm
Specification of the lens is:
$\quad$ Radius 9.30/8.60; diameter 14.00;
$\quad$ power −0.50 T5

Toric front surface lenses

These lenses can be used for both corneal and lenticular astigmatism. There are two methods of stabilization against rotation so that the front cylindrical power can be incorporated:

1. Prism ballast with or without truncation.
2. Dynamic stabilization.

Prism ballast

An example of the prism ballast toric lens is the Optima Toric (Bausch and Lomb) (Figure 7.4). It is made of hydroxyethyl methacrylate of 38% water content. It is designed without a back peripheral curve. It has a 1.25 D prism with an anterior comfort chamfer. It is available in two radii and one diameter. The cylindrical powers are minus 1.25 D and minus 1.75 D at 10° cylinder

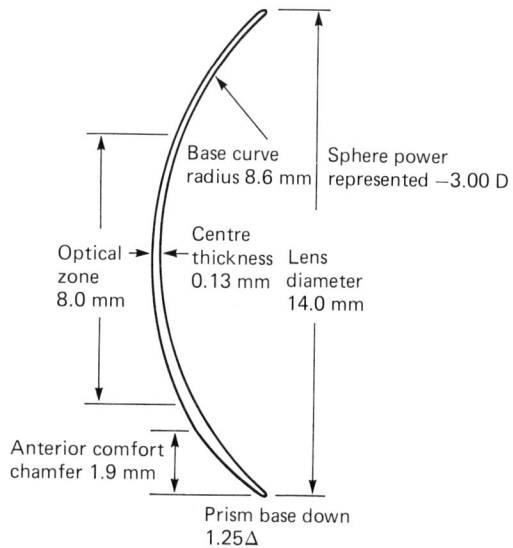

Figure 7.4 Diagram of the Optima toric soft lens

axes. Oblique cylinder axes are not obtainable. The prism is marked with three lines at 30° apart (Figure 7.5).

In fitting, an initial lens is chosen with a cylindrical power and axis as close as possible to the patient's spectacle prescription. After settling, the orientation of the centre marking of the prism is noted and the axis of the cylinder is compensated

Lens markings

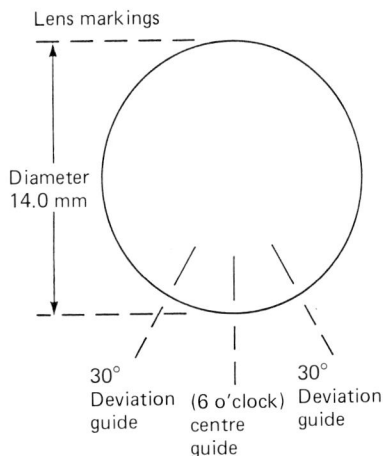

Figure 7.5 Diagram of the markings on the Optima toric soft lens

for this, after spectacle over refraction, when ordering.

A further example of prism ballast is the Hydron Z6T (Allergan) (Figure 7.6). It is manufactured from 38% water content hydroxethyl methacrylate, has a diameter of 14.0 mm and is available in four fittings. It has a centre thickness of 0.06 mm. Cylindrical powers are available up to minus 6.0 DS. Stability and orientation are controlled by peripheral prisms, eliminating the need for truncation and the optic zone of the Z6T is prism free. The standard Hydron Z6 lens can be

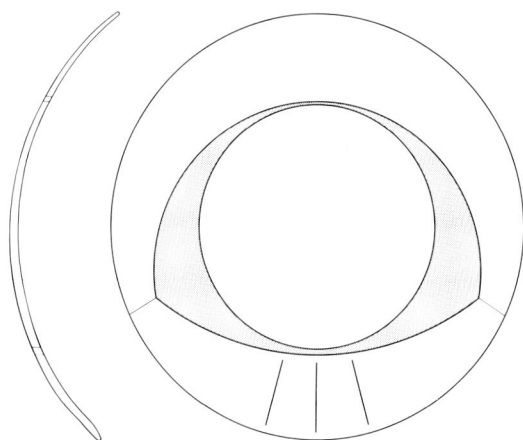

Figure 7.6 Diagram of the Hydron Z6T toric soft lens. The shaded areas represent the peripheral base down prisms

used for the fitting. Three laser markings identify the axis of the prism base.

Fitting is done using the standard Z6 lens or Z6T trial lenses. If the standard Z6 lens is used, allowance is made for the fact that Z6T lenses tend to rotate, anticlockwise in the right eye and clockwise in the left eye, by about 5°. So 5° is *subtracted* from the cylinder axis of the right eye before ordering and 5° is *added* to the cylinder axis of the left eye before ordering. If Z6T trial lenses are used, the orientation of the prism can be checked. Ordering is done on the basis of a spectacle over refraction. If the visual acuity is not optimum with the supplied lens a corrected allowance is made according to the position of the laser markings which are found in the supplied toric lens.

Dynamic stabilization

An example of this is the Torisoft lens (Ciba) (Figure 7.7). This lens is made of 38% water content hydroxyethyl methacrylate. It has two thin zones which are designed to stabilize under the lids and a thicker central optical band. The thicker optical band is marked at 0° and 180°. A trial set of six lenses is used, covering three base curves, in powers of minus 0.50 DS and minus 3.00 DS. Stabilization should be between 160° and 20° and this should be taken into consideration when ordering the axis of the required astigmatic correction. The cylindrical powers available are minus 1.00 D and minus 1.75 D.

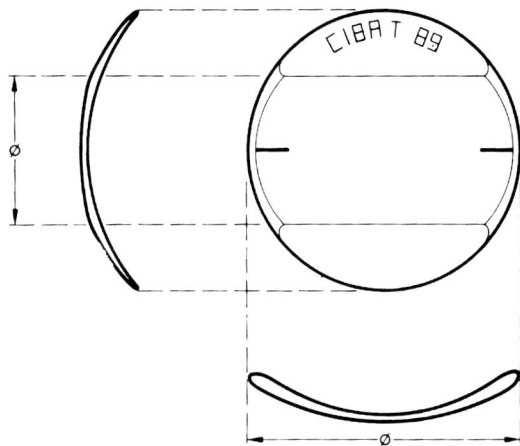

Figure 7.7 Diagram of the Torisoft toric soft lens

This lens is not successful where there is oblique astigmatism. Experience has shown that for success the astigmatism needs to be:

1. within 10° of 90° axis if the spherical power is plano to minus 3.0 DS
2. within 20° of 90° axis if the spherical power is minus 3 DS to minus 6.0 DS
3. within 15° of 180° axis, providing the spherical power is over minus 4.0 DS.

A further example of dynamic stabilization is the Lunelle Rx Toric Lens (Essilor) (Figure 7.8). It is manufactured in 70% water content material. It uses the dynamic blink action of the upper lid to stabilize the lens, making the use of prism ballast or truncation unnecessary. There are two delta-shaped profiles on the exterior surface of the lens. Stabilization is obtained by the lid pressure on the profile zones. The lens has a small aspheric peripheral curve producing a 0.50 mm edge lift. The method of manufacture enables the lens to be produced with a full front surface cylinder incorporating the two delta-shaped profiles in horizontal alignment. In order to calculate the axis of stabilization, trial lenses are engraved with two dots on the apex of the profiles. The lens is available in two diameters, each having three associated radii, and cylindrical powers are available up to minus 6.00 DS.

The profiles of the Lunelle Toric Rx Lens, in most cases, align horizontally. If they do not the

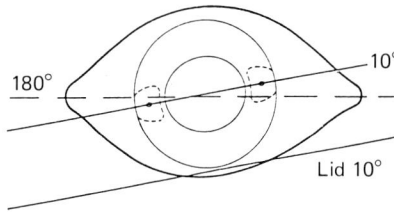

Figure 7.9 Diagram of the orientation of the Lunelle Rx toric soft lens

deviation must be taken into account when ordering the axis of the cylinder (Figure 7.9).

Dynamic stabilization usually gives better stability than prism ballast. The real difficulty occurs when there are pingeculae present, forcing the thicker profile zones into an oblique position. Unfortunately, many long-term wearers of hard corneal lenses develop these pingeculae (see Chapter 12). Intolerance of hard corneal lenses in the long term is a common finding by contact lens practitioners nowadays. They can usually be successfully fitted with soft contact lenses, but if they have induced astigmatism and pingeculae, real problems arise.

Reference

LYDON, D. (1990) Improved optics and control of astigmatism without cylinders. *Transactions of BCLA Conference*, 1990. British Contact Lens Association, London, pp 1–3.

Appendix 7.I

Equilibration of radius of curvature with surface power in dioptres for plastic of refractive index (n) of 1.4448.

Radius (mm)	Surface power (dioptres)	Radius (mm)	Surface power (dioptres)
6.00	74.13	7.00	63.54
6.10	72.92	7.10	62.65
6.20	71.74	7.20	61.78
6.30	70.60	7.30	60.93
6.40	69.50	7.40	60.11
6.50	68.43	7.50	59.31
6.60	67.39	7.60	58.53
6.70	66.39	7.70	57.75
6.80	65.41	7.80	57.03
6.90	64.46	7.90	56.30

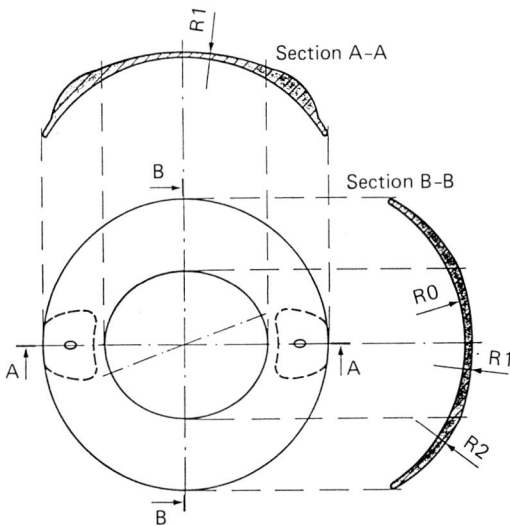

Figure 7.8 Diagram of the Lunelle Rx toric soft lens

Radius (mm)	Surface power (dioptres)	Radius (mm)	Surface power (dioptres)	Radius (mm)	Surface power (dioptres)	Radius (mm)	Surface power (dioptres)
8.00	55.60	8.50	52.33	9.00	49.42	9.50	46.82
8.10	54.91	8.60	51.72	9.10	48.88	9.60	46.33
8.20	54.24	8.70	51.13	9.20	48.35	9.70	45.86
8.30	53.59	8.80	50.55	9.30	47.83	9.80	45.39
8.40	52.95	8.90	49.98	9.40	47.32	9.90	44.93

8

Handling of contact lenses by the patient

There are many techniques of insertion and removal of contact lenses by the patient. Although the ophthalmologist will not usually be called upon to teach patients, he should know the methods. What follows is an account of standard methods. Before any procedure the hands should be washed and dried.

Hard corneal lenses

Insertion

The lens is cleaned, wetted and placed on the wet forefinger of one hand (Figure 8.1).

The ball of the thumb of the other hand is placed on the forehead with the fingers facing down and holding up the upper lid and its eyelashes (Figure 8.2). The head is held straight and both eyes are kept wide open.

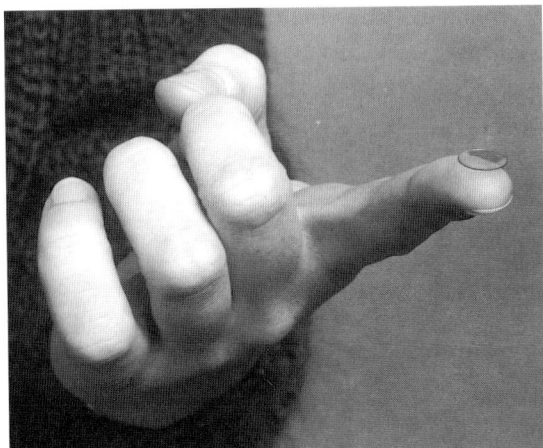

Figure 8.2

The middle finger of the hand holding the lens pulls down the lower lid and its eyelashes (Figure 8.3). The eye looks straight at the lens on the forefinger. The lens is brought gently towards the eye until it meets the cornea.

When the lens is on the cornea it is important to release the lower lid first and then the upper lid (Figure 8.4).

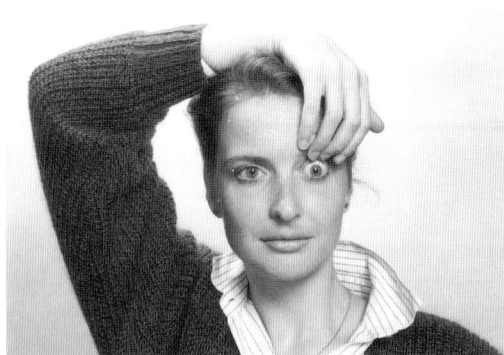

Figure 8.1

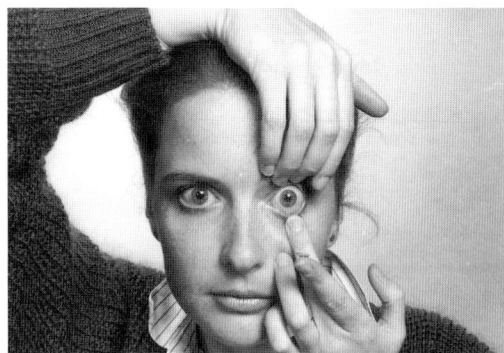

Figure 8.3

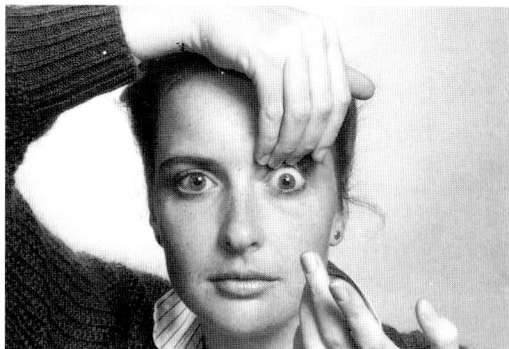

Figure 8.4

Recentring

Should the lens be displaced on to the white of the eye the following procedure should be adopted (Figure 8.5). The head is moved in the direction of the lens while the patient looks at a mirror located directly in front. This produces maximal exposure of the lens and applies whether the lens is under the upper or lower lid, or displaced laterally. The lens can be replaced on the cornea by using the forefinger to push the appropriate lid against the lens.

Removal

The head is held straight and the eyes, which are opened as widely as possible, look straight ahead (Figure 8.6). The forefinger is held vertically and the tip of it is placed on the outer corner of the eye, touching both lids and also the white of the eye at this point. The finger is pulled outwards, causing the lens to be caught between the lids. It will then pop out, or stick to the lashes, from where it can easily be removed by the forefinger and thumb. The left forefinger is used for the left

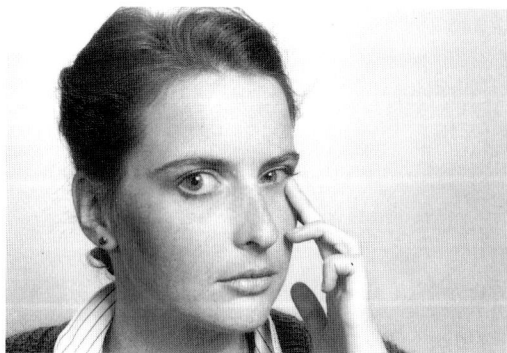

Figure 8.6

eye. If it should be necessary to blink to remove the lens the pull of the index finger should not be relaxed. The other hand should be ready to catch the lens.

Soft lenses

Insertion

The clean lens, which has been removed from its bottle containing fluid, is placed on the dry forefinger of one hand (Figure 8.7). It is orientated in the correct way if, when viewed against a light, it is the shape of a cup. If it is back to front there will be a very small lip at the edge of the lens, giving the appearance of a saucer.

The ball of the thumb of the other hand is placed on the forehead with the fingers facing down and holding up the upper lid and its eyelashes (Figure 8.8). The head is held straight and both eyes are kept wide open.

The middle finger of the hand holding the lens pulls down the lower lid and its eyelashes (Figure

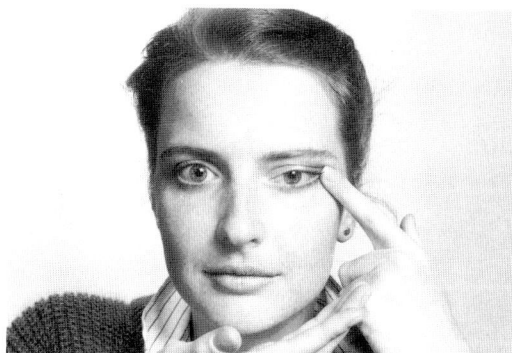

Figure 8.5

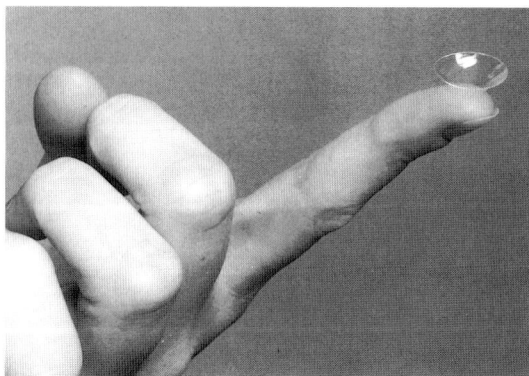

Figure 8.7

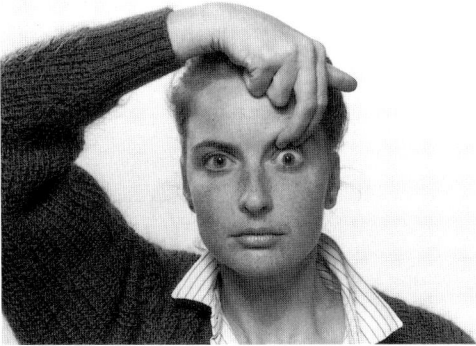

Figure 8.8

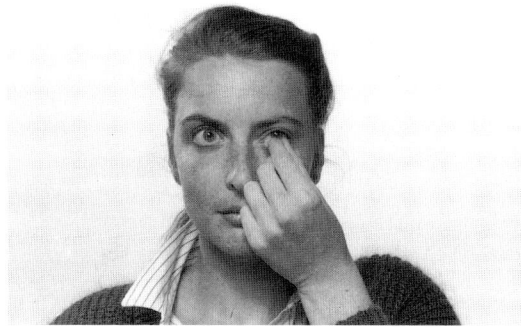

Figure 8.9

8.9). The eye looks straight at the lens on the finger. The lens is brought gently towards the eye until it meets the cornea.

When the lens is on the cornea it is important to release the lower lid first and then the upper lid.

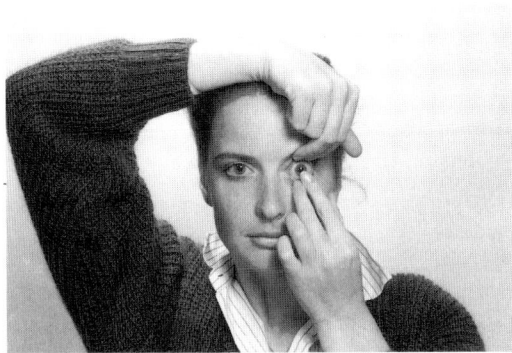

Figure 8.10

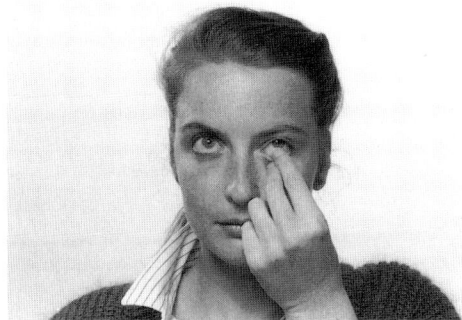

Figure 8.11

Removal

The head is held straight and the eyes, which are opened as widely as possible, look straight ahead. The forefinger is held vertically and placed on the soft lens. The patient looks up and the lens is pulled down into the lower fornix (Figure 8.10).

The lens is then pinched gently by the forefinger and thumb and removed (Figure 8.11).

Scleral lenses

Insertion

After cleaning and wetting, the lens is held by its edge with the thumb and second finger and orientated for its position on the eye (Figure 8.12).

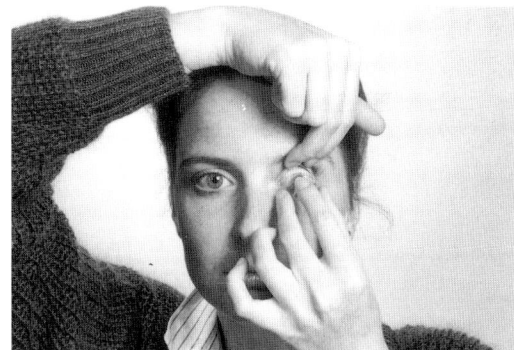

Figure 8.12

The forefinger steadies the lens. The eyes look downwards while the first two fingers of the other hand pull up the upper lid. The lens is slipped under the lid.

The other hand then releases the upper lid and moves below to pull down the lower lid so that it slips over the lens (Figure 8.13). (For photographic purposes the first hand has been lifted.)

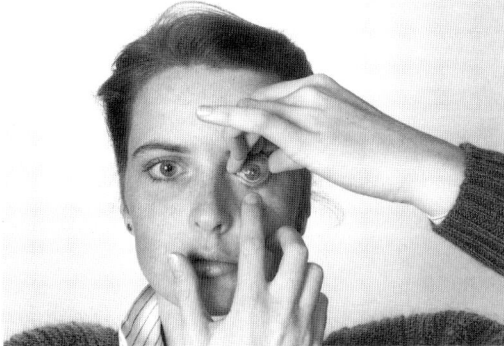

Figure 8.13

Removal

The lens is removed by looking down and pulling up the upper lid with the forefinger, so that its edge engages the edge of the lens (Figure 8.14). A little downward push by the forefinger then releases the lens from the eye and it is caught by the other hand.

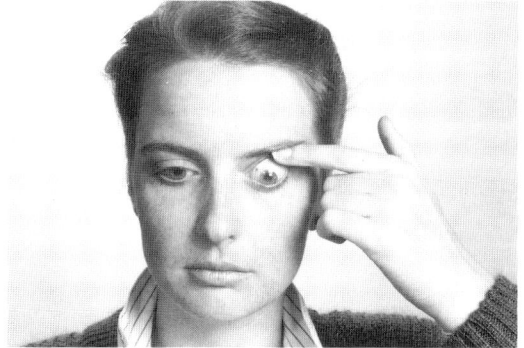

Figure 8.14

9

Care of contact lenses

Hard polymethylmethacrylate corneal lenses

Hard corneal lenses are usually cleaned with a solution which comprises a surfactant and antimicrobials and, when not in use, they are soaked in a solution containing antimicrobials. The usual antimicrobials are thiomersal, disodium edetate and chlorhexidine, and benzalkonium chloride. They, their use and abuse, will be discussed in the section of soft contact lenses. The use of thiomersal rarely gives the corneal hypersensitivity problems which are seen in soft contact lens wearers except in some cases where the lens is inserted with its concave surface filled with the solution.

Appendix 9.I is a list of preparations and their preservatives, for use with hard corneal contact lenses.

Hard corneal lenses may sometimes be seen to have surface deposit on them (Figure 9.1). This is composed of calcium and magnesium salts, or, alternatively, protein and is usually found on the concave surface of the lens. It can also be found at the junction of the lenticular portion and the carrier on the front surface of a lens. This deposit is difficult for the patient to remove. Failing return to the laboratory it can be removed in the practice setting by the use of a Professional Hard Contact Lens Cleaner (Polymer Technology Corporation, Wilmington, Mass., USA).

Scleral lenses

These lenses can be cleaned and disinfected with the same solutions as are used for hard lenses.

Gas permeable hard corneal lenses

Special cleaners are recommended for gas permeable hard corneal lenses because they are much more prone to surface deposits than polymethylmethacrylate lenses. Such cleaners are usually developed by the manufacturer of the plastic. They contain a surfactant, or a detergent, or a friction enhancing agent, such as particulate hydroxyethylmethacrylate.

Despite the use of these cleaners in the home environment, deposits are still a problem with gas permeable hard corneal lenses and they can be removed by the method advocated above for hard polymethylmethacrylate lenses.

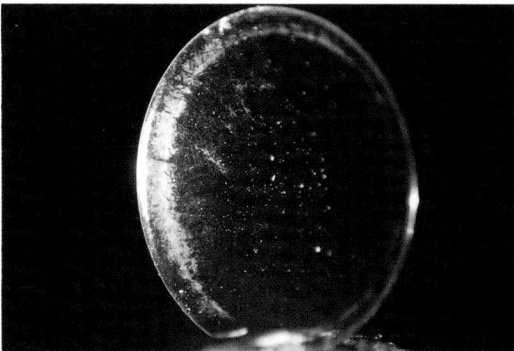

Figure 9.1 Deposit on a hard corneal lens. This may consist of calcium and magnesium salts or, alternatively, protein

Rosenthal *et al.* (1986) have shown that benz-alkonium chloride is unique in its property of strongly binding to silicone/acrylate lenses by a self-propagating mechanism that is independent of solution formulation or concentration of benzalkonium chloride. On silicone/acrylate lenses benzalkonium chloride has the potential of creating toxic surface levels and markedly reducing surface wettability. In contrast, the adsorption of chlorhexidine is limited to a low concentration level that is further reduced by solution formulation. Chlorhexidine is less strongly bound to the lens polymers and does not create a hydrophobic surface.

Chapman, Cheeks and Green (1990) have studied the uptake of benzalkonium chloride by rigid contact lenses. Fluorosilicone-acrylate polymer lenses adsorb and release the most preservative while polymethylmethacrylate lenses adsorb and release the least. The released benzylkonium chloride from hard lenses is of a sufficient concentration to be at or above the upper limits of safety.

Soft hydrophilic lenses

Soft contact lenses are usually cleaned by surfactants, proteolytic enzymes or ultrasound and disinfected by heat, chemicals or radiation. Corneal and conjunctival infections have a higher incidence in wearers of soft contact lenses than they have in wearers of hard corneal lenses and this is especially true when the soft lenses are worn on an extended basis.

Smolin, Okumoto and Nozik (1979) found that 5% of extended wear patients and 8% of aphakic extended wear patients grew potential pathogens from their conjunctival sacs. However, they also found that 21% of a group of preoperative cataract patients grew potential pathogens.

Tragakis, Brown and Pearce (1973) failed to demonstrate any change in the ocular flora with lens use. Hvding (1981) found that, compared with a control group, a significantly increased frequency of negative conjunctival cultures was found among the lens wearers. The conjunctival flora cannot be blamed for the problem of infection.

It is, however, of interest that Nicastro *et al.* (1975) have shown that methylmethacrylate can inhibit phagocytosis by rabbit alveolar macrophages.

Lens contamination

Bacteria

Probably of more importance than the conjunctival flora is the attachment of organisms to soft contact lenses. Fowler, Greiner and Allansmith (1979a) showed that under ordinary circumstances microorganisms cling to the surface of contact lenses.

Duran *et al.* (1987) found that when new unworn soft contact lenses were exposed to a suspension of 10^{-8} colony forming units per millilitre of *Pseudomonas aeruginosa*, increasing numbers of bacteria were found to attach to lenses with time. The attachment was considered to be irreversible since washing did not remove the bacteria. Slusher *et al.* (1987) pointed out that 'while medical scientific knowledge pertaining to bacterial adhesion to biomaterials has become a rapidly growing field in most areas of medicine, its significance in ophthalmic infections has not been emphasised. The designation of the contact lens itself as a suitable substratum for bacterial colonization and as a source of subsequent inoculum to compromised epithelial cells are important factors in the pathophysiology of corneal ulcer formation'.

According to Griffiths, Elliot and McTaggart (1989) bacterial adherence on surfaces can be divided into two stages. The first involves reversible attraction due to electrostatic and van der Waals forces and hydrophobic bonding. The second involves adherence of organisms due to biofilm production. The first stage was studied by Vafidis, Marsh and Stacey (1984). They wiped sterile intraocular lenses round the wound site at the time of surgery and subsequently placed the intraocular lenses in nutrient broth. In 26% of cases *Staphylococcus epidermidis* grew in the broth. The lenses were not examined under the microscope after incubation in the broth so this figure is a measure of reversibility adherent microorganisms.

The second stage was studied by Griffiths, Elliot and McTaggart (1989). Intraocular lenses were suspended in bacterial cultures of *Staph. epidermidis* by a fine wire and incubated at 37 °C for various periods of time. The lenses were then prepared for light and scanning microscopy. Griffiths *et al.* found that there was no difference in the amount of bacteria adherent to the lenses whether they were washed once, twice or three times. They also found that the number of adherent organisms increased the longer the lens remained in the broth culture.

Slusher *et al.* (1987) demonstrated polysaccharide-(biofilm)-mediated, adhesion of *Ps. aeruginosa* and *Staph. epidermidis* to the surface of extended wear soft lenses in vitro. The interaction between the biomaterial and bacterial organisms represented a favourable self-protective environment for propagation and inoculation. Gristina *et al.* (1985) stated that adhesive colonization is an almost universal quality of bacteria in natural environments which appears to be maintained by a highly anionic surface polysaccharide polymer produced by the bacteria. Thus, the soft contact lens can serve as a passive but constant substratum for bacterial colonization and as a nidus

for bacterial shedding with subsequent adhesion to damaged corneal basal epithelial cells. The bacteria then become available as a slime-enclosed, resistant, infecting inoculum for compromised corneal epithelium (Slusher *et al.*, 1987) (Figures 9.2 and 9.3).

Schwarzmann and Boring (1971) demonstrated an antiphagocytic effect of slime from a mucoid strain of *Ps. aeruginosa*.

Ruseska, Robbins and Costerton (1982) have shown that bacteria adherent to a biofilm were

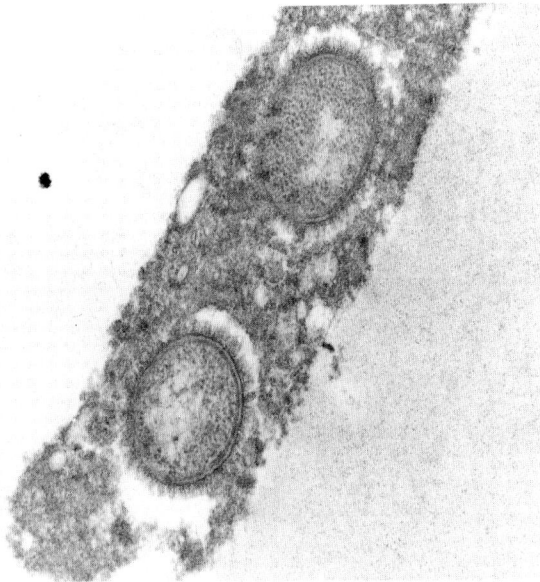

(a)

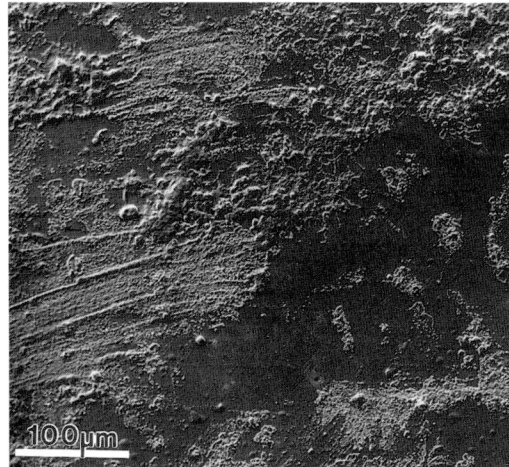

(b)

Figure 9.3 Scanning electron microscopy of bacteria on a soft contact lens (courtesy of Professor Noel Dilly). (a) Irregular biofilm on a soft contact lens showing adherent bacteria. Magnification × 230. (b) Bacterium in a biofilm on a soft contact lens showing pili. The pili are assumed to increase adherence. Magnification × 1050

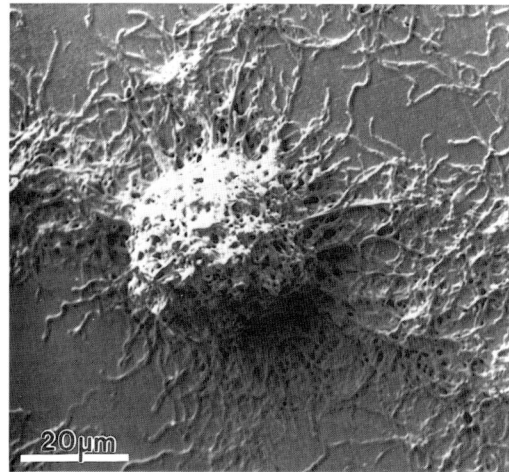

Figure 9.2 Pseudomonas in a biofilm stained with ruthenium red showing pili issuing from the bacteria. These pili are thought to secure the attachment of the bacterium to the biofilm. Adhesion to epithelial cells has been shown in vitro to depend on pili (Reichert, Das and Zam, 1983) but the relationship to the biofilm has yet to be explored. Transmission electron micrograph, magnification × 26 000. (Courtesy of Mr John Dart and Dr D.V. Seal and Editor of *Eye*, 1988, **2**; Suppl. S46–S55)

50-fold more resistant to chemical biocides than similar bacteria in their planktonic mode of growth.

Marrie and Costerton (1981) have shown that cells of *Serratia marcescens* in a biofilm adhering to a plastic surface were resistant to 2% chlorhexidine and dispersed cells were sensitive to that same concentration. The usual concentration of chlorhexidine in contact lens solutions is 0.002% to 0.004%.

Costerton, Irvin and Cheng (1981a) have suggested that the hydrated polyanionic bacterial glycocalyx acts as an ion-exchange resin in binding charged antibiotic molecules and that it thus limits their access to targets within the cells and cell envelopes.

Dart and Badenoch (1986) found that *Staph. aureus* adhered more to soft lenses than *Ps. aeruginosa* and that adherence was not affected by ocular deposits on the soft lenses. Butrus *et al.* (1990) found that contact lens surface deposits increased the adhesion of *Ps. aeruginosa*.

Dart and Seal (1988) have reviewed the pathogeneses of *Ps. aeruginosa*, including its adhesion, invasion and the role of the biofilm. In their rabbit model they found that *Ps. aeruginosa* disappeared from the corneal surface within four hours from inoculation with 10^6 bacteria unless trauma was made with a 4 mm trephine to the anterior stroma. They review the literature on pili and biofilm (Figures 9.2 and 9.3), together with that on host factors with particular reference to phagocytosis of *Pseudomonas* by polymorphonuclear leucocytes.

Miller *et al.* (1989) have recorded the presence of an extensive biofilm in the corneal tissue of one of their patients. They postulate that biofilm formation in ocular tissue by *Ps. aeruginosa* is a mechanism by which the organism may become sequestered and remain refractive to maximum therapy.

Klotz *et al.* (1989) found that ten isolates of *Ps. aeruginosa* obtained from the corneas of patients with pseudomonas keratitis adhered to soft contact lenses in significantly greater numbers than did six isolates from other body sites. They further found that isolates grown statically in broth at 37 °C formed a pellicle (biofilm) and adhered twice as much to contact lenses as did isolates grown in broth, while shaking, which did not form a pellicle. The more adherent isolates were shown to be more hydrophilic than the less

adherent bacteria. They concluded that hydrophilic interactions may significantly contribute to the ability of *Ps. aeruginosa* to adhere to contact lenses.

Wilson, Sawant and Ahearn (1991) studied the comparative efficiencies of soft contact lens disinfectant solutions against microbial films in lens cases. They found that the relative order of resistance of bacterial biofilms was as follows: *S. marcescens* was greater than *Ps. aeruginosa* which was greater than *Staph. epidermidis* which was greater than *Streptococcus pyogenes*. Air drying of biofilms for 10 hours increased the efficacy of the disinfectant solutions but drying was not enough to decrease the incidence of recovery to 0% for all solutions.

Fungi

Bernstein (1973) and Filipi, Pfister and Hill (1973) have both described the penetration of fungi into hydrophilic lenses (Figure 9.4). Wilson and Ahearn (1986) isolated fungi from 11 extended wear soft contact lenses. In two cases fungi had penetrated through the contact lens and the same fungus was cultured from corneal ulcers. In four cases fungal growth on and in the soft contact lens matrix was associated with conjunctivitis and punctate fluorescein staining of the corneal epithelium.

Acanthamoeba

Acanthamoebic corneal infection has been associated with the use of both hard and soft contact

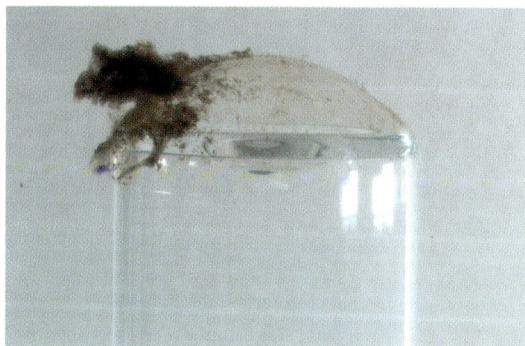

Figure 9.4 Fungal growth and penetration in a soft contact lens. The lens was removed from a patient's eye and was stored in sterile saline in a clean container for four months before this fungal growth was discovered

lenses (C.D.C., 1986). They feed on bacteria and may be adherent to bacteria and biofilm on the contact lens. Donzis *et al.* (1989) in a paper on the microbial analysis of contact lens care systems contaminated by acanthamoeba found that these organisms were found only in contact lens cases, or solutions, that also had bacterial, and in many cases, fungal contamination, suggesting that the presence of bacterial and fungal contamination within the contact lens care system may be an important element for the survival and growth of acanthamoeba. They analysed bacterial and fungal contamination within the contact lens care systems of 10 patients who had acanthamoeba detected in their care systems. Seven patients had acanthamoeba keratitis, one had pseudomonas keratitis and the remaining two were asymptomatic. Fungi were isolated in six of the contact lens care systems.

John, Desal and Sahm (1989), however, have shown, by scanning electron microscopy, that both *Acanthamoeba castellani* cysts and trophozoites can firmly adhere to unused soft contact lenses.

Kilvington and Larkin (1990) studied the quantitative adherence of a keratitis isolate of *Acanthamoeba polyphaga* to low and high water content non-ionic soft contact lenses and one type of rigid gas permeable lens was investigated. Adherence of trophozoite and cyst forms of the organism was observed in vitro and adherent amoebae counted by a plaque assay method following detachment. Trophozoites adhered to all lens types with adherence being statistically greater to high water content soft lenses. Cyst attachment occurred only to the soft lenses and not to gas permeable lenses and was significantly higher for the high water content lenses. It would have been interesting to compare non-ionic soft lenses with ionic soft contact lenses. For explanation of the terms non-ionic and ionic, see further on in this chapter.

Clinicians should be aware that acanthamoeba exists in two forms – trophozoites and cysts. Cysts are much more resistant to killing and any report on the efficiency of a disinfection method should clearly state in which form the acanthamoeba is killed.

Standard contact lens heat disinfection methods have been reported to kill *A. polyphaga* and *A. castellani* cysts and trophozoites in suspension while the organisms survived treatment with 3% hydrogen peroxide and an 0.013% alkyl triethanol ammonium chloride/0.002% thimerosal solution under conditions similar to standard soft contact lens chemical disinfection (Ludwig *et al.*, 1986). An 0.005% chlorhexidine/0.001% thimerosal solution killed *A. castellani* cysts and trophozoites but not those of *A. polyphaga* (Ludwig *et al.*, 1986).

Silvany *et al.* (1987) found sorbic acid, edetate disodium, thimerosal and potassium sorbate ineffective against *A. castellani*. They also found thimerosal-edetate, chlorhexidine edetate and hydrogen peroxide without a catalyst were effective against *A. castellani* at 24 hour exposures. Moore *et al.* (1987) express their 'great concern at the inability of most current chemical sterilization methods to kill the organism if the lens becomes contaminated'.

Moore (1988) lays much of the blame for contact-lens-associated acanthamoeba infections on home-made saline from salt tablets and distilled water which is used with heat disinfection methods. She and her colleagues were able to find acanthamoebae in open bottles of distilled water and contact lens solutions, in contact lens cases, but not in unopened bottles of distilled water, although they found bacteria and fungi in these unopened bottles.

Moore (1988) recommends heat or a four-hour soak in hydrogen peroxide without catalyst for the destruction of acanthamoebae.

Penley, Willis and Sickler (1989) evaluated 10 soft lens cleaners for anti-acanthamoeba activity. They found that Miraflow (Ciba) was the only cleaner that killed trophozoites and cysts of *A. polyphaga* and *A. castellanii* on all lenses during the cleaning and this was done in 20 seconds.

The epidemiology of acanthamoeba keratitis has been assessed (Stehr-Green, Bailey and Visvesvara, 1989). A total of 208 cases were identified in the USA at that time. Of the 138 cases who wore contact lenses and for whom information was available, 88 (64%) used saline prepared by dissolving salt tablets in distilled water.

Human immunodeficiency virus (HIV)

Human immunodeficiency virus, the aetiological agent of the acquired immune deficiency syndrome, has been found in various body fluids, including tears (Fujikawa *et al.*, 1985) and has been recovered from conjunctival epithelial cells released from high water content contact lenses worn overnight (Tervo *et al.*, 1986).

Recommendations for preventing possible transmission of HIV have been made by the United States Center for Disease and Control (1985). Briefly, these include hand washing between patients and cleaning of instruments coming into direct contact with the eye, followed by a five to ten minute exposure to:

1. a fresh solution of 3% hydrogen peroxide
2. a fresh solution containing 5000 parts per million free available chlorine – a one in ten dilution of common household bleach
3. 70% ethanol
4. 70% isopropyl alcohol.

Contact lenses used in trial fittings should be disinfected between each fitting with either:

1. commercially available contact lens disinfectant or
2. heat treatment, i.e. 78–80 °C for 10 minutes.

Vogt *et al.* (1986) found that (in the USA) all commercially available solutions tested were able to disinfect lenses exposed to HTLV III. On the other hand, Hanson *et al.* (1989) found that 70% industrial methylated spirit failed to inactivate cell-free and cell-associated HIV within 20 and 15 minutes respectively and 70% ethanol did not inactivate cell-free virus within 10 minutes. They found that fresh 2% solutions of alkaline gluteraldehyde are effective, but recommend that care should be taken that they are not too dilute or have not become stale when used for disinfecting HIV associated with organic matter.

Lens spoilation

Apart from the question of contamination with organisms there is that of lens spoilation. Fowler, Greiner and Allansmith (1979a) found that the surfaces of all worn lenses are strikingly different from those of unworn lenses. The worn lenses were covered with deposits, some forming thickened coatings, although a few areas resembled the surface of never worn lenses.

Fowler, Korb and Allansmith (1985) found that the level of deposit formation appears to be proportional to the water content of soft lenses. Refojo and Leong (1979) measured the depth of penetration of fluorescein-labelled dextrans,

serum albumin, and lysozyme into hydrogel lenses. They found that lysozyme, which is abundant in the tears, penetrated hydroxyethyl methacrylate but not glycerylmethacrylate. Serum albumin did not penetrate either of these polymers except when the former was high-hydrated.

Castillo *et al.* (1985) found that poly-2-hydroxyethylmethacrylate-methacrylic acid lenses adsorbed 30 times more lysozyme than poly-2-hydroxyethylmethacrylate lenses and that fabrication processes appeared to induce different adsorption behaviour as lathe cut poly-2-hydroxyethylmethacrylate lenses adsorbed twice the amount of protein compared with spun cast lenses of the same material. Karageogian (1976) demonstrated, with the use of an amino acid analyser, that the protein coating on worn soft contact lenses was almost entirely lysozyme.

Castillo *et al.* (1986) have studied the adsorption of mucin on soft contact lenses. They found that surface morphology (lathe cut or spun cast) was an important adsorption parameter only for reversibly adsorbed mucin. Again, lathe cut lenses adsorbed more than spun cast lenses. Mucin can irreversibly bond to hydrogel surfaces.

Protein deposits originate primarily from complex interactions between the tear film and the contact lens surface (Yoshitomo and Shuzo, 1984; Gachon, Bilbaut and Dastugue, 1985). Protein adsorption onto soft hydrophilic lenses has been studied by a variety of techniques, including standard analytical chemical procedures, histochemical staining, scanning electron and immunofluorescence microscopy and spectroscopic techniques for surface analysis (Wedler, 1977; Holly, 1979; Bilbaut, Gachon and Dastugue, 1986; Castillo *et al.*, 1985; Gudmundsson *et al.*, 1985).

Wedler *et al.* (1977) showed that all proteins found in lens deposits are also present in human tear fluid, including lactoferrin, albumin, tear specific prealbumin and lysozyme. Stone, Mowrey-McKee and Kreutzer (1984) showed that protein will preferentially deposit onto acid-containing, high water content lenses. Fowler, Korb and Allansmith (1985) demonstrated that high water content lenses have more deposits on their surfaces than low water content lenses.

Sack *et al.* (1987) found that the nature and composition of the protein film on hydrophilic soft lenses depends on the ionic character of the polymer matrix. In 1986 the Food and Drugs

Administration in the USA adopted a classification system for soft hydrophilic material:

Group I   Low water content, non-ionic matrix.
Group II   High water, non-ionic matrix
Group III Low water ionic matrix.
Group IV   High water ionic matrix.

Minarik and Rapp (1989) assayed the protein deposition on new, never worn hydrogel contact lenses incubated in artificial (protein containing) tear solution and hydrogel lenses that were returned by patients due to deposit formation. Their work suggests that it is primarily the water content of a hydrogel and secondarily its ionic nature that determines the extent of its potential contamination by proteinaceous material. Groups I and III lenses showed relatively little protein deposition because of their low water content. Within the category of low water content lenses Group III showed more protein deposition than Group I because of its greater ionicity.

The terms ionicity or ionic can be explained as follows. Saline solution consists of two types of 'ions', positively charged sodium ions (denoted Na^+) and negatively charged ions (denoted Cl^-). These split particles are equally divided and balanced in a saline solution, hence the saline solution is overall electrically neutral.

Most polymers used in contact lens manufacture are overall electrically neutral and the term 'non-ionic' is used to describe them. However, extra monomers may be added to a material to alter, or perhaps improve, certain characteristics. For instance methacrylic acid might be added to hydroxyethylmethacrylate to increase its water content and this may leave the material with an overall weak negative charge. Such a material would be termed ionic.

If a lens is made from ionic material it will be more reactive in its surface characteristics than a lens made of non-ionic material. This may mean that a wetting solution may be more attracted to it but, alternatively, it may also mean that lipids which tend to be polar in nature will also be attracted to it, favouring surface deposition and thus deterioration.

Adsorbed protein, that is, lysozyme or mucin, can be removed from lenses by enzymatic digestion by papain or trypsin and this has been found to be of practical use (Hathaway and Lowther, 1978). However, Fowler and Allansmith (1981) found that none of the commercially available (in America) cleaning regimens successfully remove all the protein contaminants from a hydrophilic lens.

Calcium deposits can accumulate on soft contact lenses, especially those that are worn on an extended wear basis. They impair the ability of the patient to wear the lenses and they blur the vision. They can be identified at the slit lamp as white crystalline protrusions of the carbonate, usually covered with mucus (Figure 9.5), or plaques of opaque deposit of the phosphate characterized by their irregular shape. They resist ordinary cleaning and when the crystalline deposits are removed they leave a defect on the lens surface which is rapidly replaced in wear by a further deposit. Tear calcium is considered to be the source of these deposits (Ruben, Tripathi and Winder, 1975).

Begley and Waggoner (1991) studied these nodular deposits on soft lenses ('jelly bumps') which are extremely difficult to remove without affecting lens quality. Scanning electron microscopy and energy dispersive X-rays were used to examine the composition of these deposits on new (two to nine weeks old) and old (greater than six months old) soft lenses. Calcium was detected in 69 of 72 nodular deposits. Calcium was found throughout the deposit but was concentrated in the basal layers, while polysaccharides (e.g. niacin) were found in newer deposits.

A small number of patients develop calcium deposits on their lenses within a short time, especially with extended wear, and the reasons for this patient predisposition are at present unknown. Tapaszto *et al.* (1988, 1989) have reviewed and highlighted the great variability of tears constituents among individuals, particularly in relation to contact lens wear.

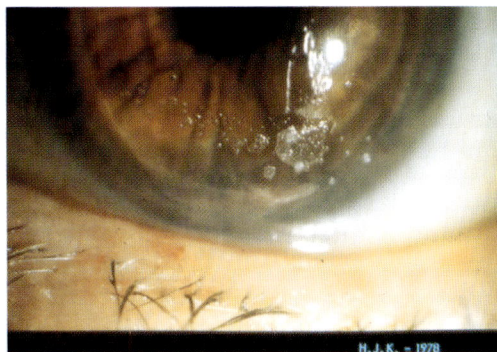

Figure 9.5 Calcium deposits on a soft lens, 'jelly bumps'

What is known is that some lenses are less likely to accumulate deposits than others. Levy (1984) has shown that the glyceryl methyl methacrylate lens (CSI, Pilkington) is less likely to acquire calcium deposits and continues to be wearable longer than the hydroxyethylmethacrylate (HEMA) lens. The stimulus for his study was the smaller pore size of glycerylmethacrylate material (1.9 nm compared with 2.5 to 3.0 nm diameter for hydroxyethylmethacrylate).

Seger, Mauger and Hill (1981) demonstrated that, although spoilation has been associated clinically with lens intolerance, neither extended wear spoilage nor common contaminants (either protein or lipid in nature) cause significant reduction in oxygen transmission per se in high water contact lenses. There are, of course, other factors which remain to be examined to elucidate the causes of intolerance of aged soft contact lenses.

Lipid deposits occur, but these can easily be removed by the action of a surfactant.

Contact lens spoilation can be caused by the use of drugs. Rifampicin which may cause a reddish discoloration of the tears (as well as sputum and urine) may produce permanent orange discoloration of soft contact lenses (Lyons, 1979) and the patient should be warned of this fact. Similar discoloration has been reported with sulphasalazine (Riley, Flegg and Mandal, 1986). Adrenaline, used as a glaucoma medication, has been reported to cause adenochrome pigment staining of soft lenses (Sugar, 1974). Although the pigment is within the lenses it may be cleared with hydrogen peroxide (Miller, Brooks and Mobilia, 1976). Fluorescein stains soft lenses yellow and in some of the higher water content lenses it is irreversible. In others the staining gradually fades.

The ophthalmologist should ascertain that there is not a contact lens in the eye before instilling fluorescein. An eye should be rinsed with saline, if fluorescein has been used, before a soft contact lens is inserted.

The high molecular weight dimer of fluorescein, fluorexan, which is distributed as an 0.35% solution in isotonic saline (Fluoresoft, Holles Laboratories Inc., Cohasset, Massachusetts, 02025, USA) (Refojo, Miller and Fiore, 1972) does not readily stain hydrophilic soft contact lenses. It has not found much favour with contact lens practitioners.

Goldmann applanation tonometry can be performed with sodium benoxinate 0.4% alone without fluorescein and without the cobalt light and gives comparable results suitable for routine assessment of the ocular tension.

Minute particles of iron that cannot easily be seen with the slit lamp may be blown against soft contact lenses and adhere. They give rise to rust spots.

Soft contact lenses may be inspected, to some extent, when on the patient's eye, but more thorough inspection is conveniently done with the use of a lens lift (see Figure 2.5) and the slit lamp. Alternatively, the lens lift can be used with retroillumination and surgical binocular operating spectacles.

Lastly, soft contact lenses may absorb ophthalmic preparations and their preservatives. A ubiquitous preservative in ophthalmic preparations is benzalkonium chloride. This preservative is known to cause physiological and morphological disturbances in the corneal epithelium (Green and Tonjum, 1971; Tonjum, 1975). Chapman, Cheeks and Green (1990) measured the uptake and washout of benzalkonium chloride by representative hard and soft contact lenses using a radioactive tracer. High-water content contact lenses absorbed greater quantities of benzalkonium chloride than did the low-water content lenses and these soft lenses released it slowly. Hard contact lenses took up a much smaller quantity of benzalkonium chloride, but released it more rapidly. Fluorosilicone-acrylate polymer lenses adsorbed and released the most preservative, while polymethylmethacrylate adsorbed and released the least. The released benzalkonium chloride from either soft or hard lenses was found to be of a sufficient concentration to be at or above the upper limits of safety.

In clinical practice the incorporation of benzalkonium chloride as a preservative in ophthalmic preparations used concurrently with contact lenses seldom leads to problems. It is, however, important not to treat a patient with an ophthalmic preparation which contains a preservative to which the patient has become hypersensitive. A list of ophthalmic preparations and their preservatives can be found in Appendix 7.II.

Deproteinization

This can be performed by proteolytic enzymes and several preparations are available on the commerical market. Some preparations contain stabilized papain (Primecare by Smith & Nephew, Hydrocare by Allergan and Soft Lens Care Tablets by Bausch & Lomb). Another preparation contains a protease, a pronase and a lipase, together with EDTA (Amiclair by Abatron Ltd). Yet another contains pancreatin BP 2.5 mg per tablet, equivalent to not less than 3.5 units protease activity (Clen-zym, Alcon). These substances are used for gas permeable as well as soft lenses and weekly treatment is usually advocated.

Ultrazyme (Allergan) contains subtilisin A, an enzyme that works in combination with the hydrogen peroxide preparation Oxysept 1 (Allergan) to remove protein deposition. Deproteinization and disinfection is thus a one step process in which the Ultrazyme tablet is added to the Oxysept 1. Allergan claim that the addition of Ultrazyme to Oxysept 1 results in an alkaline pH which has been shown to enhance the disinfecting power of the peroxide solution.

Dernstein *et al.* (1984) have described a case of local ocular anaphylaxis to papain enzyme in a contact lens cleaning solution. The patient developed IgE-mediated sensitization and subsequent ocular angioedema and conjunctivitis from papain contained in a commercial contact lens cleaning solution. Serum specific IgE and positive cutaneous prick tests to papain and chymopapain were detected. They point out that recognition of this route of papain-induced sensitization may be important in those patients undergoing chemonucleolysis with chymopapain, who may be at greater risk to develop a systemic allergic reaction after injection of this enzyme.

Cleaning

Cleaning usually means the employment of a surfactant or detergent or friction enhancer such as particulate polyhydroxymethylmethacrylate. There are many cleaners on the commercial market.

It is preferable to avoid thimerosal because this may be the only route in an ocular hypersensitivity reaction.

One cleaner (Miraflow by Ciba) uses isopropyl alcohol as a base which in itself is bacteriostatic and amoebicidal. Ghajar, Houlsby and Chavez (1989) found that Miraflow had greater antimicrobial activity than five other leading proprietary

cleaners when tested against two Gram-negative and on Gram-positive bacteria, a yeast and a fungus. The work of Penley, Willis and Sickler (1989) on the amoebicidal activity of Miraflow has already been referred to in this chapter. Miraflow contains no preservative.

Disinfection

Heat disinfection

This can be performed in a commercially available unit which usually heats the lenses immersed in saline within a container to a temperature of about 78–80 °C in 10 minutes and then allows them to cool. Early units surrounded the lens container with a water bath, but later units have dispensed with this.

Busschaert, Good and Szabocsik (1978) demonstrated experimentally that exposure to 80 °C temperature for 10 minutes and 75 °C for five minutes were both satisfactory for moist heat disinfection when the initial load was 10^9 organisms. The figure 10^9 is significant for contact lens disinfection. It represents an order of magnitude estimate of the number of bacteria that may be present per millilitre of solution on a contact lens. This presumes microbial dimensions of average magnitude and that the storage saline for the contact lenses is uncontaminated. As part of their study Busschaert, Good and Szabocsik (1978) established D and z values for many of the microorganisms used. The D value is the time required to kill 90% of an inoculum or, expressed in another way, to reduce the organism population by one log. The D value determines the probability of survival as a function of time and is influenced by many environmental factors including pH, tonicity, nutrients and the age of the bacterium. The temperature change in degrees centigrade required to change the D value by a factor of ten is called the z value.

Liubinas, Swenson and Carney (1987) have examined the basic concepts associated with thermal disinfection of contact lenses and have described the mathematical models used to predict the probability of survival of microorganisms as applied to ocular pathogens. They have established the time–temperature profiles of several commercially available heat disinfection units and have evaluated their performance in comparison to both current and proposed standards. They point out that sterilization is the process of destroying all forms of microbial life. Disinfection is the process of destroying infectious agents. It does not imply sterilization. Sanitization, which is the reduction of the microbial population to safe levels as judged by public health standards, is the most common result of disinfection. They recommend a revised standard with the disinfecting temperature to exceed 70 °C for five minutes, but not to exceed 80 °C. They suggest that this will minimize possible lens degradation resulting from excessive heat exposure. They did not investigate the effect of the units on acanthamoeba.

Martin, McDougal and Loskoski (1985) monitored the rate of inactivation of 10 μl of AIDS virus concentrate when subjected to 56 °C. In an attempt to simulate the protection from heat disinfection that might be provided by serum protein they diluted the concentrate with human serum. No viral activity was detectable after 10 minutes at 56 °C. One unit can be obtained which cleans lenses ultrasonically before sterilizing (Sonasept, made by S.M.C. Technology Ltd, 8th Floor, Yan Nin Industrial Building, 8 Fung Yip Street, Hong Kong). The locally appointed retail agent there is Vision Plus Optical Co. Ltd, 339 Hennesy Road, Hong Kong. Tests conducted by Professor G.L. French at the Chinese University of Hong Kong showed that the cleaner appears to be effective against heavy inocula of a range of organisms, as specified by the American Food and Drug Administration, including aspergillus spores giving D values of up to 2.5 minutes. These results were quoted in the accompanying literature with the instrument purchased by the author.

Phillips, Badenoch and Copley (1989) found that the unit functioned safely at the soft low water contact lens cycle, when challenged with *Pseudomonas aeruginosa* and *Candida albicans*, but did not function safely against these organisms at the lower temperatures of the hard contact lens cycle or the soft high water contact lens cycle. He found the timing device to be inaccurate.

Kilvington (1989) tested this machine and found that it was effective against pathogenic acanthamoeba cysts only on the soft low water content contact lens cycle. This resulted in 100% kill of a cyst inoculum of 1×10^6. The other two cycles (soft high water content and hard lens cycles) were not effective, resulting in the recovery of viable cysts after disinfection treatment.

In the context of vascular prosthetic graft material, Tollefson *et al.* (1987) found that ultrasonic oscillation (sonication) could disrupt surface biofilms and increase the recovery of adherent microorganisms. Ludwig *et al.* (1986) have shown that acanthamoeba organisms are only consistently killed by heat. They report that standard contact lens heat disinfection kills *Acanthamoeba polyphaga* and *A. castellani* cysts and trophozoites in suspension. Lindquist *et al.* (1987) found heat disinfection effective against *A. castellani* and *A. polyphaga*.

Warhurst (personal communication, 1988) notes that there is little published data on the effect of heat on acanthamoeba. In his experience 30 minutes pasteurization, by the holder method, is required to eradicate acanthamoeba cysts. Contact lens heat sterilizing units use the flash method of pasteurization whereby the fluid in the container is brought to a certain temperature, the electric current is switched off and the fluid is allowed to cool.

Bernstein, Stow and Maddox (1973) have questioned the effectiveness of 'aseptization' with standard soft lens thermal units. They found that 11 of 25 unopened, previously asepticized lens cases contained bacterial organisms.

Heat disinfection has disadvantages and shortcomings. Gruber (1981) has reported that the heat disinfection method shortens contact lens life, is incompatible with extended wear lenses and possibly coagulates deposits on the lens surface. Certain soft contact lenses on the market (e.g. Hydrocurve II, Pilkington Barnes Hind) are destroyed by heat treatment and the manufacturers warn against its use. Tragakis, Brown and Pearce (1973) reported the survival of *Aspergillus fumigatus* after 15 minutes of boiling. Pitts and Krachmer (1979) found that with the thermal disinfection system in a random sample from the home environment 34.5% of contact lenses were contaminated.

Microwave

Rohrer *et al.* (1986) have used standard 2450 MHz irradiation to achieve sterilization of hydrophilic contact lenses contaminated with a variety of bacterial, fungal and viral corneal pathogens. The contact lenses became dehydrated in approximately two minutes. Rehydration with normal saline restored their shape and appearance. The time necessary to prohibit all growth of the bacterial and fungal organisms studied ranged from 45 seconds to eight minutes. All viral contaminants were completely inactivated after four minutes of microwave exposure. Refractive properties were unaffected after 101 exposures to microwaves for ten minutes. Slit lamp examination and scanning electron microscopy disclosed minute particles on the surface of these contact lenses but no damage to the lens matrix from irradiation. Perhaps because of these particles a human volunteer complained of slight discomfort after wearing a treated lens. The technique involved placing radar absorbent material in the oven as a parallel load (Rohrer and Bulard, 1985).

Kerr (1985) recommends that the lenses are first cleaned with a surfactant agent and then thoroughly rinsed in unit dose buffered saline. The lenses should then be transferred to lightly closed individual cases, or vials, each containing about 15 ml of unit dose buffered saline. The containers should not, of course, have metallic components. The vials should then be placed in a microwave unit and the saline within allowed to reach boiling point. The unit should then be immediately shut off and the lenses allowed to cool. They may then be considered to be aseptisized and ready to be worn. With experience the time taken to reach boiling point in a particular microwave oven will be known.

Harris *et al.* (1989) have evaluated the effectiveness and convenience of microwave irradiation as a method of disinfecting soft contact lenses. Soft contact lenses from each of four Food and Drug Administration (FDA) categories (discussed earlier in this chapter) were placed in sterile vials and immersed in 2 ml of saline which had been contaminated with one of three common species of bacteria (*Pseudomonas aeruginosa*, *Serratia marcescens* and *Staphylococcus aureus*). The sterile glass vials had two or three small holes placed in each vial screw cap to act as steam vents. The contaminated lens vials were placed in a standard 600 W microwave oven and exposed to microwave irradiation times ranging from 30 to 180 seconds. Significant reductions in bacteria colony counts were found after 30 seconds of microwave irradiation. Few of the bacteria survived 60 seconds of microwave exposure and none survived 90 seconds. Unfortunately, these authors did not evaluate the effectiveness of microwaves against acanthamoeba trophozoites and cysts.

More recently, Harris *et al.* (1990) have evaluated the effectiveness of an in-office microwave disinfection procedure. They used a standard 2450 MHz 650 W Philips model 7440P microwave oven with a rotating glass plate to ensure even microwave exposure to all contact lens cases. The lenses were put, with sterile saline, in Ciba AOSept cases which had a vent pore at the top of the case. This acted as a steam vent and prevented the case from cracking under the intense boiling produced by microwave irradiation. They found that none of the six Food and Drug Administration test challenge microorganisms survived two minutes or longer of microwave exposure. Their findings indicated that microwave irradiation can be a convenient, rapid and effective method of disinfecting a number of soft contact lenses and, thus, was adaptable as an in-office soft contact lens disinfection procedure.

Ultraviolet irradiation

A unit named the Aquasteril combines ultraviolet disinfection with ultrasonic cleaning. It is manufactured by Optelec, 6 Rue des Chalets, 94450 Lemeil-Brevannes, France. It is distributed in England by Specialist Optical, 57 Dukes Wood Drive, Gerrards Cross, Bucks., SL9 7L7. It is claimed that studies at the Pasteur Institute showed that the system destroys contact lens organisms, streptococcus, salmonella, staphylococcus, *Escherichia coli* and *Vibrio cholerae* and that studies at the Centre Hospitalier Aire, Toulouse, have shown adequate fungicidal action. The cleaning bath does not exceed 37 °C and so does not present any problems of molecular change to the matrix, nor does it affect the optical parameters of the lenses.

The distributors of the Aquasteril supply a further report on the efficacy of the instrument from the Centre for Contact Lens Research at the University of Waterloo, Canada. The study tested *Escherichia coli*, *Pseudomonas aeruginosa*, *Staphylococcus aureus*, *Serratia marcescens*, *Aspergillus fumigatus* and *Candida albicans*. The unit was found to be effective against the four bacteria and *Aspergillus fumigatus*, but not against *Candida albicans* when contact lenses were not placed in the cups. When these studies were repeated with a contact lens in each cup, weak growth was observed after 24 hours' incubation in all three tubes from one machine for the organisms *Escherichia coli* and

Serratia marcescens. No growth was observed for the other two machines. It was concluded that the first machine was under powered.

Kessler *et al*. (1989) have investigated a device which uses an ultraviolet light source to achieve disinfection of hydrophilic lenses. The device provided a source of energy at a wave length of 254 nm with 450 μW/cm^2 of radiation at 2.5 cm. They subjected contact lenses of high and low water content to continued ultraviolet exposure for up to 48 hours and no changes in their characteristics were found. They studied the efficacy of the device in sterilizing saline solutions contaminated with a number of ATCC (American Type Collection Culture) bacterial and fungal pathogens per Food and Drugs Administration protocol for approval of contact lens solutions. All bacterial species tested achieved greater than five log units of killing and fungal cultures demonstrated greater than two log units of killing within 30 minutes.

Dolman and Dobrogowski (1989) have tested ultraviolet light of wave length 253.7 nm and intensity 1100 μW/cm^2 for its germicidal activity against contact lenses and storage solutions contaminated with various corneal pathogens. They found that the exposure time necessary to reduce a concentration of organisms from 10^6/ml to less than 10/ml was 30 seconds for *Staphylococcus aureus*, 60 seconds for *Pseudomonas aeruginosa* and 84 seconds for *Candida albicans*. The time necessary to sterilize a suspension of 10^4/ml *Acanthamoeba polyphaga* was less than three minutes. Four brands of soft contact lenses were exposed to ultraviolet light for over eight hours without changing their appearance, comfort or refraction. They point out that the major drawback of ultraviolet light disinfection is that the system depends on a high transmission of germicidal ultraviolet light by the contact lenses and solutions. Because preserved saline and some other contact lens solutions transmit ultraviolet light poorly, and can impair its potency, such solutions should not be used in this system. Some contact lenses tested also transmitted 253.7 nm ultraviolet light poorly.

Scanlon (1991) has questioned the efficacy of the Aquasteril instrument. It uses a 253.7 nm mercury steam lamp in common with the instrument used by Dolman and Dobrogowski. Scanlon found that the intensity of the three Aquasteril machines he tested varied considerably. The intensity at 4 mm from the fluid in the cups of the instrument varied from 0.956 μW/m^2 to 44.32 μW/m^2 depending on which machine was used and the number of cycles for which it had been used. One of the three machines was considerably better than the other two. The intensities of these machines compared unfavourably with the quoted intensity of 1100 μW/m^2 given for the instrument used by Dolman and Dobrogowski. Scanlon (1991) attributes the fall in output of the Aquasteril machines with continued use either to a crazing, which he observed in the window between the UV lamp and the cups, or to a fall in the output of the UV lamp itself.

Palmer, Scanlon and McNulty (1991) studied the efficacy of the Aquasteril instrument with a range of microbial challenge organisms. There was a 90% kill (one log unit) of *Staphylococcus aureus*, a 50% kill of *Pseudomonas aeruginosa*, a 33% kill of *Serratia marcescens*, a 23% kill of *Micrococcus luteus* and a 25% kill of *Candida albicans*.

Kilvington and Scanlon (1991) studied the efficacy of the Aquasteril instrument against acanthamoeba isolates and found that the survival rate for both cysts and trophozoites was between 85% and 95%.

Chemical disinfection

The great disadvantage of this method is that the patient can become hypersensitive to the chemicals used, particularly thimerosal. This latter antimicrobial is popular because it is fungistatic as well as bactericidal and does not bind to lens plastic. One of the breakdown products of thimerosal is ethyl mercuric chloride, which is highly toxic and is used in agriculture as a pesticide.

With soft contact lens use, preservatives are in contact with the eye for several hours. Furthermore, the concentration of these chemicals at the lens–eye interface, posteriorly, may be higher than it is anteriorly, and cannot be evaluated by models in the laboratory. The chemicals in common use are thiomersal, chlorhexidine and disodium edetate.

Thimerosal   Thimerosal (also thiomersalate, thiomersal, mercurothiolate and sodium ethyl mercurithiosalicylate) is bacteriostatic and fungistatic. For contact lens solutions the concentration varies between 0.001 and 0.004%. Its use in cosmetics and toiletries is restricted in Great Britain under the Cosmetic Products Regulations 1978 (SI 1978 No. 1354). Now that there is awareness of a large hypersensitivity problem with thiomersal it has been replaced by sorbic acid in one cleaner (Pliagel, Alcon).

Connor, Blocker and Pitts (1989) have reported 92% survival of acanthamoeba cysts after 24 hours in thimerosal 0.002%.

Chlorhexidine Chlorhexidine is a disinfectant which is effective against a wide range of vegetative Gram-positive and Gram-negative bacteria. It is ineffective against acid-fast bacteria, bacterial spores, fungi and viruses. It is more effective against Gram-positive than Gram-negative bacteria, some species of *Pseudomonas* and *Proteus* being relatively less susceptible. Chlorhexidine is most active at a neutral or slightly alkaline pH, but its activity is reduced by organic matter. It is usually used in concentrations of 0.002 to 0.005%.

The widespread use of chlorhexidine can be attributed to its high antimicrobial efficiency (Davies, 1978) and its relatively low level of irritation observed when solutions are used with hydrogel lenses (Browne, Anderson and Charves, 1974, 1975; Callender, 1978)

Chlorhexidine binds to polyhydroxyethylmethacrylate. Levels of preservative are accumulated within the polymer that are significantly in excess of the values predicted for the relevant concentration of surrounding solution (Plaut, Meakin and Davies, 1980).

Ludwig *et al*. (1986) have shown that acanthamoeba organisms may resist chemical and peroxide disinfection.

Davies *et al*. (1988) dispute the observations of Ludwig *et al*. (1986) and have shown that chlorhexidine, in properly formulated solutions (500, 15 000 and 1 000 000 parts per ml) kills cysts of both *Acanthamoeba castellani* and *A. polyphaga* within four hours.

Connor, Blocker and Pitts (1989) have reported 25% survival of acanthamoeba cysts after 24 hours in chlorhexidine 0.01% and 42% survival after 24 hours in chlorhexidine 0.001%.

Green *et al*. (1980) showed, in experiments on rabbits, that chlorhexidine digluconate, at concentrations likely to be found in the tear film following desorption from soft contact lenses, produced little effect on the epithelium of corneas perfused across the epithelial surface for three hours. They

also found that, at clinically relevant concentrations, no endothelial changes occurred after that period of time.

Phinney *et al*. (1988) have again drawn attention to the cytotoxic effect of chlorhexidine which is the active antiseptic agent in Hibiclens. They reported five cases of corneal oedema caused by accidental preoperative ocular exposure to this preparation. Between two and five weeks after exposure stromal and epithelial oedema developed in all patients. The corneal oedema resolved in three patients in approximately six months, leaving mild stromal scarring and reduced endothelial cell counts. The corneal oedema in the other two patients progressed to diffuse bullous keratopathy, which eventually required penetrating keratoplasty. Endothelial toxicity to high concentrations of chlorhexidine was demonstrated in rabbits by Green *et al*. (1980). It is tempting to speculate whether the endothelial changes seen in long-term wearers of contact lenses, both hard and soft, are, in fact, due to anoxia as supposed. The ubiquitous use of chlorhexidine with contact lenses over long periods may have implications so far as the corneal endothelium is concerned.

Chlorhexidine is known to sensitize skin (Ljunnggren and Moller, 1972) and its use in alcohol aerosol sprays has been associated with occupational asthma in nurses (Waclawski, McAlpine and Thompson, 1989).

Disodium edetate Disodium edetate (EDTA, sodium edetate, disodium dihydrogen edetate, disodium edathamal and disodium tetracemate) is a chelating agent which forms complexes with divalent and trivalent metals, completely changing the properties of these ions in solution. It is included in nearly all contact lens solutions, the usual concentration being 0.1%. Its chelating action inhibits the growth of some bacteria by making certain trace elements, required for growth, unavailable, or by complexing with metals within the cell wall of the bacterium.

Disodium edetate is used to remove traces of heavy metals from pharmaceutical preparations and so improve their stability. Disodium edetate also acts by removing traces of heavy metals which often catalyse autoxidation reactions. Its use is reviewed by Lachman (1968).

Sorbic acid Sorbic acid has antibacterial and antifungal properties. It is active against moulds and yeasts and, to a lesser degree, against bacteria. It is not effective above about pH 6.5. The optimum pH is about 4.5. Its fungistatic activity is increased by the addition of acids and sodium chloride. *Bacillus cereus* is resistant to sorbic acid. Sorbic acid tends to be used mainly in cleaners for contact lenses to replace thimerosal. Its antimicrobial action would appear to be too weak for use in storage solutions.

Polyquad   A further preservative, Polyquad (Alcon) has been introduced in the USA. It is a high molecular weight, quaternary compound which is soluble in water. It has a molecular weight of approximately 5000, which is significantly greater than that of current preservatives used with soft contact lenses (thimerosal 405, chlorhexidine 359 and sorbic acid 112). The high molecular weight, together with its molecular configuration, prevent the adsorption of Polyquad into the pores of the soft contact lens matrix. Polyquad has been shown to have a broad spectrum of antimicrobial activity, but the spectrum has not been disclosed. Lindquist *et al.* (1988) found that chemical disinfection by means of quaternary ammonium compounds was ineffective in eradicating acanthamoeba organisms from contact lenses of patients. Polyquad is claimed to have a low capacity to cause ocular irritation. Lopez, Calleja and Claramonte (1992) have reported a study of 14 non-oxidizing disinfecting systems available in Spain. These systems contained, among other things, chlorhexidine, EDTA, trimerosal, Polyquad, polyaminopropyl biguanide and alkyl triethanol ammonium chloride. They were found to be only weakly active against *Acanthamoeba culbertsoni*. Ten to 50% of the pathogens survived an eight hour exposure.

Chemical sterilization has the disadvantage that it may not be effective. Tragakis, Brown and Pearce (1973) found that *P. vulgaris* survived after two hours of treatment with chlorhexidine and thimerosal. Donzis *et al.* (1987) examined the contact lens care systems of 100 asymptomatic patients who used hard or soft contact lenses. Sixteen of 126 bottles (13%) of commercial contact lens care solutions were contaminated, but contamination was not found in bottles of preserved solutions that were opened and used for less than 21 days. All 12 bottles of home-made saline were contaminated with bacteria and acanthamoeba was isolated from two of these bottles. Pseudo-

monas was found in the care systems of 12 patients. Bacillus species, which form spores resistant to heat, were found in the care systems of seven patients. Endotoxin, which is also resistant to heat, was detected in nine of the 35 care systems.

In a prospective study of 24 contact lens patients with culture- or histopathology-proven microbial keratitis, Bowden *et al.* (1989) found that failure to follow standard recommendations regarding contact lens care was widespread (21 of 24, 88%). In the majority of patients (20 of 24, 83%) bacterial contamination of the contact lens case and/or solutions was present. Almost two-thirds (15 of 24, 62%) of patients used solutions that were more than three months old. Cosmetic extended wear patients were most likely (7 of 8, 88%) to use solutions that were more than three months old and very likely (6 of 8, 85%) to have contaminated solutions.

Donzis, Mondino and Weissman (1988) reported two cases of soft contact lens wearers who developed keratitis associated with Bacillus contamination of their contact lens care systems. One case developed a corneal ulcer caused by *B. subtilis* and the other, diffuse, punctate corneal opacities associated with *B. cereus* contamination in the contact lens and lens case compartment. The contact lens cases of both patients contained Bacillus spores that survived multiple heat disinfection treatments. Three different contact lens chemical disinfection systems used for the minimum recommended time failed to kill the Bacillus organisms. Only prolonged exposure to 3% hydrogen peroxide effectively eradicated both Bacillus species in their study. Turner (1983) has reported that hydrogen peroxide is sporicidal to Bacillus organisms with sufficient exposure.

Richardson *et al.* (1977) have drawn attention to the loss of antibacterial preservatives from contact lens solutions during storage. They attribute this to their sorption by polyethylene and polypropylene containers which may lead to almost complete loss of preservative on storage.

Holland *et al.* (1989) have reported that the production of biofilm may provide a mechanism for bacterial survival in contaminated topical eye medications associated with ocular infections despite the presence of preservatives. Their isolates were predominantly Pseudomonas. Bacteria were found in biofilm or glycocalyx inside the caps, on the inside walls and inner bases of bottles studied.

Oxidizing systems

Hydrogen peroxide The disinfecting mechanism of hydrogen peroxide is not completely understood, but there is evidence that free radicals are formed in the presence of trace amounts of metallic ions that originate from any bacteria present. These free radicals then act directly on the cell wall of the invading organism, probably destroying it through oxidation with resultant cell death (Janoff, 1979).

Wilson, Sawant and Ahearn (1991) found that hydrogen peroxide was more effective against biofilms than disinfectant solutions formulated with chlorhexidine gluconate or polyquaternium or polyaminopropyl biguanide. Hydrogen peroxide is used at 3% concentration for a recommended 20 minutes in one system and 10 minutes in another. Penley *et al*. (1985) investigated this system and found that *Serratia marcescens* survived for the usual standard treatment time of 10 minutes. Silvany *et al*. (1987) found hydrogen peroxide without a catalyst was effective against *Acanthamoeba castellani* after 24 hour exposure. *A. polyphaga* and *A. castellani* cysts and trophozoites have been shown to survive treatment with 3% hydrogen peroxide (Ludwig *et al*. 1986). Lindquist *et al*. (1988) found hydrogen peroxide disinfection universally ineffective in eradicating acanthamoeba organisms as the protozoans were readily recovered from the treated lenses. Connor, Blocker and Pitts (1989) have reported 100% survival of acanthamoeba cysts after one hour in 3% hydrogen peroxide.

Brandt, Ware and Visvesvara (1989) studied the viability of acanthamoeba cysts in ophthalmic solutions used with contact lenses. Disinfectants, as expected, were the most effective of all tested solutions in killing acanthamoeba cysts. Survival times, in these disinfectant solutions, ranged from six hours to 14 days. Five of the solutions contained chlorhexidine, thimerosal, EDTA mixtures. A sixth peroxide solution (Lensept, American Optical) was tested. In it, cysts of all three species of acanthamoeba (*A. castellanii*, *A. polyphaga* and *A. culbertsoni*) survived for six hours, but not 24 hours.

Lowe, Vallas and Brennan (1992) found that 3% hydrogen peroxide when used over longer disinfecting periods (i.e. a minimum of 2.4 hours) gave adequate performance against fungi.

In addition to the effects of oxidation, hydrogen peroxide seems to cause dimensional changes in a soft lens. This 'sucking and squeezing' effect adds to the cleaning potential (Janoff, 1979). After treatment with this agent lenses swell. It may take more than the 10 minutes of neutralization used by one system for the lens to regain its previous dimensions and in this condition it is fragile.

There are a number of peroxide systems on the commercial market. One system (Septicon, Ciba) uses 3% hydrogen peroxide for 20 minutes, followed by immersion in a solution containing thimerosal. A catalyst (a platinum-coated disc) is used to convert the hydrogen peroxide to water and oxygen. Since the incorporation of thimerosal in the neutralizing solution rather defeats the object of the system, this solution is often replaced by sterile buffered unpreserved normal saline (Kerr, 1982), either in individually packed containers or from a pressurized can.

A second system (Ten Ten, Ciba) uses sodium pyruvate to neutralize the hydrogen peroxide. The lens is soaked for 10 minutes in hydrogen peroxide and 10 minutes in sodium pyruvate.

A third system (Oxysept, Allergan) uses catalase to neutralize the hydrogen peroxide and, again, the recommended soaking times are 10 minutes in each solution.

It must be borne in mind that these systems use hydrogen peroxide which incorporates stabilizers, the nature of which appears to be a trade secret since one contact lens solution manufacturer told the author that they did not know the nature of the chemicals incorporated in the hydrogen peroxide which they bought from their supplier. These stabilizers are compatible with contact lens materials but, in the experience of the author, may give hypersensitivity reactions in the cornea and conjunctiva. Hydrogen peroxide solutions, not intended for contact lens use, are usually dispensed at a concentration of 3%.

The British Pharmacopoeia allows up to 0.25% of suitable stabilizers. Acetanilide, benzoic acid, hydroxyquinoline and phenacetin have been used. The acidity is regulated by dilute phosphoric acid or dilute sulphuric acid. The author has known patients to use the BP formulation for contact lens disinfection without problems.

Sack, Harvey and Nunes (1989) carried out chemical analysis on clinically obtained hazy white hydrogel lenses that had been exposed to hydrogen peroxide disinfection. Analysis revealed that hazing was a surface phenomenon limited to high water content, ionic matrix, hydrogels (Type IV), the type associated with the deposition of large amounts of lysozyme. Hazing proved independent of the presence of hydrogen peroxide, but dependent on the interaction of lens bound lysozyme and stannate anion, the latter derived from sodium stannate present in the disinfectant as a stabilizing agent. Only Type IV hydrogels have a sufficient number of anionic binding sites and are of sufficient porosity to allow the penetration of lysozyme. No other protein is small enough to penetrate the hydrogel matrix or basic enough to have a marked affinity for the lens and to provide binding sites for the stannate anion.

Tripathi and Tripathi (1989) have drawn attention to the possible dangers of the continued use of hydrogen peroxide. They point out that neutralization may not always be complete and residual concentrations of 100 parts per million and less were found by Paugh, Brennan and Efron (1988) to elicit comfort responses similar to those experienced with physiological saline, suggesting that the corneal tissues of patients could be exposed to residual peroxide without inducing discomfort that would otherwise serve as an alerting signal.

Tripathi and Tripathi (1989) demonstrated deleterious effects on the corneal epithelium in vitro by hydrogen peroxide at concentrations as low as 30 parts per million. They are concerned that by adding exogenous peroxide repeatedly to the anterior surface of the cornea, in effect, the corneal tissues are bathed with at least trace amounts of the agent both anteriorly and posteriorly. They point out that the role of the highly toxic hydroxyl radical OH, which is produced from hydrogen peroxide, has expanded greatly and includes the pathogenesis of ocular disorders such as cataracts, ocular haemorrhage, degenerative retinal damage, retinopathy of prematurity and photic retinopathy.

Furthermore, hydrogen peroxide can also directly damage DNA and this mode of injury has led investigators to conclude that this agent may be capable of causing a number of corneal disorders.

Chlorine-releasing compounds One of these systems (Softab by Alcon) uses sodium dichloroiso-cyanurate which, when dissolved in saline solution, releases available chlorine. This is said to disinfect lenses over a period of four hours. After rinsing in saline the lenses are ready to wear. The manufacturers state that the tablet of sodium dichloroisocyanurate does not contain binding material or stabilizers. They do, however, recommend the use of a surfactant cleaner prior to treatment of the lenses. The tablets release 12 parts per million of chlorine and it has been stated that a concentration of 360 parts per million are necessary to get a toxicity reaction to chlorine in the corneal epithelium. Ferreira *et al.* (1991) found that the antimicrobial activity of Softab was well within the requirements set down in both the British and American standards for disinfecting solutions. Lowe, Vallas and Breunan (1992) found that Softab failed to meet the Food and Drugs Administration (USA) standard for bacteria.

Beekhuis *et al.* (1992) have investigated the use of Softab for trial lenses in the practice situation. They found it to be effective against a standard range of bacteria. Even when used without a cleaning step, the efficacy was good. For disinfection of contact lenses contaminated by a high load of Aspergillus, Softab did not completely meet expectations. Their virological investigation is interesting. Softab will not inactivate non-enveloped viruses such as poliovirus or adenovirus. Enveloped viruses are effectively eliminated by Softab. In their study they used herpes simplex virus (type 1). Schunk and Schweisfurth (1989) have shown it to be effective against human immunodeficiency virus (HIV).

An alternative system (Aerotab by Sauflon Pharmaceuticals Ltd) uses parasulphondichloramide benzoic acid (Halazone). Again the tablet releases chlorine when dissolved in water and hypochlorous acid (HOCl) is formed. It is generally accepted that this chemical is responsible for the biocidal activity. Formulations which are slightly acid give optimum biocidal activity. Lowe, Vallas and Brennan (1992) found it a poor fungicide. Rosenthal *et al.* (1992) found that Aerotab demonstrated minimal activity against both *C. albicans* and *Fusarium solani* even after 24 hours of exposure. The Aerotab formulation includes an effervescent base consisting of sodium carbonate and adipic acid.

Copley (1989) has studied the properties of the two organic chlorine-releasing systems present at that time on the Australian market. He found that both performed to international standards on properly cleaned lenses. However, he found that soiled lenses may severely reduce the efficiency of such agents. This finding is particularly pertinent in the case of high water content, high ionic, disposable lenses at present on the market. Chlorine-releasing compounds are often prescribed for the disinfection of these lenses in the UK. These lenses soil with protein with extreme rapidity (Leahy, Mandell and Lin, 1989).

Harf (1991) found that a solution of chlorine-based tablets had an amoebicidal effect on trophozoites, but the concentration used and the duration of contact (four hours) were insufficient to kill cysts. The use of chlorine-releasing compounds for contact lens disinfection has not been approved by the FDA in the USA.

Appendix 9.III is a list of preparations and their preservatives for use with soft contact lenses.

Autoclave For the busy contact lens practitioner an autoclave is helpful for sterilizing (rather than pasteurizing) a large number of lenses at one time. Unfortunately, not all autoclaves are suitable. They can be classified as follows.

1 Porous load autoclave This autoclave heats to 134 °C for three minutes and is used for dressings, towels, gowns and surgical instruments. It is unsuitable for contact lenses as the heat will not penetrate the containers and sterilization will be incomplete. There is also the danger of the containers exploding as the first stage is the withdrawal of air from the autoclave chamber.

2 Fluids autoclave This autoclave heats to 121 °C for 15 minutes. There are three types.

A AIR BALLASTED This autoclave can be used for contact lenses as it is used extensively for the sterilization of fluids in sealed bottles. It is needed for plastics. Air is injected during the cycle and after the heat is withdrawn to equilibrate the pressures within and without the containers, to prevent them exploding.

Unfortunately, these autoclaves are large with a chamber capacity of about 5 cubic feet (0.14 m^3). They are not portable and cannot be put on a desk top and they are, thus, not really suitable for contact lens clinic use.

B NORMAL AUTOCLAVE This autoclave is not air ballasted and is not suitable for sterilizing fluids in bottles or contact lenses in containers.

C NORMAL AUTOCLAVE WITH SLOW EXHAUST Slow exhaust autoclaves are normal autoclaves which have been modified to maintain the inside pressure after the cycle has ended. The pressure only goes down to atmospheric levels once all the steam has condensed. This autoclave is especially suitable for contact lens sterilization as it is portable and can be obtained in desk top size. A suitable instrument is the Napco 8000, obtainable from T.I.S. Services, 10 Chawton Park Road, Alton, Hampshire.

3 Low temperature steam and formaldehyde autoclave These heat to 70 °C for a validated time with formaldehyde and are designed for surgical instruments. They are not applicable to contact lenses.

Dry heat sterilizer These heat to a minimum of 180 °C for not less than 30 minutes, a minimum of 170 °C for not less than one hour, or a minimum of 160 °C for not less than two hours. These sterilizers are considerably cheaper than autoclaves and may be used for heat stable, non-aqueous preparations and certain types of containers, but they are unsuitable for fluid or contact lenses in sealed bottles because of the risk of the bottles exploding and the high temperatures generated.

Preservative-free saline in aerosol cans This is a convenient method of dispensing saline which is often used in conjunction with heat disinfection and chemical disinfection. Riordan-Eva, Eykyn and Kerr-Muir (1988) have described a case of *Pseudomonas aeruginosa* suppurative keratitis in a contact lens wearer associated with the use of an aerosol of preservative free saline. *Pseudomonas aeruginosa* pyocine type 10c was isolated from the right eye, the surface of the right contact lens, the top of the aerosol can of preservative free saline, and the contents of the can obtained by direct puncture. There was no growth from the contents of another sample can from the same manufacturer's batch. The patient used a chlorine-release tablet system in association with the preservative free saline. During his travels his aerosol can of preservative free saline was stored in a wash bag, together with wet face cloths. The cap was often found to be off the can.

Disposable contact lenses

Disposable extended wear hydrogel contact lenses, intended to be worn continuously for one or two weeks, and then discarded, have been introduced. Claims have been made that these lenses will reduce the risk of infections caused by non-compliance with good lens care, since no cleaning or disinfection is required. Furthermore, the risks associated with ageing lenses, including cracks or surface defects which might cause microtrauma to the cornea and thus penetration of organisms, might be avoided. Lowther (1991) examined the incidence of edge and surface defects in Acuvue and SeeQuence disposable lenses. Two hundred and forty lenses of each brand were studied. Fifty four of the Acuvue lenses (22.5%) had some sort of defects such as nicks, rough edges, scratched surfaces and edge tears. Six of the SeeQuence lenses examined (2.5%) had defects. These defects can, presumably, act as a nidus for bacterial multiplication.

A further advantage is claimed in the avoidance of chemicals used as preservatives in contact lens solutions, which might give toxic or hypersensitivity reactions. Unfortunately, for economic reasons, these lenses are advertised for extended wear with all that implies so far as the increased incidence of suppurative keratitis is concerned.

Killingsworth and Stern (1989) and Rabinowitz, Pflugfelder and Goldberg (1989) have both reported cases of pseudomonas keratitis associated with their use and Dunn *et al*. (1989) have reported four further cases of suppurative keratitis. The latter authors pointed out that the premarket study of Acuvue (Johnson and Johnson) disposable hydrogel contact lenses (etafilcon 55% water content) consisting of 733 patients followed up for eight months of wear, found an overall complication rate of only 5.6% and no corneal ulcers were noted. The author has personally seen two cases of suppurative keratopathy associated with their use in patients who previously wore daily wear lenses with no trouble. A number of such cases have been seen at Moorfields Eye Hospital, including one case of acanthamoeba keratitis (Ficker *et al*., 1989).

Heidemann *et al*. (1990) have reported three cases of acanthamoeba keratitis in disposable contact lens wearers and all three were non-compliant. Disposability does not guarantee compliance.

Buehler *et al*. (1992) have drawn attention to the increased risk of ulcerative keratitis among disposable contact lens users. In their study they found that daily wear soft lens users had the lowest risk of developing ulcerative keratitis and they were assigned a risk of 1.0. Relative to this, users of gas permeable lenses had a risk of 1.3 and users of extended wear soft lenses a risk of 6.3. Disposable soft lens users had the highest risk of developing ulcerative keratitis. Their relative risk was 19.4.

Care of contact lens cases

Larkin, Kilvington and Easty (1990) have studied the contamination of contact lens storage cases by acanthamoebae and bacteria in 102 asymptomatic lens wearers. Cases were shaken and opened under aseptic conditions. All solution was transferred to a sterile universal container. A sterile cotton-wool swab, moistened with sterile unpreserved saline, was then rubbed over the internal surface of the case and the tip added to the universal container. The contents of the container were then mixed in a vortex mixer for 10 seconds and divided for bacterial and amoebal studies. Forty three cases had significant counts of viable bacteria and only 40 cases had negligible counts. Seven had contamination by acanthamoebae, of whom six also had significant bacterial counts. They found that contamination by *Serratia marcescens*, a recognized corneal pathogen, was significantly associated with chlorhexidine disinfection and in this context the paper by Marrie and Costerton (1981), quoted earlier in this chapter, is pertinent.

Larkin, Kilvington and Easty (1990) found contamination in the cases of patients using all disinfection methods and solutions. Similar bacteria contaminated hard and soft lens cases. The lower rate of bacterial contamination, which they found in soft lens cases, reflected the use of hydrogen peroxide or heat disinfection by 38 patients in this group. They found that these methods were more effective in reducing bacterial contamination. Acanthamoeba contamination in lens storage cases was more prevalent than expected and numerically significant bacterial contamination was found in to coexist in most instances. This suggested that bacteria may support acanthamoeba. These organisms feed on bacteria, or cell nuclei, and this may possibly enhance their virulence. Six of the seven patients from whose cases acanthamoeba was isolated complied with lens hygiene instructions; only one patient prepared 'home-made' saline solutions. None of these seven patients used chlorhexidine or hydrogen peroxide.

Guidelines have not been established for the care of contact lens cases. Strong disinfectants, which are commercially available for domestic use, are not advised, first because of the possibility of catastrophic accidents when they come in contact with the eye and, secondly, because small residual amounts, left after their use, may cause problems. The author has seen such problems.

Scrubbing with soap and water, or water alone, cannot be advised because the scrubbing brush could be a source of contamination and tap water is a source of acanthamoeba. Dr David Seal (personal communication) has found that bathroom tap water coming from a storage tank is much more offensive in this respect than mains water coming from the tap in the kitchen.

The problem with contact lens cases is not so much the container for the fluid, but inaccessible areas such as a catalytic disc, the inside of the screw top and its soft plastic insert.

It would be too expensive to soak the case in the hydrogen peroxide of the contact lens disinfecting system, but ordinary 3% hydrogen peroxide, obtainable from a chemist, is a possibility for disinfecting the case prior to the use of a proprietary disinfecting system.

Microwave disinfection is another possibility and this could be done after the case was scrubbed in tap water. This could be part of an evening routine before the lenses were removed and put into the case for disinfection. Boiling the case would be simpler, but compliance with this instruction would be poor. Much more research has to be done on this subject.

Dr David Seal (personal communication) has pointed out that Gram-negative bacilli (e.g. coliforms and *Ps. aeruginosa*) do not survive in dry conditions and he suggests that the case be dried thoroughly with a disposable paper towel after the lenses have been inserted in the morning.

Frequent renewal of the contact lens case is desirable. Perhaps we need daily disposable cases.

Contact lenses and corneal infections

There has been an alarming increase in reports of serious contact lens-related infections (Krachmer and Purcell, 1978; Galentine *et al.*, 1984; Alfonso *et al.*, 1986; Ormerod and Smith, 1986). In this last report from a major referral centre 70% of all recently infected corneal ulcers occurred in contact lens wearers. The major risk would appear to be that of corneal inoculation with available biofilm coated microorganisms from the contact lens surface. Corneal defences are perhaps weakened by the fact that lens wear affects corneal physiology. All contact lenses lead to some relative oxygen deprivation of the cornea. Extended wear exacerbates this problem since the cornea has to rely on oxygen from the conjunctival capillaries during sleep. Aswad, Barza and Baum (1989) have shown, on the basis of findings in an experimental model (the rabbit), that extended eyelid closure is a risk factor for pseudomonas keratitis.

There are other possible factors such as changes in pH, temperature, blink rate and tear composition. Acute and chronic changes in the corneal surface are seen with lens use (Barr and Schlossler, 1980; Schlossler and Woloschak, 1981; Bergmanson and Chu, 1982). Hyndiuk (1981) has drawn attention to microscopic breaks in the corneal surface epithelium that occur with lens wear. These may act as avenues for the inoculation of microorganisms.

Hamano *et al.* (1985), in a study of 66 000 patients followed up for one year, noted that the corneal ulcer rates were 3.2 per 10 000 patient-years for daily wear soft contact lens wearers and 3.0 per 10 000 patient-years for daily wear rigid gas permeable lens wearers.

MacRae *et al.* (1991) analysed clinical data on 22 739 contact lens wearers who were studied and whose lenses were approved under 48 manufacturer-sponsored studies for the Food and Drug Administration between 1980 and 1988. They found that the incidence of corneal ulcers was one in 1923 patient-years in the daily wear soft contact lens group and one in 1471 patient-years in the daily wear rigid gas permeable group.

Poggio *et al.* (1989) conducted a prospective study in five New England states to estimate the incidence of ulcerative keratitis among those who use cosmetic extended wear and daily wear soft contact lenses. To obtain a numerator for each estimate of incidence, they surveyed all practising ophthalmologists in the study area to identify all new cases diagnosed over a four-month study period. To provide the denominator they conducted a survey of 4178 households to estimate the number of persons who wore each type of contact lens.

The annualized incidence of ulcerative keratitis was estimated to be 20.9 per 10 000 persons (0.21%) using extended wear soft contact lenses for cosmetic purposes and 4.1 per 10 000 persons (0.04%) using daily wear soft contact lenses. The annualized incidence in hard contact lens wearers was 2.0 per 10 000 wearers (0.04%) and in rigid gas permeable lenses, 4 per 10 000 wearers (0.08%). Neither the figures for hard contact lens wearers nor those for rigid gas permeable wearers were significantly different from the incidence for soft daily wear lenses. Female users of daily wear lenses had an estimated incidence of 3.1 per 10 000 and male users an estimated incidence of 6.1 per 10 000 – a difference which was statistically significant. The estimated incidences for extended wear users, between male and female, was not significant.

Schein *et al*. (1989), in a companion study, carried out in six major eye centres around the country, found that 38% of those who used extended wear lenses wore them only during the day and 11% of those who used daily wear lenses wore them overnight, at least occasionally. Thus the relative risk of ulcerative keratitis changes considerably when actual overnight use is taken into account. Poggio *et al*. (1989) estimate the risk of extended wear, taking this factor into account, to be 2 to 3 per 10 000 for daily wear (0.02–0.03%) and 22 to 32 per 10 000 for extended wear lenses (0.22–0.32%).

The risk for overnight wear is then 10 times to 15 times as great for extended wear and, for users of daily wear lenses who sometimes wear them overnight, nine times the risk for users of such lenses who did not (Schein *et al*., 1989). In this latter study smokers were estimated to have about three times the risk of non-smokers.

Glynn *et al*. (1991), in a prospective study, evaluated the incidence of ulcerative keratitis among aphakic contact lens wearers in New England. Six hundred and twelve ophthalmologists participated in the study over a period of four months. The estimated annual incidence

rates were 181 and 25.9 cases per 10 000 wearers for extended and daily wear, respectively. Aphakic extended wear patients are seven times more likely to have ulcerative keratitis than their daily wear counterparts. Compared to cosmetic wearers of the same type, aphakic extended wear and daily wear users are 8.7 and 6.3 times more likely to have ulcerative keratitis.

Dart, Stapleton and Minassian (1991) have done a case-control study of 91 cases of keratitis seen at Moorfields Eye Hospital; included were 60 contact lens users. Relative risks and population attributable risk percentages for keratitis were estimated for different causes and for the different types of contact lenses. The relative risk for overnight wear soft lenses was found to be 21, for daily wear soft lenses 3.6 and for polymethylmethacrylate hard lenses 1.3, compared with gas permeable hard lenses.

MacRae *et al*. (1991), when analysing premarket studies performed for the Food and Drug Administration, found that aphakic extended wear soft lens users were nine times more likely to develop a corneal ulcer when compared to the soft daily wear cosmetic users.

Currently available care systems disinfect or pasteurize contact lenses but they rarely sterilize them. What is missing is hard data on the effectiveness of these systems, both in the laboratory and properly used in the home situation.

Manufacturers do not appear to have to state against which organisms their products are effective. Their submissions to the regulating authorities in the UK are confidential and ophthalmologists who are members of advisory committees are not allowed to study the manufacturers' submissions, except within the committee chamber.

Ophthalmologists and opticians, who have to recommend these solutions, cannot even check the methodology by which the manufacturers' conclusions were reached. It is left to a very small body of interested workers, outside the commercial field, to write papers and dispute the effectivity of various systems.

A further problem arises, since the bacterial pathogens are firmly adherent to an inert surface, is that bacterial cells recovered by routine sampling procedures (e.g. swabbing) may not include all or any of the representatives of the bacteria adherent to contact lenses and contact lens cases after exposure to commercial sterilizing systems. It is these bacteria rather than the bacteria in the surrounding solution that are important. The type of mistake that can be made is illustrated by the fact that for years *Streptococcus mutans* was believed to predominate in dental plaque because it was the organism most often recovered and cultured by routine methods. Now careful direct sampling of the plaque has shown that *Strep. mutans* is only a minor component of that typical biofilm population.

Many solutions on the market were approved long before the importance of biofilm was recognized only a few years ago.

The contact lens wearing public should be made aware that there is a certain risk in wearing contact lenses just as there is in many human preoccupations such as crossing the road or driving a car. Adequate precautions should be taken and these precautions include the prompt assessment of an uncomfortable or painful eye by a doctor of medicine with ophthalmological training without delay (see Chapter 13 on suppurative keratitis). If the eye is painful, it is not conjunctivitis!

References

ALFONSO, E., MANDELBAUM, S., FOX, M.J. *et al.* (1986) Ulcerative keratitis associated with contact lens wear. *American Journal of Ophthalmology*, **101**, 429–433

ASWAD, M.I., BARZA, M. and BAUM, J. (1989) Effect of lid closure on contact lens-associated Pseudomonas keratitis. *Archives of Ophthalmology*, **107** 1667–1670

BARR, J.T. and SCHLOSSLER, J.P. (1980) Corneal endothelial response to rigid contact lenses. *American Journal of Optometry and Physiological Optics*, **57**, 267–272

BEEKHUIS, W.H., EGGINK, F.A.G.J., VREUGDENHIL, W., PLATENKANP, G. and BUITENWERF, J. (1992) Disinfection of trial mid water content soft contact lenses in the practice: the efficacy of sodium dichloroisocyanurate. *Journal of the British Contact Lens Association*, **15**, 3, 103–107

BEGLEY, C.G. and WAGGONER, P.J. (1991) An analysis of nodular deposits on soft contact lenses. *Journal of the American Optometric Association*, **62**, 3, 208–214

BERGMANSON, J.P.G. and CHU, L. (1982) Corneal response to rigid contact lens wear. *British Journal of Ophthalmology*, **66**, 667–675

BERNSTEIN, H.N. (1973) Fungal growth into a Bionite hydrophilic contact lens. *Annals of Ophthalmology*, **5**, 317–322

BERNSTEIN, H.N., STOW, M.N. and MADDOX, Y. (1973) Evaluation of the 'Aseptization' procedure for the Softlens hydrophilic contact lens. *Canadian Journal of Ophthalmology*, **8**, 575–576

BILBAUT, T., GACHON, A.M. and DASTUGUE, B. (1986) Deposits on soft contact lenses. Electrophoresis and scanning electron microscopic examinations. *Experimental Eye Research*, **43**, 153–165

BOWDEN, F.W., COHEN, E.J., ARENTSEN, J.J. and LAIBSON, P.R. (1989) Patterns of lens care practices and lens product contamination in contact lens associated microbial keratitis. *CLAO Journal*, **15**, 1, 49–54

BRANDT, F.H., WARE, D.A. and VISVESVARA, G.S. (1989) Viability of Acanthamoeba cysts in ophthalmic solutions. *Applied and Environmental Microbiology*, **55**, 5, 1144–1146

BROWNE, R.K., ANDERSON, A.N. and CHARVEZ, B.W. (1974) Solving the solution problem. *The Optician*, **167**, 19–24

BROWNE, R.K., ANDERSON, A.N. and CHARVEZ, B.W. (1975) Ophthalmic response to chlorhexidine digluconate in rabbits. *Toxicology and Applied Pharmacology*, **32**, 3, 621–627

BUEHLER, P.O., SCHEIN, O.D., STAMLER, E.F. and VERDIER, D.V. (1992) The increased risk of ulcerative keratitis among disposable contact lens users. *Investigative Ophthalmology and Visual Science*, **33**, 1209

BUSSCHAERT, S.C., GOOD, R.C. and SZABOCSIK, J. (1978) Evaluation of thermal disinfection procedures for hydrophilic contact lenses. *Applied and Environmental Microbiology*, **35**, 618–621

BUTRUS, S.I., KLOTZ, S.A., CHARLOTTESVILLE, V.A. and SHREVEPORT, L.A. (1990) Contact lens surface deposits increase the adhesion of *Pseudomonas aeruginosa*. *Current Eye Research*, **9**, 8, 717–724

CALLENDER, M. (1978) A comparison of soflens (polymacon) wearer sensitivity to thermal or cold disinfecting systems. *Contact Lens Journal*, **7**, 2–6

CASTILLO, E.J., KOENIG, J.L., ANDERSON, J.M. and LO, J. (1985) Protein adsorption on hydrogels. II. Reversible and irreversible interactions between lysozyme and soft contact lens surfaces – methacrylic acid. *Biomaterials*, **6**, 338–345

CASTILLO, E.J., KOENIG, J.L., ANDERSON, J.M. and JENTOFT, N. (1986) Protein adsorption on soft contact lenses III Mucin. *Biomaterials*, **7**, 9–16

C.D.C. (1986) Acanthamoeba keratitis associated with contact lenses. *Morbidity, Mortality Weekly Report*, **35**, 405–408

CHAPMAN, J.M., CHEEKS, L. and GREEN, K. (1990) Interactions of benzalkonium chloride with soft and hard contact lenses. *Archives of Ophthalmology*, **108**, 2, 244–246

CONNOR, C.G., BLOCKER, Y. and PITTS, D.G. (1989) The disinfection of Acanthamoeba cysts. *Investigative Ophthalmology and Visual Science*, **30**, 3 (Suppl.), 41

COPLEY, C.A. (1989) Chlorine disinfection of soft contact lenses. *Clinical and Experimental Optometry*, **72**, 1, 3–7

COSTERTON, J.W., IRVIN, R.T. and CHENG, K.J. (1981a) The bacterial glycocalyx in nature and disease. *Annual Review of Microbiology*, **35**, 299–324

DART, J.K.G. and BADENOCH, P.R. (1986) Bacterial adherence to contact lenses. *The CLAO Journal*, **12**, 4, 220–224

DART, J.K.G. and SEAL, D.V. (1988) Pathogenesis and therapy of *Pseudomonas aeruginosa* keratitis. *Eye*, **2** (Suppl.), S46–S55

DART, J.K.G., STAPLETON, F. and MINASSIAN, D. (1991) Contact lenses and other risk factors in microbial keratitis. *Lancet*, **ii**, 650–653

DAVIES, D.J.G. (1978) Antimicrobial agents as preservatives in pharmaceutical and cosmetic products. Agents as preservatives in eye drops and contact lens solutions. *Journal of Applied Bacteriology*, **44**, 3 (Suppl.), 19–28

DAVIES, D.J.G., ANTHONY, Y., MEAKIN, B.J., KILVINGTON, S. and WHITE, D. (1988) Anti-acanthamoeba activity of cholorhexidine and hydrogen peroxide. *Transactions of BCLA International Contact Lens Congress*, London, May, 1988. *BCLA Journal*, **5**, 60–62

DERNSTEIN, D.I., GALLACHER, J.S., SNAD, M. and DERNSTEIN, I.L. (1984) Local ocular anaphylaxis to papain enzyme contained in a contact lens cleansing solution. *Journal of Allergy and Clinical Immunology*, **74**, 3, 250–260

DOLMAN, P.J. and DOBROGOWSKI, M.J. (1989) Contact lens disinfection by ultraviolet light. *American Journal of Ophthalmology*, **108**, 665–669

DONZIS, P.B., MONDINO, B.J. and WEISSMAN, B.A. (1988) Bacillus keratitis associated with contaminated contact lens care systems. *American Journal of Ophthalmology*, **105**, 195–197

DONZIS, P.B., MONDINO, B.J., WEISSMAN, B.A. and BRUCKNER, D.A. (1987) Microbial contamination of contact lens care systems. *American Journal of Ophthalmology*, **104**, 4, 325–333

DONZIS, P.B., MONDINO, B.J., WEISSMAN, B.A. and BRUCKNER, D.A. (1989) Microbial analysis of contact lens care systems contaminated with acanthamoeba. *American Journal of Ophthalmology*, **108**, 53–56

DUNN, J.P., MONDINO, B.J., WEISSMAN, B.A., DONZIS, P.B and KIKKAWA, D.Ø. (1989) Corneal ulcers associated with disposable contact lenses. *American Journal of Ophthalmology*, **108**, 113–117

DURAN, J.A., REFOJO, M.F., GIPSON, I.K. and KENYON, K.R. (1987) Pseudomonas attachment to new hydrogel contact lenses. *Archives of Ophthalmology*, **105**, 106–109

FERREIRA, J.T., KRIEL, F., VAN DER MERWE, D. and PHEIFFER, G. (1991) Efficacy of chlorine disinfection of soft contact lenses. *Optometry and Visual Science*, **68**, 9, 718–720

FICKER, L., HUNTER, P., SEAL, D.V. and WRIGHT, P. (1989) Acanthamoeba keratitis with disposable contact lens wear. *American Journal of Ophthalmology*, **108**, 4, 453

FILIPI, J.A., PFISTER, R.M. and HILL, R.M. (1973) Penetration of hydrophilic contact lenses by *Aspergillus fumigatus*. *American Journal of Optometry*, **50**, 7, 553–557

FOWLER, S.A. and ALLANSMITH, M.R. (1981) The effect of cleaning soft contact lenses. A scanning electron microscopic study. *Archives of Ophthalmology*, **99**, 1382–1386

FOWLER, S.A., GREINER, J.V. and ALLANSMITH, M.A. (1979a) Attachment of bacteria to soft contact lenses. *Archives of Ophthalmology*, **97**, 659–660

FOWLER, S.A., GREINER, J.V. and ALLANSMITH, M.A. (1979b) Soft contact lenses from patients with giant papillary conjunctivitis. *American Journal of Ophthalmology*, **88**, 1056–1061

FOWLER, S.A., KORB, D.R. and ALLANSMITH, M.R. (1985) Deposits on soft contact lenses of various water contents. *CLAO Journal*, **11**, 124–127

FUJIKAWA, L.S., PALESTINE, A.G., NUSSENBLATT, R.B., SALA-HUDDIN, S.Z., MASUR, H. and GALLO, R.C. (1985) Isolation of human T-lymphocyte virus type III from the tears of a patient acquired immunodeficiency syndrome. *Lancet*, **ii**, 529–530

GACHON, A.M., BILBAUT, T. and DASTUGUE, B. (1985) Adsorption of tear proteins on soft contact lenses. *Experimental Eye Research*, **40**, 105–116

GALENTINE, P.G., COHEN, E.J., LAIBSON, P.R. *et al*. (1984) Corneal ulcers associated with contact lens wear. *Archives of Ophthalmology*, **102**, 891–894

GHAJAR, M., HOULSBY, R.D. and CHAVEZ, G. (1989) Microbiological evaluation of Miraflow. *Journal of the American Optometric Association*, **60**, 8, 592–595

GLYNN, R.J., SCHEIN, O.D., SEDDON, J.M. *et al*. (1991) The incidence of ulcerative keratitis among aphakic contact lens wearers in New England. *Archives of Ophthalmology*, **109**, 1, 104–107

GREEN, K., LIVINGSTONE, V., BOWMAN, K. and HULL, D.S. (1980) Chlorhexidine effects on corneal epithelium and endothelium. *Archives of Ophthalmology*, **98**, 7, 1273–1278

GREEN, K. and TONJUM, A.M. (1971) Influence of various agents on corneal permeability. *American Journal of Ophthalmology*, **72**, 897–905

GRIFFITHS, F.G., ELLIOT, T.S.J. and MCTAGGART, L. (1989) Adherence of *Staphylococcus epidermidis* to intraocular lenses. *British Journal of Ophthalmology*, **73**, 402–406

GRISTINA, A.G., OGA, M., WEBB, L.X. *et al*. (1985) Adherent bacterial colonization in the pathogenisis of osteomyelitis. *Science*, **228**, 990–993

GRUBER, E. (1981) Hot or cold care systems for hydrophilic lenses. *Contact Lens Intraocular Lens Medical Journal*, **7**, 339–340

GUDMUNDSSON, O.G., WOODWARD, D.F., FOWLER, S.A. *et al*. (1985) Identification of proteins in contact lens surface deposits by immunofluorescence microscopy. *Archives of Ophthalmology*, **103**, 196–197

HAMANO, H., KITANO, J., MITSUNAGA, S., KOJIMA, S. and KISSLING, G.E. (1985) Adverse effects of contact lens wear in a large Japanese population. *CLAO Journal*, **11**, 141

HANSON, P.J.V., GOR, D., JEFFRIES, D.J. and COLLINS, J.V. (1989) Chemical inactivation of HIV on surfaces. *British Medical Journal*, **298**, 862–864

HARF, C. (1991) Efficacy of contact lens disinfecting solutions for prevention of Acanthamoeba keratitis. *Reviews of Infectious Diseases*, **13** (Suppl. 5), S413

HARRIS, M.G., KIRBY, J.E., TORNATORE, C.W. and WRIGHT-NOUR, J.A. (1989) Microwave disinfection of soft contact lenses. *Optometry and Visual Science*, **66**, 2, 82–86

HARRIS, M.G., RECHBURGER, J., GRANT, T. and HOLDEN, B.A. (1990) In-office microwave disinfection of soft contact lenses. *Optometry and Visual Science*, **67**, 2, 129–132

HATHAWAY, R.A. and LOWTHER, G.E. (1978) Soft lens cleaners: their effectiveness in removing deposits. *Journal of the American Optometric Association*, **49**, 259–226

HEIDEMANN, D.G., VERDIER, D.D., DUNN, S.P. and STAMLER, J.F. (1990) Acanthamoeba keratitis associated with disposable contact lenses. *American Journal of Ophthalmology*, **110**, 630–634

HOLLAND, S.P., MILLER, D., CHUANG, E. *et al*. (1989) Biofilm. A method of bacterial survival in contaminated topical medications associated with ocular infections. *Investigative Ophthalmology and Visual Science*, **30**, 3, (Suppl.), Abstract 36, 503

HOLLY, F.J. (1979) Protein and lipid adsorption by acrylic hydrogels and their relation to water wettability. *Journal of Polymer Science*, **66**, 409–417

HVDING, G. (1981) The conjunctival and contact lens bacterial flora during lens wear. *Acta Ophthalmologica (Copenhagen)*, **59**, 387–401

HYNDIUK, R.A. (1981) Experimental Psuedomonas keratitis. *Transactions of the American Ophthalmological Society*, **79**, 541–546

JANOFF, L.E. (1979) The effective disinfection of soft contact lenses using hydrogen peroxide. *Contacto*, **23**, 1, 37–40

JOHN, T., DESAL, D. and SAHM, D. (1989) Adherence of *Acanthamoeba castellani* cysts and trophozoites to hydrogel contact lenses. *Invest. Ophthalmology and Visual Science*, **30**, 3 (Suppl.), Abstract 8, 480

KARAGEOGIAN, H.L. (1976) Use of amino acid analyser to illustrate the efficacy of an enzyme preparation for cleaning hydrophilic lenses. *Contacto*, **20**, 5–10

KERR, C. (1982) Solutions? The case for hydrogen peroxide. *Optician*, **184**, 14–16

KERR, C. (1985) Contact Lens Monthly. *Optician*, 1 February, 14

KESSLER, A.I., NIRANKARI, Y.S., TITTEL, P.G. and RICHARDS, R.D. (1989) An ultraviolet light disinfection device for hydrophilic contact lenses: efficacy against multiple bacterial pathogens. *Investigative Ophthalmology and Visual Science*, **30**, 3 (Suppl.), Abstract 13, 481

KILLINGSWORTH, D.W. and STERN, G.A. (1989) Pseudomonas keratitis asssociated with the use of disposable contact lenses. *Archives of Ophthalmology*, **107**, 795–796

KILVINGTON, S. (1989) Moist-heat disinfection of pathogenic Acanthamoeba cysts. Letters. *Applied Microbiology*, **9**, 187–189

KILVINGTON, S. and LARKIN, D.F.P. (1990) Acanthamoeba adherence to contact lenses and removal by cleaning agents. *Eye*, **4**, 4, 589–593

KILVINGTON, S. and SCANLON, P. (1991) Efficacy of an ultraviolet light contact lens disinfection unit against Acanthamoeba keratitis isolates. *Journal of the British Contact Lens Association*, **14**, 1, 9–11

KLOTZ, S.A., BUTRUS, S.I., MISRA, R.P. and OSATO, M.S. (1989) The contribution of bacterial surface hydrophobicity to the process of adherence of *Pseudomonas aeruginosa* to hydrophilic contact lenses. *Current Eye Research*, **8**, 2, 195–202

KRACHMER, J.H. and PURCELL, J.J., JR (1978) Bacterial corneal ulcers in cosmetic contact lens wearers. *Archives of Ophthalmology*, **96**, 57–61

LACHMAN, L. (1968) Antioxidants and chelating agents as stabilisers in liquid dosage forms. *Drugs and Cosmetic Industry*, **102**, 36–148, 43–149

LARKIN, D.F.P., KILVINGTON, S. and EASTY, D.L. (1990) Contamination of contact lens storage cases by Acanthamoeba and bacteria. *British Journal of Ophthalmology*, **74**, 133–135

LEAHY, C.D., MANDELL, R.B. and LIN, S.T. (1989) Do disposable lenses solve the problems of extended wear? *Contact Lens Spectrum*, **4**, 4, 25–28

LEVY, B. (1984) Calcium deposits on glyceryl methyl methacrylate and hydroxyethyl methacrylate contact lenses. *American Journal of Optometry and Physiological Optics*, **61**, 9, 605–607

LINDQUIST, T.D., DOUGHMAN, D.T., RUBENSTEIN, B. and MOORE, J.W. (1987) Acanthamoeba infected hydrogel contact lenses: susceptibility to disinfection. ARVO Abstracts. *Investigative Ophthalmology and Visual Science*, **28** (Suppl.), 371

LINDQUIST, T.D., DOUGHMAN, D.T., RUBENSTEIN, B., MOORE, J.W. and CAMPBELL, R.C. (1988) Acanthamoeba-contaminated hydrogel contact lenses; susceptibility to disinfection. *Cornea*, **7**, 4, 300–303

LIUBINAS, J., SWENSON, G. and CARNEY, L.G. (1987) Thermal disinfection of contact lenses. *Clinical and Experimental Optometry*, **70**, 1, 8–14

LJUNNGGREN, B. and MOLLER, H. (1972) Eczematous contact allergy to chlorhexidine. *Acta Dermato-Venereologica*, **52**, 308–310

LOPEZ, A., CALLEJA, M. and CLARAMONTE, P. (1992) Effect of non-oxidising contact lens disinfection systems on *Acanthamoeba culbertsoni*. *Contactalogia*, **14**, 2, 68–73

LOWE, R., VALLAS, V. and BRENNAN, N. (1992) Comparative efficacy of contact lens solutions. *CLAO Journal*, **18**, 1, 34–40

LOWTHER, G.E. (1991) Evaluation of disposable lens edges. *Contact Lens Spectrum*, **6**, 1, 41–43

LUDWIG, I.H., MEISLER, D.M. RUTHERFORD, I., BICAN, F.E., LANGSTON, R.H.S. and VISVESVARA, G.S. (1986) Susceptibility of Acanthamoeba to soft contact lens disinfection systems. *Investigative Ophthalmology and Visual Science*, **27**, 626–628

LYONS, R.W. (1979) Orange contact lenses from rifampicin. *New England Journal of Medicine*, **300**, 372–373

MACRAE, S., HERMAN, C., STULTING, D. *et al*. (1991) Corneal ulcer and adverse reaction rates in premarket contact lens studies. *American Journal of Ophthalmology*, **111**, 457–465

MARRIE, T.J. and COSTERTON, J.W. (1981) Prolonged survival of *Serratia marcescens* in chlorhexidine. *Applied and Environmental Microbiology*, **42**, 1093–1102

MARTIN, L.S., MCDOUGAL, J.S. and LOSKOSKI, S.L. (1985) Disinfection and inactivation of the human T-lymphotrophic virus type III/lymphadenopathy – associated virus. *Journal of Infectious Diseases*, **152**, 400–403

MILLER, D., BROOKS, S.M. and MOBILIA, E. (1976) Adenochrome staining of soft contact lenses. *Annals of Ophthalmology*, **8**, 65–67

MILLER, D., HOLLAND, S.P., SONG, D., ALFONSO, E., COSTERTON, J.W. and RUSESKA, I. (1989) Role of glycocalyx (biofilm) in persistent and recurrent *Pseudomonas aeruginosa* ocular infections. *Investigative Ophthalmology and Visual Science*, **30**, 3 (Suppl.), Abstract 92, 196

MINARIK, A.V. and RAPP, J. (1989) Protein deposits on individual hydrophilic contact lenses: effects of water and ionicity. *CLAO Journal*, **15**, 3, 185–188

MOORE, M.B. (1988) Editorial: Acanthamoeba keratitis. *Archives of Ophthalmology*, **106**, 1181–1183

MOORE, M.B., MCCULLEY, J.P., NEWTON, C. *et al*. (1987) Acanthamoeba keratitis: a growing problem in soft and hard contact lens wearers. *Ophthalmology*, **94**, 12, 1654–1661

NICASTRO, J.F., SHOJI, H., ROVERE, G.D. *et al*. (1975) Effects of methylmethacrylate on *S. aureus* growth and rabbit alveolar macrophage phagocytosis and glucose metabolism. *Surgery Forum*, **26**, 501–503

ORMEROD, L.D. and SMITH, R.E. (1986) Contact lens associated microbial keratitis. *Archives of Ophthalmology*, **104**, 79–83

PALMER, W., SCANLON, P. and MCNULTY, C. (1991) Efficacy of an ultraviolet light contact lens disinfection unit against microbial pathogenic organisms. *Journal of the British Contact Lens Association*, **14**, 1, 13–16

PAUGH, J.R., BRENNAN, N.A. and EFRON, N. (1988) Ocular response to hydrogen peroxide. *American Journal of Optometry and Physiological Optics*, **65**, 91–98

PENLEY, C.A., LLABRES, C., WILSON, L. and AHEARN, D. (1985) Efficacy of hydrogen peroxide disinfection systems for soft contact lenses contaminated with fungi. *CLAO Journal*, **11**, 65–68

PENLEY, C.A., WILLIS, S.W. and SICKLER, S.G. (1989) Comparative antimicrobial efficacy of soft and rigid gas permeable contact lens solutions against acanthamoeba. *CLAO Journal*, **15**, 4, 257–260

PHILLIPS, A.J., BADENOCH, P. and COPLEY, C. (1989) Ultrasound cleaning and disinfection of contact lenses: a preliminary report. Transactions of *BCLA Conference*, Birmingham, 1989, no. 6, 20–23

PHINNEY, R.B., MONDINO, B.J., HOFBAUER, J.D. *et al*. (1988) Corneal ŏedema related to accidental Hibiclens exposure. *American Journal of Ophthalmology*, **106**, 210–215

PITTS, R. and KRACHMER, J. (1979) Evaluation of soft contact lens disinfection in the home environment. *Archives of Ophthalmology*, **97**, 470–472

PLAUT, B.S., MEAKIN, B.J. and DAVIES, D.J.G. (1980) On the anomalous sorption behaviour of chlorhexidine with poly (2 hydroxyethyl methacrylate). *Journal of Pharmacy and Pharmacology*, **32**, 525–532

POGGIO, E.C., GLYNN, R.J., SCHEIN, O.D. *et al*. (1989) The incidence of ulcerative keratitis among users of daily wear and extended wear soft contact lenses. *New England Journal of Medicine*, **321**, 12, 779–783

RABINOWITZ, S.M., PFLUGFELDER, S.C. and GOLDBERG, M. (1989) Disposable extended-wear contact lens-related keratitis. *Archives of Ophthalmology*, **107**, 1121

REFOJO, M.F., MILLER, D. and FIORE, A.S. (1972) A new fluorescent stain for soft hydrophilic lens fitting. *Archives of Ophthalmology*, **87**, 275–277

REFOJO, M.F. and LEONG, F. (1979) Microscopic determination of the penetration of proteins and polysaccharides into poly (hydroxyethyl methacrylate) and similar hydrogels. *Journal of Polymer Science: Polymer Symposium*, **66**, 227–237

REICHERT, R.W., DAS, N.E. and ZAM, Z.S. (1983) Adherence properties of Pseudomonas pili to epithelial cells of the human cornea. *Current Eye Research*, **2**, 289–293

RICHARDSON, N.E., DAVIES, D.J.G., MEAKIN, B.J. and NORTON, D.A. (1977) Loss of antibacterial preservatives from contact lens solutions during storage. *Journal of Pharmacy and Pharmacology*, **29**, 717–722

RILEY, S.A., FLEGG, P.J. and MANDAL, B.K. (1986) Contact lens staining due to sulphasalazine. *Lancet*, i, 972

RIORDAN-EVA, P., EYKYN, S.J. and KERR-MUIR, M.G. (1988) *Pseudomonas aeruginosa* corneal ulcer associated with an aerosol can of preservative-free saline. Case report. *Archives of Ophthalmology*, **106**, 11, 1506

ROHRER, M.D. and BULARD, R.A. (1985) Microwave sterilisation. *Journal of the American Dental Association*, **110**, 194–198

ROHRER, M.D., TERRY, M.A., BULARD, R.A., GRAVES, D.C. and TAYLOR, E.M. (1986) Microwave sterilisation of hydrophilic contact lenses. *American Journal of Ophthalmology*, **101**, 49–57

ROSENTHAL, P.R., CHOU, M.H., SALAMONI, J.C. and ISRAEL, S.C. (1986) Quantative analysis of chlorhexidine gluconate and benzalkonium chloride adsorption on silicone/acrylate polymers. *CLAO Journal*, **12**, 1, 43–50

ROSENTHAL, R.A., SCHLITZER, R.L., MCNAMEE, L.S., DASSANAYAKE, N.L. and AMASS, R. (1992) Antimicrobial activity of organic chlorine releasing compounds. *Journal of the British Contact Lens Association*, **15**, 2, 81–84

RUBEN, M., TRIPATHI, R.C. and WINDER, A.F. (1975) Calcium deposition as a cause of spoilation of hydrophilic soft contact lenses. *British Journal of Ophthalmology*, **59**, 141–148

RUSESKA, I., ROBBINS, J. and COSTERTON, J.W. (1982) Biocide testing against corrosion-causing oilfield bacteria helps control plugging. *Oil and Gas Journal*, 8 March, 253–264

SACK, R.A., JONES, B., ANTIGNANI, A. *et al*. (1987) Specificity and biological activity of the protein deposited on of the hydrogel surface. *Investigative Ophthalmology and Visual Science*, **28**, 842–849

SACK, R.A., HARVEY H. and NUNES, I. (1989) Disinfection associated spoilage of high water content, ionic matrix hydrogels. *CLAO Journal*, **15**, 2, 138–145

SCANLON, P. (1991) Presidential address to British Contact Lens Society, 1990, Microbiological aspects of combined ultrasonic contact lens disinfection units. *Journal of the British Contact Lens Association*, **14**, 2, 55–59

SCHEIN, O.D., GLYNN, R.J., POGGIO, E.C., SEDDON, J.M., KENYON, K.R. and the Microbial Keratitis Study Group. (1989) The relative risk of ulcerative keratitis among users of daily wear and extended wear soft contact lenses. *New England Journal of Medicine*, **321**, 12, 773–778

SCHLOSSLER, J.P. and WOLOSCHAK, M.J. (1981) Corneal endothelium in veteran PMMA contact lens wearers. *International Contact Lens Clinic*, **8**, 19–22

SCHUNK, T. and SCHWEISFURTH, R. (1989) Desinfektionsleistung oxidierender Hygeinesysteme bei organische Belastung auf Kontaktlinsen. *Contactologia*, **11**, 90–95

SCHWARZMANN, S. and BORING, J.R., III. (1971) Antiphagocytic effect of slime from a mucoid strain of *Pseudomonas aeruginosa*. *Infection and Immunity*, **3**, 762–767

SEGER, R.G., MAUGER, T.F. and HILL, R.M. (1981) Oxygen and the aging hydrogel. *International Contact Lens Clinic*, **8**, 15–18

SILVANY, R.E., WOOD, T.S., BOWMAN, R.W. and MCCULLEY, J.P. (1987) The effect of preservatives in contact lens solutions on two species of acanthamoeba. *ARVO Abstracts Investigative Ophthalmology and Visual Science*, **28** (Suppl.), 371

SLUSHER, M.M., MYRVIK, Q.N., LEWIS, J.C. and GRISTINA, A.G. (1987) Extended wear lenses, biofilm and bacterial adhesion. *Archives of Ophthalmology*, **105**, 110–115

SMOLIN, G., OKUMOTO, M. and NOZIK, R.A. (1979) The microbial flora in extended wear soft contact lens wearers. *American Journal of Ophthalmology*, **88**, 543–547

SUGAR, J. (1974) Adenochrome pigmentation of hydrophilic lenses. *Archives of Ophthalmology*, **91**, 11–12

STEHR-GREEN, J.K., BAILEY, T.M. and VISVESVARA, G.S. (1989) The epidemiology of acanthamoeba keratitis in the USA. *American Journal of Ophthalmology*, **107**, 331–336

STONE, R.P., MOWREY-MCKEE, M.F. and KREUTZER, P. (1984) Protein. A source of lens discolouration. *Contact Lens Forum*, **9**, 33–41

TAPASZTO, I., KOLLER, A., TAPASZTO, Z. and TAPASZTO, B. (1988/89) Biochemical changes in the human tears of hard and soft lens wearers. *Contact Lens Journal*, **16**, no. 9, 233–236; **16**, no. 10, 265–268; **17**, no. 1, 5–8; **2**, 37–40, **10**, 316–322

TERVO, T., LAHDEVIRTA, J., VAHERI, A., VALLE, S-L. and SUNI, J. (1986) Recovery of HTLV – III from contact lenses. *Lancet*, i, 379–380

TOLLEFSON, D.F., BANDYK, D.F., KAEBNICK, H.W., SEABROOK, G.R. and TOWNE, J.B. (1987) Surface biofilm disruption. *Archives of Surgery*, **122**, 38–43

TONJUM, A.M. (1975) Effects of benzalkonium chloride upon the corneal epithelium studied with scanning electron microscopy. *Acta Ophthalmologica*, **53**, 358–365

TRAGAKIS, M.P., BROWN, S.I. and PEARCE, D.B. (1973) Bacteriologic studies of contamination associated with soft contact lenses. *American Journal of Ophthalmology*, **75**, 496–499

TRIPATHI, B.J. and TRIPATHI, R.C. (1989) Hydrogen peroxide damage to human corneal epithelial cells in vitro. Implications for contact lens disinfection systems. *Archives of Ophthalmology*, **107**, 1516–1519

TURNER, F.J. (1983) Hydrogen peroxide and other oxidant disinfectants. In *Disinfection, Preservation and Sterilisation* (Block, S.S., ed.), 3rd edn. Lea and Febiger, Philadelphia, pp. 240–250

UNITED STATES CENTERS FOR DISEASE CONTROL (1985) Recommendations for preventing possible transmission of human T-lymphotrophic virus type III/lymphadenopathy associated virus from tears. *Morbidity and Mortality Weekly Report*, **34**, 533–534

VAPIDIS, G.C., MARSH, R.J. and STACEY, A.R. (1984) Bacterial contamination of intraocular lens surgery. *British Journal of Ophthalmology*, **68**, 8, 520–523

VOGT, M.W., NO, D.D., DAKAR, G.R., GILBARD, J.P., SCHOOLEY, R.T. and HIRSCH, M.S. (1986) Disinfection of contact lenses after contamination with HTLV III. *Ophthalmology*, **73**, 6, 771–774

WACLAWSKI, E.R., MCALPINE, L.G. and THOMPSON, N.C. (1989) Occupational asthma in nurses caused by chlorhexidine and alcohol aerosols. *British Medical Journal*, **298**, 929–930

WEDLER, F.C. (1977) Analysis of biomaterials deposited on soft contact lenses. *Journal of Biomedical Materials Research*, **11**, 525–535

WEDLER, F.C., ILLMAN, B.L., HORENSKY, D.S. *et al*. (1987) Analysis of protein and mucin components deposited on hydrophilic contact lenses. *Clinical and Experimental Optometry*, **70**, 59–68

WILSON, L.A. and AHEARN, D.G. (1986) Association of fungi with extended wear soft contact lenses. *American Journal of Ophthalmology*, **101**, 434–436

WILSON, L.A., SAWANT, A.D. and AHEARN, D.G. (1991) Comparative efficiencies of soft contact lens disinfectant solutions against microbial films in lens cases. *Archives of Ophthalmology*, **109**, 1155–1157

YOSHITOMO, J. and SHUZO, I. (1984) Studies on the interaction between contact lens and tear fluid (VIII). Phenomenon of human tear lysozyme and lactoferrin adsorption onto contact lens materials. *Journal of the Japanese Contact Lens Society*, **26**, 225–229

Appendix 9.I

Preparations for use with hard contact lenses

Alcon
Clens (C) BKC 0.02, Pliagel (C) Sorbic Acid 0.1, Soaclens (S/D) BKC 0.01.

Allergan
Clean-n-Soak (C & S/D) PMN 0.004, LC65 (C) THM 0.001 EDTA, Total (S/D & W) BKC 0.004 PVA 2.5, Liquifilm Wetting (W) BKC 0.004 PVA 2.0.

Barnes Hind
Cleaning and Soaking (C) BKC 0.01, Titan (C) BKC 0.02, Intensive Cleaner (C) THM 0.001, Soquette (S/D) BKC 0.01, Wetting and Soaking (S/D) BKC 0.005, Wetting (W) BKC 0.004, BKC 0.005, One Solution (C, W, S & D) BKC 0.01.

Bausch & Lomb
Bausch & Lomb cleaning (CHX), Bausch & Lomb Wetting & Soaking (CHX).

Boots
Cleaning, Soaking and Wetting CHX 0.06 BKC 0.004 EDTA 0.128.

CIBA Vision Contactasol
Contactaclean (C) Contactasoak (S) and Contactasol (W) all contain BKC 0.004, CHX 0.006 EDTA 0.128. 02 Care* (C) BKC 0.005 EDTA 0.12.
*Specifically for use with Menicon 02 gas permeable lenses.
Complete Care Solution (C, W, S & D) BKC 0.01, disodium edetate 0.06.

Polymer technology
The Boston Lens Cleaner (C), Boston Lens Wetting and Soaking Solution (S & D & W) CHX 0.006 EDTA 0.6.

Sauflon Pharmaceuticals
Stericlens (C & W) THM 0.004, EDTA 0.1, Sterisoak (S/D) BKC 0.002 CHB 0.4 EDTA 0.1.

Smith & Nephew
Transol (W), Transoak BKC 0.01 EDTA 0.2 and Transdrop (RW) BKC 0.004.

Key to use of preparations
(C) Cleaning; (S/D) soaking and disinfecting; (W) wetting; (RW) rewetting.

Key to antimicrobials
BKC: Benzalkonium chloride; CHX: chlorhexidine digluconate; THM: thiomersal (thimerosal); PVA: polyvinyl alcohol; CHB: chlorbutol; PMN: phenylmercuric nitrate; EDTA: sodium edetate.

Appendix 9.II

Ophthalmic preparations

Product	Manufacturer	Preservative
Acetylcysteine	M	BAC
Adrenaline neutral 0.1, 0.5, 1%	M	CHA
Albucid 10, 20 & 30%	NIC	SPC
Amechol (methacholine) 2.5%	M	PMN
Amethocaine 1%	M	PMA
Atropine 0.25 & 2.0%		
Atropine 1%	RID	BAC
B.J.6	THR	CHA
	MAC	CHD
Benoxinate 0.4%	M	CHA
Benoxinate & fluorescein	M	PMN
Betamethasone	RID	BAC
Betamethasone & neomycin	RID	THM

Carbachol (Isopto) 3%	ALC	BAC
Chloramphenicol	M	PMN
	M	THM
	SHP	PMN
Clobetasone	GLA	BAC
Cocaine 4%	M	CHA
	MAC	PMN
Cocaine & homatropine	MAC	CHA
Cyclopentolate 0.5% & 1%	M	BAC
Cyclopentolate (Mydrilate) 0.5% & 1%	WBP	BAC
Dendrid	ALC	BAC
Dexamethasone Soln. 0.1%	ALC	BAC
Dipivefrin (Propine)	ALC	BAC & EDTA
Disodium edetate (EDTA) 0.37%	M	THM
Eppy	S & N	PMA
Eserine 0.25 & 0.5%	M	BAC & SOM
Eumovate	GLA	BAC
Eumovate N	GLA	BAC
F3T (trifluorothymidine)	M	BAC
FML & FML-N	ALL	BAC
Fluometholone	ALL	BAC
Ganda 1 + 0.2, 3 + 0.5, 5 + 0.05 & 5 + 1	S & N	BAC
Gentamicin forte	M	THM
Genticin	KW	BAC
Glycerin 10, 30 & 50%	M	THM
Guanethidine (Ismelin 5%)	ZYM	BAC
Homatropine 1 & 2%	KW	BAC
Homatropine 1%	KW	BAC
Hydrocortisone 1% & w.neomycin	RID	PMN
Hyoscine 0.25 & 0.5%	M	CHA
Hyoscine 0.25%	RID	BAC
Hypromellose	EVA	BAC
Hypromellose	SHP	BAC
Hypromellose	M	BAC
Hypromellose (alkaline)	M	BAC
Kerecid (IDU 0.1%)	ALL	BAC
IDU 0.1%	M	BAC
Ismelin 5% (guanethidine)	ZYM	BAC
Isopto alkaline	ALC	BAC
Isopto carpine 0.5, 1, 2, 3 & 4%	ALC	BAC
Isopto epinal 0.5 & 1%	ALC	BAC
Isopto frin	ALC	BAC
Isopto plain	ALC	BAC
Lachesine 1%	M	PMN
Liquifilm tears	ALL	BAC

Maxidex	ALC	BAC
Maxitrol	ALC	BAC
Methicillin	M	PMN
Methylcellulose 1%	M	PMN
Mydriacyl 0.5 & 1%	ALC	BAC
Mydrilate 0.5 & 1%	WBP	BAC
Natamycin 5%	M	BAC
Neomycin	THR	PMA
Neosporin	WEL	THM
Normal Saline (isotronic saline)	M	THM
Ocusol (sulphacetamide & zinc)	BOO	CET
Opticrom	FIS	EDTA/BAC
Otrivine-Antistin	ZYM	BAC
Penicillin	M	PMN
Phenylephrine 0.12%	ALL	BAC
Phenylephrine 5 & 10%	M	BAC
		EDTA
		SOM
Phenylephrine 10%	RID	BAC
Phospholine iodide 0.06, 0.125	AYE	CHB
& 0.25%		Boric Acid
Physostigmine (Eserine)	M	BAC
0.25 & 0.5%		SOM
Pilocarpine 0.1 to 6%	M	BAC
Pilocarpine 0.5 & 1%	EVA	BAC
0.5, 1, 2, 3 & 4%	KIR	BAC
1, 3 & 4%	MAC	BAC
Pilocarpine 4% + Eserine 1/4%	M	BAC & SOM
Pilocarpine 4% + Eserine 1/2%	RID	BAC
PVP (polyvinylpyrrolidone) 0.5%	M	THM & EDTA
Polytrim	WEL	THM
Potassium ascorbate 10%	M	SOM & EDTA
Prednisolone 0.0003, 0.0001,	M	BAC
0.003, 0.01, 0.03, 0.1 & 0.3%		
Prednisoline forte 1%	ALL	BAC & EDTA
Predsol	GLA	BAC
Predsol N	GLA	THM
Propine	ALL	BAC & EDTA
Simplene 1% (adrenaline)	S & N	BAC
Sodium cromoglycate 2%	FIS	BAC
Sofradex	ROU	THM
Soframycin	ROU	PMN
SNO-Pilo 1, 2, 3 & 4%	S & N	BAC
Sulphacetamide 10%	KW	THM
Sulphacetamide 10, 20 & 30%	M	SOP & SOM
Sulphacetamide & zinc	M	PMN
Tears naturale	ALC	BAC & EDTA
Thymoxamine 0.2%	M	PMN

Timoptol 0.25 & 0.5%	MSD	BAC
Tropicamide 0.5% & 1%	ALC	BAC
Vasocon-A	COO	BAC & EDTA
Vista-Methasone	RID	BAC
Vista-Methasone N	RID	THM
Zincfrin	ALC	BAC
Zinc sulphate	RID	PMN
Zinc & adrenaline	M	PMN
HPMC 1 & 2%	M	BAC

Eye ointments with preservative:

Genticin	NIC	MHB & PHB
Lacri-Lube	ALL	CHB

Eye drops without preservative

Acetyl cystine 5 & 10%	M
Achromycin ophthalmic suspension	LED
Ami-Dose (N-saline)	ABA
Atropine 1%	M
Chloramphenicol	M
Clotrimazole 1% in arachis oil	M
Cyclopentolate 1%	M
Dexamethasone solution 0.1%	M
Disodium edetate 0.37%	M
Econazole 1% in arachis oil	M
F$_3$T 1%	M
Gentamicin 0.3%	M
Glycerin 100%	M
Homatropine 1 & 2%	M
Hydroxyamphetamine 1%	M
Hypromellose	M
IDU 0.1%	M
L-cysteine 0.1	M
Miconazole 1% in arachis oil	M
Paraffin liquid	MAC
Penylephrine 10%	M
Pilocarpine 0.5–6%	M
Potassium ascorbate 10%	M
Prednisolone 0.01, 0.03, 0.1 & 0.3%	M
Sodium chloride 0.9% (N-saline)	ABA
All Minims drops	S & N

Key to preservatives
BAC – Benzalkonium chloride; CET – Cetrimide; CHA – Chlorhexidine acetate; CHB – Chlorbutanol; CHD – Chlorhexidine digluconate; EDTA – Disodium edetate; MHB – Methylhydroxybenzoate; PHB – Propylhydroxybenzoate; PHE – Phenylethanol; PMA – Phenylmercuric acetate; PMN – Phenylmercuric nitrate; SOM – Sodium metabisulphite; SOP & SPC – Sodium pentachlorophenate; THM – thiomersal.

Key to manufacturers
ABA = Abatron; ALC = Alcon; ALL = Allergan; ARM = Armour; AYE = Ayerst; BOO = Boots; COO = CooperVision; EVA = Evans; FIS = Fisons; GLA = Glaxo; KW = Kirby Warwick; LED = Lederle; MAC = Macarthys; MSD = Merck Sharp & Dohme; M = Moorfields Eye Hospital; NIC = Nicholas; RID = Richard Daniel; ROU = Roussell; StM = St Mary's Hospital; SAU = Sauflon; SHP = Shering Plough; S & N = Smith & Nephew; THR = Thornton Ross; WBP = W P Pharmaceuticals; WEL = Wellcome; WOH = Western Ophthalmic Hospital; ZYM = Zyma.

Artificial tear preparations

Major component	Trade name	Preservative
		Unit dose
Hydroxypropyl methylcellulose	Isopto Alkaline	BAC
	Isopto Plain	BAC
	SNO tears	BAC + EDTA
Polyvinyl alcohol and cellulose ester	Hypotears PVA & PEG	BAC
	Liquifilm wetting solution	BAC & EDTA
Other polymeric systems	Tears Naturale (Alcon)	BAC & EDTA

Appendix 9.III

Preparations for use with soft contact lenses

Abatron
Amidose Saline (R) N/A Amiclair Enzyme Tabs (Protease, Lipase and Pronase).

Alcon
Preflex (DC) THM 0.004, Pliagel (DC) Sorbic acid 0.1, Flexcare;
Flexsol (S & D) & Normol (R) THM 0.001 & CHX 0.005, Softabs Tabs (S/D) Chlorine (DIC),
Salettes Aerosol (buffered) N/A & Alcon Aerosol Saline (unbuffered) N/A, Clen-zym (Pancreatin).

Allergan Hydrocare
Cleaning & Soaking (DC) & (S & D) THM 0.001 QUAT 0.013, LC 65 (DC) NA EDTA, Hydrocare Fizzy Protein Removing Tablets (Papain), Lens Plus Unpreserved saline, Oxysept 1 3% H_2O_2, Oxysept 2 (Catalase).

Barnes Hind
Cleaner No. 4 (DC) THM 0.001, Intensive Cleaner Solution (C) THM 0.001, Hexidin (S & D) THM 0.002 & CHX 0.003, Perform 1 (H_2O_2) & Perform II (Sodium thiosulphate neutralizer) – unpreserved solutions.

Bausch & Lomb
Daily Cleaner (DC) Sorbic acid, Saline Aerosol N/A, Soflens Protein Tabs (Papain),
Optim-eyes (CHX), only available with B & L lenses and contraindicated with high water ionic materials.

Boots
Daily cleaner Soaking (S & D) and Comfort Drops (RW) THM 0.0025 CHX 0.0025 & EDTA.

CIBA vision
Hydroclean (DC); Hydrosoak (S & D) and Hydrosol (RW) THM 0.0025 CHX 0.0025 EDTA 0.128, 0.5 Pyruvate and N-saline, Solar Saline Aerosol N/A,
Lensept (C) H_2O_2 3%, Lensrins (& catalyst) (R) THM 0.001 EDTA 0.1, Miraflow (DC) IPA, 10:10 Hydrogen peroxide and sodium pyruvate neutraliser. Clerz (RW) Unit dose N/A.

Sauflon Pharmaceuticals
Sterisolv (DC) THM 0.004 EDTA 0.1, Sterisal 2 (S & D) THM 0.002 CHX 0.002 EDTA 0.1, Aerosol Saline N/A,
Aerotabs tablets (S & D) Chlorine (Halazone).

Smith & Nephew
Prymeclean (C) CHX 0.002, Prymesoak (S & D) CHX 0.002.

Key to function of preparation
B, Boiling; R, rinsing; S & D, soaking and disinfecting; DC, daily cleaner; RW, rewetting.

Key to antimicrobial present
CHB – Chlorbutol; CHX – Chlorhexidine digluconate; DIC – dichloroisocyanurate; EDTA – Sodium edetate; IPA – isopropyl alcohol; PMN – Phenylmercuric nitrate; QUAT – quaternary ammonium base; THM – Thiomersal (Thimerosal); NA – no antimicrobial present.

10

Refraction problems related to contact lens wear

Hard corneal contact lenses

Problems arise when the hard corneal contact lens wearer requires a spectacle prescription. Opinions are divided as to how long the lens wear should be discontinued before the refraction is carried out. The time usually quoted is from one to three days, but may even be as much as two weeks. There seems to be little reasoned thought associated with the choice of these time periods. It seems pointless to prescribe a pair of spectacles which will only be of use after a delayed period. In the opinion of the author the hard corneal contact lenses should be removed in the consulting room and the refraction should then proceed after 15 minutes (Figure 10.1). If the subjective responses indicate an inability to distinguish between moderate dioptric changes in both sphere and cylinder and also in cylinder axis then it is futile to continue with the refraction as it will not be reliable. In this case the patient's whole contact lens status needs to be re-evaluated and no spectacle prescription will be satisfactory until it is. If the refraction is straightforward, the patient should be asked to return not having worn the contact lenses for 24 hours – any period of 24 hours. If this second refraction is similar to the first refraction, glasses should be ordered. There is a high probability of patient satisfaction regardless of whether he (or she) continues to wear his lenses on a regular or intermittent basis.

If the patient intends to discontinue hard corneal contact lens wear he must be warned of the possibility of unpredictable changes in the refraction over the course of perhaps a year. If the second refraction is quite different, or not straightforward, and if there is difficulty in distinguishing moderate dioptric changes in sphere or cylinder, or cylinder axis, then the contact lenses need to be re-evaluated and no spectacle prescription will be satisfactory.

It should be pointed out to the patient that it is only by long-term discontinuation of contact lens wear that the stability of his spectacle correction can be evaluated. Most contact lens wearers are not prepared to discontinue lens wear on a long-term basis.

This procedure, which the author recommends, can be justified on a pathophysiological basis.

The purpose of the 15-minute interval is to eliminate any small degree of transient spectacle blur which may exist. It also allows time for the eyes to be examined prior to the refraction.

The particular concern is so-called spectacle

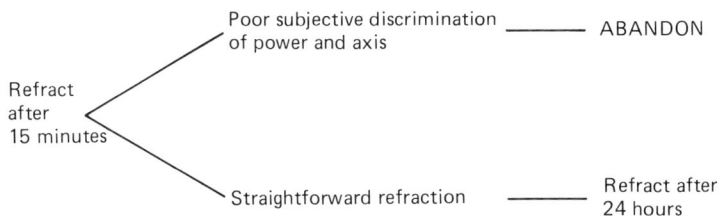

Figure 10.1 Refraction after 15 minutes

blur. This is a blurring of vision which may be experienced when spectacle wear is resumed. It is measured as a loss in Snellen spectacle acuity compared with the prefitting acuity *or* a loss in spectacle acuity compared with the contact lens acuity and this loss is often the same in both cases.

Spectacle blur may be refractive or absolute (Figure 10.2). Refractive blur implies that it can be eliminated by a new prescription. Absolute blur implies that no alteration of the spectacle prescription will restore the acuity.

Transient spectacle blur will have disappeared within 15 minutes. It manifests itself as altered spherical power, usually in a more minus direction. It is due to a change in corneal shape.

In a famous paper, 'The Fort Dix Report', Rengstorff (1965) pointed out that the changes in corneal shape were more complex than mere moulding. In other words, flat or steep as a corneal lens might be, fitting it might cause either an increase or a decrease in astigmatism. Carney (1975) showed that the change in corneal shape after two hours of corneal lens wear could have at least two causes. One was an unevenly distributed corneal thickness and the other a mechanical moulding of the shape.

Wilson *et al.* (1990), on the basis of a study of seven eyes of four patients, suggest that rigid contact lens decentration is a risk factor for corneal warpage. Using computer-assisted topographic analysis, they noted that the topographic abnormalities correlated with the decentred resting position of the contact lens on the cornea. The warpage topography, for each of the corneas, was characterized by a relative flattening of the cornea

underlying the resting position of the contact lens.

Mandell and Polse (1971) showed that visible corneal oedema, or central corneal clouding (Korb, 1963), as they refer to it, was related to an increase in corneal thickness in that area of cornea.

Visible corneal oedema must be looked for in a special way in wearers of hard corneal lenses (see Figure 12.1):

1. The room must be dark.
2. The microscope must not be used.
3. Direct the slit lamp beam at the limbus at an angle of 45° to the optical axis of the patient.
4. Observe the cornea at an angle of 90° to the slit lamp beam from a distance of 25 cm (10 inches).
5. Observe the cornea against the darkness of the pupil and try to elicit a change in the transparency of the cornea from one area to another.

The cornea is observed against the darkness of the pupil and an effort is made to try to elicit a change in the transparency of the cornea from one area to another (see Figure 12.2). If the corneal contact lens rides high on the cornea, it may help, in the elucidation of the sign, if the eye looks down. Likewise, if the corneal contact lens rides low, the eye should look up.

With practice small amounts of oedema become visible. (If the pupils are small and it is necessary to prove a point the pupils may be dilated and this should be done before the lenses are removed.) This is the first examination which should be done once the contact lenses are re-

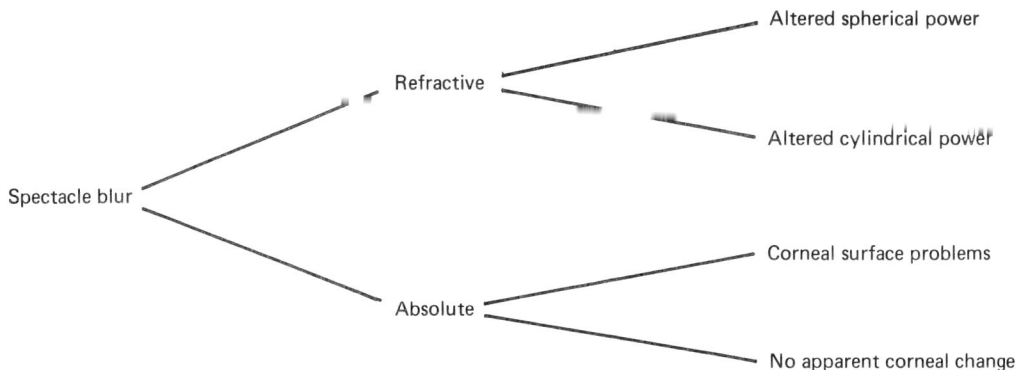

Figure 10.2 Spectacle blur

moved in the 15 minutes before the refraction is performed. The sign disappears rapidly.

If oedema is seen one should not proceed with the refraction. In this case the contact lenses need to be re-evaluated. At this time surface changes may be seen on the cornea. These may blur the spectacle refraction – absolute spectacle blur. They may be due to oedema which can produce a friable epithelium, or corneal surface irregularity caused by the deposition of sediment on the back surface of the contact lens, or abrupt transition of its posterior curves. Surface changes in the cornea demand an examination of the contact lenses at the slit lamp.

The transient reversible changes which occur early and perhaps on a day-to-day basis are altered spherical power and corneal surface changes.

Chronic changes can occur with long-term corneal lens wear and will also given rise to spectacle blur. The author contends that the majority of cases in which there are profound corneal changes will show up within a 24-hour period of discontinuing contact lens wear.

The problems can be listed as follows:

1. Altered or altering spherical power.
2. Increased or altering cylindrical power.
3. Decreased or decreasing spectacle acuity.
4. Keratoconus.

A substantial number of long-term wearers of hard corneal contact lenses develop these problems, although frank keratoconus is rare.

It is interesting to speculate on why these changes occur. Cremer-Bartels (1977) showed that the biosynthesis of keratan sulphate in the corneal stroma of rabbits is inhibited by the removal of the epithelium. It could be that the biosynthesis is interrupted in the presence of an oedematous epithelium. Keratan sulphate plays a role in the dehydration of the corneal stroma.

Polse (1972) has shown that only those wearers who demonstrated an increase in corneal thickness when lenses were worn throughout the day showed significant corneal fluctuations when lens wear was discontinued. He noted that these changes could last for several weeks after lens wear had been discontinued. In the author's experience the changes can go on for many months.

Altered spherical power may be in the direction of emmetropia. An example is shown in Figure 10.3, where, for simplicity, only the changes in

J.K. (D.O.B. 1938)

1956	$\dfrac{-3.0}{-0.50}_{10}$ = 6/5
3rd April, 1977	Lens wear stopped
7th April, 1977	−0.75 = 6/9
21st April, 1977	$\dfrac{-0.25}{-0.50}_{90}$ = 6/9
19th May, 1977	$\dfrac{-0.25}{-0.50}_{115}$ = 6/6 pt
23rd June, 1977	$\dfrac{-0.25}{-0.50}_{110}$ = 6/6
22nd August, 1977	$\dfrac{-0.25}{-1.25}_{115}$ = 6/6
3rd March, 1978	$\dfrac{-}{-1.75}_{95}$ = 6/5 −2

Figure 10.3 Altered spherical power in the direction of emmetropia and increase in cylindrical power after ceasing hard corneal lens wear

the right eye are considered. This patient was fitted with hard corneal lenses in 1956 and the refraction at that time is recorded. He became intolerant to hard corneal lenses in April, 1977, and stopped wear. He lost his spherical myopia, but after four months moderate astigmatism developed. He ceased to wear corneal lenses altogether.

Occasionally bizarre changes in the spectacle refraction are seen, as shown in the case of a high myope in Figure 10.4. Again, only the right eye changes are shown as both eyes behaved in a similar manner.

The development of increased cylinder, together with some diminution of spectacle acuity can be seen in the case recorded in Figure 10.5.

D.M. (D.O.B. 1940)

1960	$\dfrac{-11.25}{-3.00}_{180}$ = 6/18
1960	Hard corneal lenses fitted
19th May, 1980	−7.50 = 6/12 Contact lens wear stopped
7th June, 1980	$\dfrac{-18.00}{-2.00}_{70}$ = 6/9

Figure 10.4 Bizarre changes in refraction in a high myope after ceasing hard corneal lens wear

C.M. (D.O.B. 1947)

1963	$\dfrac{-2.75}{-0.50}$ 180
2nd Feb., 1976	$\dfrac{-4.0}{-1.0}$ 50 = 6/9 − 1 (immediately on removal of CL)
	Lens wear stopped
1st April, 1976	$\dfrac{-2.75}{-2.50}$ 180 = 6/5
17th May, 1979	$\dfrac{-3.0}{-3.0}$ 175 = 6/5

Figure 10.5 Increased cylindrical refraction with some decrease in acuity after ceasing hard corneal lens wear

J.K. (D.O.B. 1946)

1965	$\dfrac{-3.75}{-1.50}$ 180
1967	Corneal lenses fitted
13th August, 1979	$\dfrac{-4.50}{-0.25}$ 135 = 6/6 pt (immediately on removal of CL)
	Contact lens wear stopped
17th August, 1979	$\dfrac{-2.25}{-0.50}$ 175 = 6/5 pt
8th Oct., 1979	$\dfrac{-3.0}{-0.50}$ 110 = 6/5 pt
29th Oct., 1979	$\dfrac{-3.50}{-0.50}$ 90 = 6/6 pt
24th Jan., 1980	$\dfrac{-3.75}{-0.50}$ 90 = 6/6
10th March, 1980	$\dfrac{-4.0}{-0.50}$ 90 = 6/6

Figure 10.6 Fluctuation of spectacle refraction after ceasing hard corneal lens wear

Again only the details for the right eye are shown. Both eyes behaved in like manner. This girl was forced to discontinue hard corneal lenses because of increasing three and nine o'clock corneal infiltrates. The development of a substantial degree of astigmatism was a tragedy for her. She is an artist and writer and could not tolerate the astigmatic correction. She was so intolerant that for everyday use she prefered a spherical correction with consequently much diminished acuity. Now that toric soft contact lenses have reached such a high degree of perfection it is probable that they are the best way to manage such cases. Harstein (1965) has described the development of up to 8.5 dioptres of astigmatism. The fluctuation of spectacle correction can be demonstrated in the case recorded in Figure 10.6. Again, only the right eye is shown. This man developed intolerance to his hard corneal lenses after 14 years. It will be noted that five months after cessation of wear he had regained his spherical prefitting refraction of 1965. It can also be seen that he has lost one dioptre of astigmatism. His astigmatism is now against the rule instead of with it, as it was formerly. These changes cannot be predicted. He has now been fitted with soft lenses. These seldom cause spectacle blur.

The development of frank keratoconus in corneal lens wearers was first described by Harstein (1965). Harstein and Becker (1970) subsequently proposed that those cases which developed keratoconus had low scleral rigidity as demonstrated by the Friedenwald nomograms devised for glaucoma investigation. Macsai, Varley and

Kratchmer (1990) carried out a retrospective review of 398 eyes of 199 patients with keratoconus and this revealed 106 eyes of 53 patients (47 with PMMA lenses, three with soft lenses and three with gas permeable lenses) with an association between contact lens wear and the development of keratoconus. The absence of keratoconus at the time of contact lens fitting was confirmed by slit lamp examination, keratometry readings and manifest refraction. Keratoconus was diagnosed in these patients after a mean of 12.2 years of contact lens wear. This group was compared with patients with sporadic keratoconus with either no history of contact lens wear or a history of contact lens wear after the diagnosis. The patients in the group studied were older at the time of diagnosis, had central versus decentred cones and had a tendency towards flatter corneal curvatures. These authors believe that contact lens wear is a factor that can lead to keratoconus.

The present author has seen a number of cases of keratoconus which have developed in hard contact lens wearers. It cannot be denied that these patients might have been predestined to develop the disease if they had not been wearing contact lenses. The author has been impressed by the mild and non-progressive nature of the keratoconus in these patients.

Corneal distortion and warping has received considerable attention in the contact lens literature. Suggestions have been put forward on how to avoid it. Arner (1977) and Rengstorff (1977) suggest slow withdrawal of corneal lenses. Lee (1979) advises the fitting of patients with gas permeable lenses with similar parameters to their existing lenses.

Gas permeable hard contact lenses are generally available. They are permeable to oxygen and carbon dioxide. With conventionally accepted standards of fitting they do not induce corneal oedema. They are said to produce little or no spectacle blur (Reich, 1975; Mackie, 1978; Sarver, Polse and Harris, 1977). Nevertheless, the same procedure should be adopted as is outlined at the beginning of this chapter, when refracting patients so fitted for spectacles. It is evident that corneas vary in their response to oxygen deprivation and there is always the question of the fitting. If there is insufficient movement of the contact lens the contribution of oxygen from the tears may be grossly reduced and the transmission through the lens may then not be sufficient.

Many, as yet unsubstantiated, reports are appearing in the literature to the effect that their continued use overcomes the problems of unstable vision, increased astigmatism and corneal warpage induced by hard corneal lens wear.

In the present state of our knowledge the author feels that it is now unjustifiable to fit young people with hard non-gas permeable corneal lenses for cosmetic reasons when gas permeable lenses are readily available and reliable.

The question is often posed whether hard corneal lenses prevent the progress of myopia. There is no doubt that it is most unusual for myopic patients to need increases in the power of hard corneal lenses which they are wearing, but there are occasions when this does occur. The author has found increases to be necessary in some children and teenagers and has also seen it, frequently, in cases of high myopia. It is interesting that hypermetropic patients often need an increase in their contact lens correction as they become older, so not all features which determine the refraction are stabilized by hard corneal lenses. In an extensive thesis, Holden (1970), points out that corneal topography recovers very

slowly after a period of hard corneal lens wear and that in the case of a wearer of many years' duration it would take perhaps a year of non-wear to establish any permanency in the refractive effects.

Soft lenses

Soft lenses rarely cause problems with spectacle blur either on a transient or chronic basis in the absence of visible corneal pathology. However, the author has seen a few cases of rapidly advancing myopia associated with recent adoption of soft lens wear. This is reversed after discontinuing lens wear for two or three weeks. The increased myopia can usually, but not always, be prevented by fitting thinner, more gas transmissible lenses. Grosvenor (1975) reported on the development of increased myopia, together with changes in corneal curvature, in patients newly fitted with soft contact lenses. He associated this with a steep lens–cornea relationship, overwearing of lenses and inadequate blinking habits. This was at a time before the ready availability of thin, highly gas transmissible lenses. In a recent study on the highly gas transmissible Scanlens 75, worn monocularly by 19 patients for an average of 5.4 years, Rengstorff and Nilsson (1985) found no significant differences in refraction, keratometry or visual acuity between the experimental and control eyes seven days after lens removal.

Scleral lenses

Scleral lenses rarely cause chronic spectacle blur unless there are pathological changes such as vascularization in the cornea, in which case the acuity with the lens may be diminished. They are, however, notorious for producing transient spectacle blur – a condition known as Sattler's veil. This condition is due to corneal oedema. It is interesting that the oedema produced by hard corneal lenses requires a special examination technique, as described, to detect it, whereas that produced by scleral lenses looks like any other corneal oedema such as that found in acute glaucoma or bullous keratopathy.

One further distinction can be made. Patients

S.H. (D.O.B. 1960)

18th Jan., 1985	$\dfrac{-3.25}{-1.50}$ 175	= 6/6
30th Jan., 1985	Fitted Saturn lenses	
17th Sept., 1986	Contact lens wear stopped	
18th Sept., 1986	$\dfrac{-4.50}{-1.00}$ 165	= 6/5 pt
25th Sept., 1986	$\dfrac{-3.50}{-1.00}$ 170	= 6/5
2nd Oct., 1986	$\dfrac{-3.25}{-1.00}$ 180	= 6/5

Figure 10.7 Refractive changes after ceasing wear of a Saturn lens

with marked oedema under a corneal contact lens rarely see coloured haloes around lights, whereas the patient with oedema under a scleral contact lens almost always reports this phenomenon. Oedema under a corneal contact lens does not diminish the contact lens acuity whereas oedema under a scleral lens does, often necessitating the removal of the lens, following which the acuity usually recovers rapidly.

Saturn lenses

One final word should be said about Saturn lenses (Pilkington). These are lenses with a hard gas permeable centre and a soft hydrophilic periphery. They are useful in the correction of corneal astigmatism. The author has some experience of these lenses and they do cause spectacle refractive changes which he has not had the opportunity to investigate. An illustrative example of the changes produced by these lenses is shown in Figure 10.7. These lenses have been superceded by SoftPerm lenses.

References

ARNER, R.S. (1977) Corneal deadaptation – the case against abrupt cessation of contact lens wear. *Journal of the American Optometric Association*, **48**, 3, 339–341

CARNEY, L.G. (1975) The basis for corneal shape change during contact lens wear. *American Journal of Optometry and Physiological Optics*, **52**, 445–454

CREMER-BARTELS, G. (1977) The effect of the corneal epithelium on the biosynthesis of keratan sulphate in the stroma with regard to curvature variations important for wearing contact lenses. *Klinische Monatsblatter fur Augenheilkunde*, **171**, 6, 981–986

GROSVENOR, T. (1975) Changes in corneal curvature and subjective refraction of soft contact lens wearers. *American Journal of Optometry and Physiological Optics*, **52**, 405–413

HARSTEIN, J. (1965) Corneal warping due to contact lenses. *American Journal of Ophthalmology*, **60**, 6, 1103–1104

HARSTEIN, J. and BECKER, B. (1970) Research into the pathogenesis of keratoconus. *Archives of Ophthalmology*, **48**, 728–729

HOLDEN, B.A. (1970) A study of the development and control of myopia and the effects of contact lenses on corneal topography. *Ph.D. Thesis*, The City University, London, November, 1980

KORB, D.R. (1963) Corneal transparency with emphasis on the phenomenon of central circular clouding. *Encyclopedia of Contact Lens Practice.*, **4**, Suppl. 20, Appendix B, 106–115

LEE, J.M. (1979) Regression of induced irregular astigmatism in hard lens wearers refit with CAB lenses. *Review of Optometry*, June, 54–56

MACKIE, I.A. (1978) Experience with Silafocon A (Polycon) gas permeable hard corneal lenses. *Journal of the British Contact Lens Association*, **1**, 3, 17–25

MACSAI, M.S., VARLEY, G.A. and KRATCHMER, J.H. (1990) Development of keratoconus after contact lens wear. *Archives of Ophthalmology*, **108**, 534–538

MANDELL, R.B. and POLSE, K.A. (1971) Corneal thickness changes accompanying central corneal clouding. *American Journal of Optometry*, **48**, 2, 129–132

POLSE, K.A. (1972) Changes in corneal hydration after discontinuing contact lens wear. *American Journal of Optometry*, **49**, 511–516

REICH, L.A. (1975) The RX-56 gas permeable hard contact lens. *Contacto*, **19**, 12–18

RENGSTORFF, R.H. (1965) The Fort Dix Report – a longitudinal study of the effects of contact lenses. *American Journal of Optometry and Archives of the American Academy of Optometry*, **42**, 3, 153–163

RENGSTORFF, R.H. (1977) Astigmatism after contact lens wear. *American Journal of Optometry and Physiological Optics*, **54**, 11, 787–791

RENGSTORFF, R.H. and NILSSON, K.T. (1985) Long-term effects of extended wear lenses: changes in refraction, corneal curvature and visual acuity. *American Journal of Optometry and Physiological Optics.*, **62**, 1, 66–68

SARVER, M.D., POLSE, K.A. and HARRIS, M.G. (1977) Patient responses to gas permeable hard (Polycon) contact lenses. *American Journal of Optometry*, **54**, 4, 195–200

WILSON, S.E., LIN, D.T.C., KLYCE, S.D., REIDY, J.J. and INSLER, M.S. (1990) Rigid contact lens decentration: a risk factor for corneal warpage. *CLAO Journal*, **16**, 3, 177–182

11

Adverse reactions to scleral lenses

It is strange that the hard scleral lens which so compromised the oxygen requirements of the cornea should have been so apparently free of serious acute complications compared with the modern highly gas permeable soft contact lens, which is also really a scleral lens. Perhaps this was because it made the patient very aware when something was wrong and so it was removed. It has also to be borne in mind that comparatively few people wore these lenses in their heyday and many fewer still do now. Furthermore, tolerance in terms of hours per day was often much less than is common in modern corneal and soft contact lenses.

Sattler's veil

The main problem with the scleral lens is corneal hypoxia. This produces corneal oedema due to the inhibition of aerobic glycolysis (Smelser and Chen, 1955). Corneal epithelial oedema gives rise to the patient seeing coloured haloes (Sattler's veil). These haloes are identical to those seen in acute glaucoma. When the haloes are present the corneal epithelium can be observed to be cloudy and oedematous. This can be seen at the slit lamp without special techniques, which is not the case with hard corneal and soft lenses. The patient will usually know how long he can wear his lenses before the haloes occur. Eyes vary in their susceptibility to oedema, but haloes are very common to scleral lens wearers. Although corneal oedema is produced by hard corneal and soft contact lenses, hard corneal wearers never experience haloes and soft lens wearers seldom do. Removing the scleral lens usually clears the symptoms in about 15 minutes. Repeated corneal oedema will eventually lead to corneal vascularization over a period of time.

Corneal vascularization

Vascularization is commonly associated with scleral lens wear. It can be superficial or deep. It may suddenly appear after years of wear and be associated with lipid keratopathy. With or without the lipid keratopathy, it markedly reduces the spectacle acuity, but not necessarily the contact lens acuity. The corneal changes may be gross with tufting of vessels and involvement of the whole cornea. The vascularization is related to continuing corneal hypoxia.

Corneal opacification

Corneal opacification can be related to areas of drying under a static bubble (Mackie, 1971) (Figure 11.1). The opacification occurs hand in hand with localized corneal vascularization much in the manner of a pterygium. It can also occur at the apex of the cornea in response to hard corneal touch and continual breakdown of the central corneal epithelium. It is also associated with lipid keratopathy.

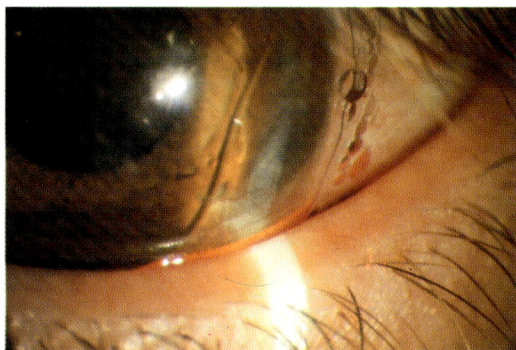

Figure 11.1 Corneal scarring in relation to a static bubble under a fenestration. In the long term opacification and vascularization have resulted – a pseudo pterygium

Giant papillary conjunctivitis

This condition occurs with scleral lenses. Discomfort and discharge occur, but itching after removal and blurred vision are not often experienced. The author has seen conjunctival scarring after many years of scleral lens use. This scarring is not a feature of soft lens or hard corneal lens giant papillary conjunctivitis. It is said that only plastic lenses and not glass lenses cause it, but this is open to debate. Certainly glass lenses are less likely to cause it. Often the giant papillae are buried in a grossly thickened palpebral conjunctiva.

Treatment

The obvious treatment is to withdraw the scleral lens and after the eye has settled to fit a soft lens, or perhaps a hard corneal lens. Patients who have worn scleral lenses for a long time do not usually take well to this procedure, but it may be necessary. It may be that no other type of contact lens can be fitted and the patient may be reliant on the scleral lens for adequate visual acuity. In this case sodium chromoglycate 2% can be used four or five times daily and when the new more potent mast cell stabilizers become available they may be much more effective.

Systemic tetracycline 250 mg twice daily or doxycycline 100 mg on alternate days should be tried over a period of many months for their anti-inflammatory rather than their antibiotic action. If this is not effective, bacterial cultures and sensitivity can be done and an appropriate antibiotic, such as erythromycin, or cephalexin, can be used in a dose of 250 mg twice daily. Whether it is necessary for the resident bacterial flora in these eyes to be sensitive to the antibiotic or not for therapeutic effect, is something that has yet to be clinically assessed.

References

MACKIE, I.A. (1971) Localised corneal drying in association with dellen, pterygia and related lesions. *Transactions of the Ophthalmological Society of the UK*, **91**, 129–145

SMELSER, G.K. and CHEN, D.K. (1955) Physiological changes in the cornea induced by contact lenses. *Archives of Ophthalmology*, **53**, 676–679

12

Adverse reactions to hard corneal lenses

The problems associated with hard corneal lenses can mostly be related to the development of corneal oedema as a result of coverage of the cornea and the inhibition of aerobic glycolysis (Smelser and Chen, 1955), or to the development of abnormal blinking mechanisms brought about by wearing the lenses. The conjunctival problems are probably related to constant minor trauma in susceptible individuals.

Corneal oedema

The oedema of the corneal epithelium produced by a corneal lens is typically localized and has been shown to be extracellular in type (Smelser and Chen, 1955). It is accompanied by stromal swelling (Mandell, Polse and Fatt, 1970; Bergmanson and Chu, 1982). Gas permeable hard lenses, that is, lenses which allow the transmission of oxygen and carbon dioxide through their substance, have greatly helped to eliminate corneal oedema in clinical practice, but it must be remembered:

1. that many hard lenses worn are still of the non-permeable type.
2. that the transmissibility of a gas permeable lens depends not only on the material but on its thickness and this may be of such a magnitude that the lens is hardly permeable.
3. that a poorly fitted (for example, dropping) gas permeable lens can still produce oedema.

A characteristic hazing of the cornea found after corneal contact lens wear was first reported by Korb (1962) and described in more detail by Korb and Exford (1968). They referred to it as 'central circular clouding' and drew attention to a unique area of changed epithelial transparency appearing 'off white' in colour and most readily observed when silhouetted against the dark background of the pupil. The 'off white' could be bluish or yellowish, depending upon the light reflected from the iris. The affected area of the cornea corresponded in location to the positioning of the corneal lens. The area of involvement was generally related to the overall size and the optic zone diameter (BOZD) of the lens and varied from less than 1 mm to as much as 8 mm in diameter. Other authors have referred to the condition as 'large round oedema', 'small round oedema' and 'gross circumscribed oedema'.

Corneal oedema in contact lens wearers is recognized at the slit lamp by using the technique of sclerotic scatter (Figure 12.1):

1. The room must be dark.
2. The microscope must not be used.
3. Direct the slit lamp beam at the limbus at an angle of 45° to the optical axis of the patient.
4. Observe the cornea at an angle of 90° to the beam from a distance of 25 cm (10 inches).
5. Observe the cornea against the darkness of the pupil and try to elicit a change in the transparency of the cornea from one area to another (Figure 12.2).

The oedema is easier to see if the pupil is large and it may be expedient to dilate the pupil before the lens is removed. The oedema must be looked for immediately after the lens is removed. This method of examination by *sclerotic scatter* is rarely used in modern slit lamp technique, but it is

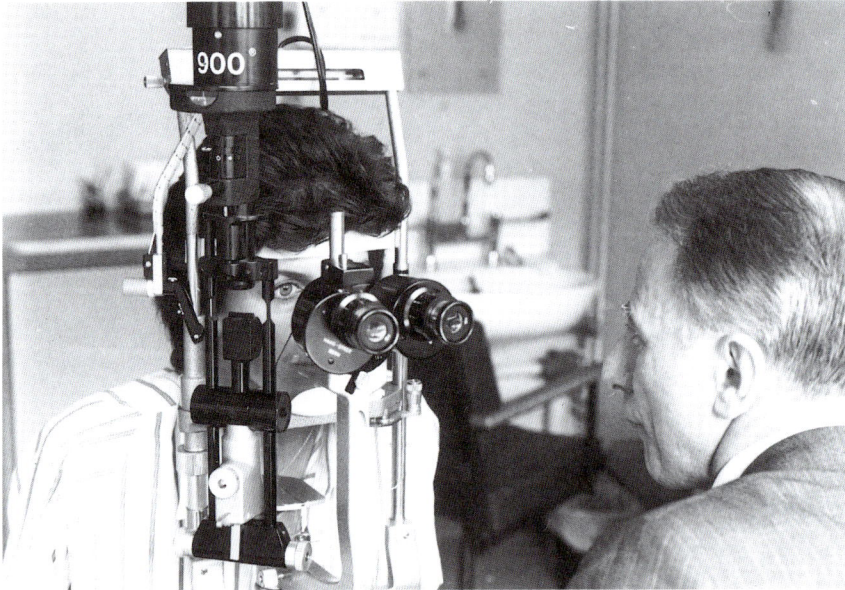

Figure 12.1 Examining for corneal oedema by the technique of sclerotic scatter. The room must be dark. The microscope must not be used. The slit lamp beam is directed at the limbus at an angle of 45° to the optical axis of the patient. The cornea is observed at an angle of 90° to the slit lamp beam from a distance of 25 cm

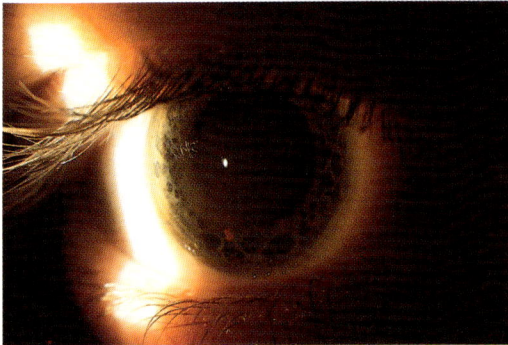

Figure 12.2 Examination of the cornea by sclerotic scatter. The photograph shows gross oedema (the grey area) in an asymptomatic hard corneal lens wearer who had worn lenses for five years

described in many old manuals and is an extremely useful preliminary examination in all external eye disease cases. The oedema is responsible for a number of hard corneal lens problems. It must however be emphasized that oedema is seldom a problem related to hard corneal lens wear in the aphakic eye. The aphakic cornea has been shown not to swell to the same extent under conditions of oxygen lack (Korb, Richmond and Herman, 1980), although the oxygen consumption of the aphakic cornea is comparable to the phakic eye (Holden, Mertz and Guillon, 1980).

Corneal deformation

Spectacle blur occurs when the corneal lens is removed and spectacles are worn. It is presumably due to corneal deformation and is measured as a loss in Snellen visual acuity in spectacles compared with the prefitting acuity, or a loss of acuity compared with the contact lens acuity. Spectacle blur can be relative or absolute depending upon whether or not the acuity can be restored by a new refraction.

Corneal deformation has been reviewed by Phillips (1990). Spectacle blur and corneal deformation are dealt with in detail in Chapter 10.

Corneal lens intolerance

Corneal oedema is responsible for a considerable amount of corneal contact lens intolerance. It may, however, be asymptomatic. Often there is a change from being symptomatic to asymptomatic for no evident reason. It may remain asymptomatic for a prolonged time after commencing contact lens wear. Sometimes the change from asymptomatic to symptomatic may be brought about by some incident such as losing a lens and having it replaced, some minor infective systemic illness, or a change in the place of work.

Corneal oedema can be associated with flushing of the areas of the face prone to rosacea, that is, the nose, cheeks, forehead and chin (Figure 12.3). This flushing is often related to the time the lenses are worn. It is also related to the ambient oxygen conditions. In a smoky, stuffy room this tendency to flushing will be increased. Patients with the rosacea diathesis, or established rosacea, are more prone to this reaction. Rosacea is a common factor in hard corneal lens intolerance.

Syndrome of Lansche and Lee

Corneal oedema can give rise to the complication described by Lansche and Lee (1960a, 1960b). Their paper was entitled 'Acute complications from corneal contact lenses, a recurring and serious problem in the command'. It was not really a serious problem. By 'serious' Lansche and Lee meant that it was getting them up too often in the middle of the night in their roles as ophthalmologists in the United States Army. The complication is sometimes referred to as the 'overwear syndrome', but this is 'save face' terminology used by the contact lens fitter. It is also known as the 'two o'clock in the morning' syndrome.

The syndrome is due to the development of corneal oedema while the lenses are worn and the subsequent breakdown of the corneal epithelium which usually occurs about two hours after re-

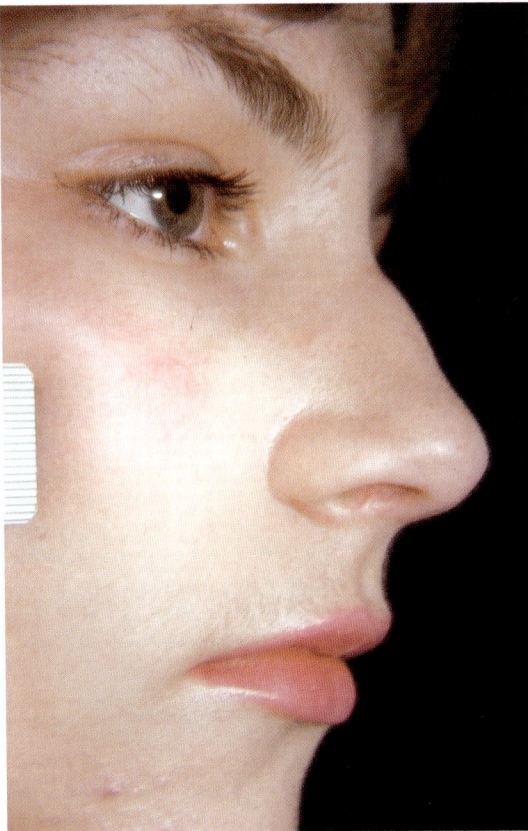

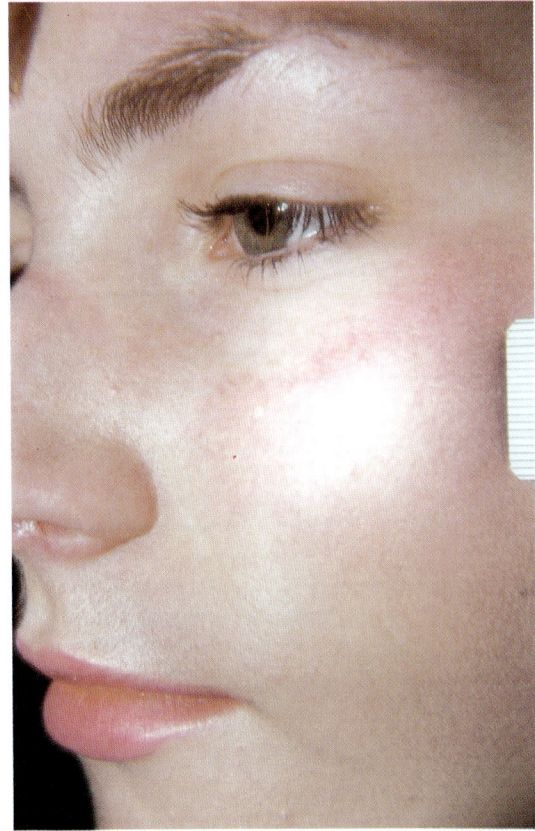

Figure 12.3 Flushing of the cheeks in association with corneal oedema caused by a hard corneal contact lens. The subject had worn a hard PMMA lens in the left eye for four hours. Compare the vascularity of the patient's left cheek with that of the right

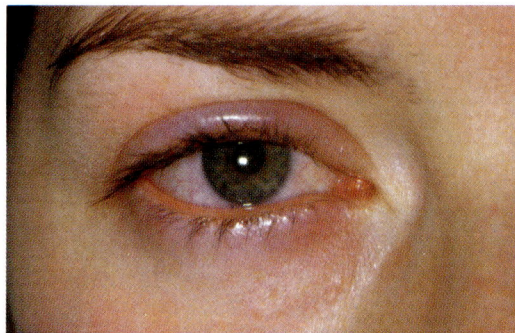

Figure 12.4 Swelling and oedema of the lids next day after an episode of the syndrome of Lansche and Lee the previous night

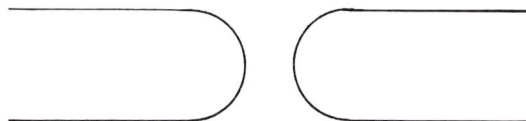

Figure 12.5 Bi-funnelled fenestration in a hard corneal lens

moving the contact lenses by which time the patient has often fallen asleep. On waking, there is agonizing pain, photophobia and blepharospasm. The vision is blurred and the eyes flood with tears if the lids can be opened. When local anaesthetic is instilled so that the cornea can be inspected it is often seen that the symptoms are out of proportion to the signs. The central epithelium usually stains with fluorescein to some extent. The epithelium usually heals within 12 hours with no residual signs, by which time the patient is symptom free. The condition may be uniocular or binocular.

A feature of the condition is marked swelling and oedema of the lids (Figure 12.4). Sometimes lid swelling occurs without the history of agony during the night. This sign may be misinterpreted, particularly in patients presenting at an external eye disease clinic or casualty department.

Treatment

Cyclopentolate 1% drops are used to counteract ciliary spasm. Atropine should not be used because its effect on the visual acuity is too prolonged. Gentamicin or tobramycin eye ointment are used as broad spectrum antibiotics. These patients are often in a very distressed state. It is often described as the worst pain they have ever had to endure. At this stage a sedative is very useful. Two eye pads are applied to the eye and these are kept in place by a two inch (5 cm) crepe bandage to the head.

The condition will recur if radical steps are not

taken to eliminate the oedema produced by the lens. Sometimes a recurrent erosion problem appears after one or more of these episodes. The simplest way of eliminating the oedema is to fenestrate the lens with one or two holes which must be central, or not more than 2.5 mm apart at the centre and the holes must be at least 0.3 mm wide. They should be bi-funnelled (Figure 12.5). This, however, results in visual disturbance in about 30% of hard corneal lens wearers. The second and more modern approach is to refit the lens in gas permeable material.

Exposure problems

Three and nine o'clock keratopathy

Exposure problems are produced by hard corneal lenses because of their effect on the normal pattern of blinking. Normal blinking invokes Bell's phenomenon and eye closure is almost totally effected by the upper lid (Ponder and Kennedy, 1927). During normal blinking, the lower lid moves in a nasal direction, an action which facilitates the transfer of the mucus thread in the inferior fornix to the inner canthus. The upper lid is an applicator of mucus to the ocular surface. Lemp *et al.* (1971) have shown that when the corneal epithelium is wiped free of mucus it becomes hydrophobic. Without its mucus coat, the cornea dries and dellen may form. In the long term, vascularization and infiltrates may develop at the site of these dellen (Mackie, 1971). An alternative explanation, and perhaps one more in line with contemporary thinking, is that the first stage in the formation of a dellen is the drying of mucus on the corneal surface. Litt, Wolf and Khan (1977) have shown that mucus dries rapidly and re-hydrates very slowly, that is, mucus which has dried hard in half an hour may take 50 hours to re-hydrate in normal saline (Figure 12.6). The

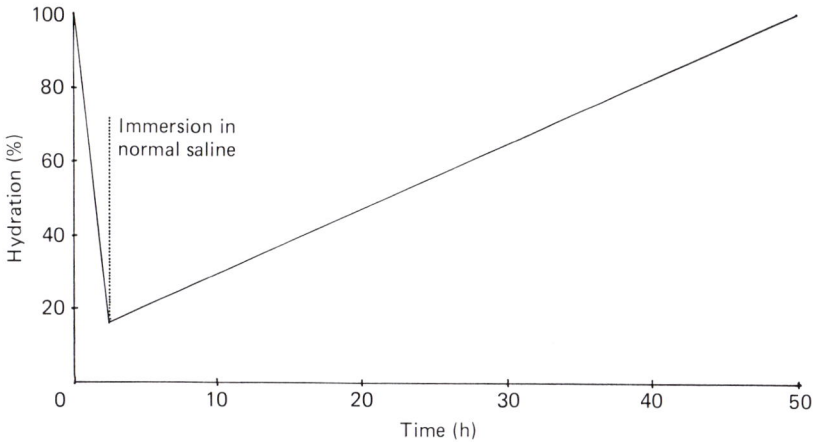

Figure 12.6 Approximate graph after Litt, showing dehydration of mucus in air and rehydration in normal saline

wearing of corneal contact lenses can cause the breakdown of normal blinking. Blinking can become sphincter like so that as the upper lid descends the lower lid rises to meet it. In this circumstance Bell's phenomenon ceases (Mackie, 1971) and closure is seldom complete, allowing the limbal areas at three o'clock and nine o'clock, which are not covered by lens or lid at any time, to become dry.

Another abnormal type of blinking is flick blinking, which occurs when the upper lid descends only as far as the superior edge of the corneal contact lens and then retracts. This is particularly common when the corneal lenses centre, or drop, on the surface of the cornea and when there is a tendency to upper lid retraction. This situation usually leads to marked problems of exposure at the three o'clock and nine o'clock positions of the limbus.

The deposition of dried ocular mucus on the front of the corneal lens during wear (greasing) is a sign of abnormal blinking. As already noted, Litt, Wolf and Khan (1977) have shown that mucus dries rapidly in air but re-hydrates very slowly in normal saline. Periods of non-blinking, or non-coverage of the lens by the top lid may allow ocular mucus to dry. Because of its physical properties the mucus may not be re-hydrated and wiped off the lens by the upper lid. The patient may learn that conscious blinking may even increase blurring and so an abnormal blinking pattern is reinforced.

Three and nine o'clock staining

These lesions, consisting of confluent erosions which are seen on either side of the cornea at the limbus, stain freely with fluorescein and rose bengal (Mackie, 1966) (Figure 12.7). They are often situated somewhat lower than the three and nine o'clock axis and extend on to adjacent conjunctiva. Their severity increases with time and this becomes associated with localized ciliary injection (Figure 12.8). The patient will complain of red eyes (Mackie, 1966). These signs must be looked for immediately after periods of wear.

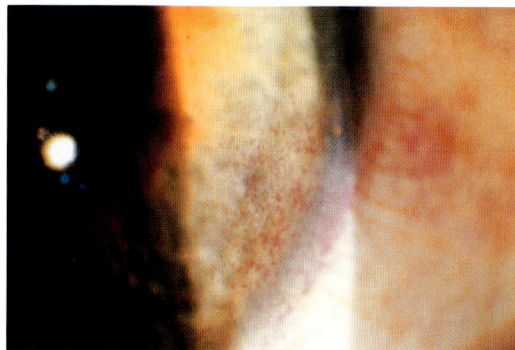

Figure 12.7 Three and nine o'clock staining of the cornea and conjunctiva, with rose bengal

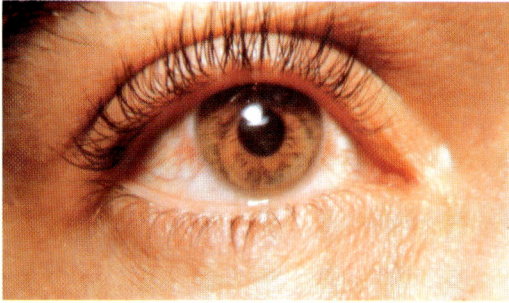

Figure 12.8 Three and nine o'clock localized ciliary injection

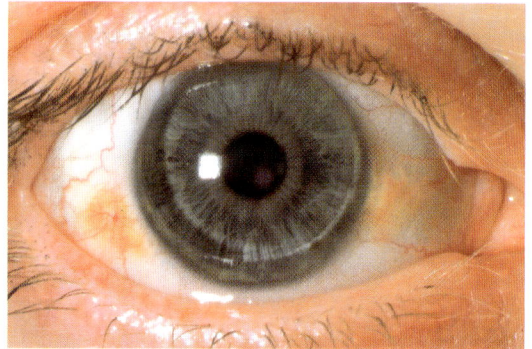

Figure 12.10 Marked pingueculae formation in a woman of 30 years of age after 14 years of hard corneal lens wear

Dellen formation

Sometimes the area of the staining is seen to be depressed and this depression extends on to the conjunctiva. Sometimes the depression is marked and a true dellen is seen (Mackie, 1971) (Figure 12.9).

Pingueculae formation

Sometimes the cornea is spared and only the conjunctiva adjacent to the three and nine o'clock areas dries. Over many years this can lead to the formation of ugly yellow pingueculae. This is seen from time to time in young people of around 30 years of age who have worn hard corneal lenses for 10–15 years (Figure 12.10).

Three and nine o'clock infiltrates

With long-term subjection of an eye to three and nine o'clock erosions, infiltrated lesions may develop at the site of the erosions (Mackie, 1966, 1971; Stainer *et al.*, 1981) (Figures 12.11 and 12.12). These can be flat and involve the cornea only or can be elevated above the corneal and conjunctival surfaces. The appearance is often that of a true pterygium.

Many patients who are wearing soft contact lenses will have worn hard corneal lenses in the past which may have induced corneal scars associated with three and nine o'clock epithelial erosions. These scars are often flat and lightly vascularized (Figure 12.13). It is important not to misinterpret these scars as indicating progressive corneal disease associated with soft contact lenses.

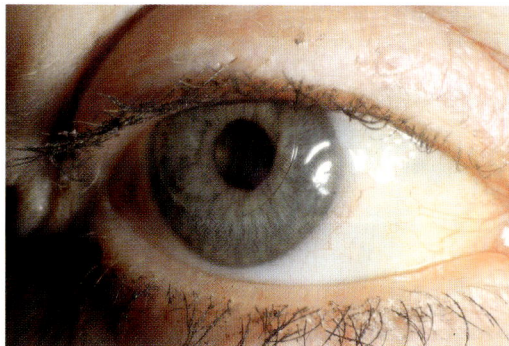

Figure 12.9 Dellen in association with three and nine o'clock staining

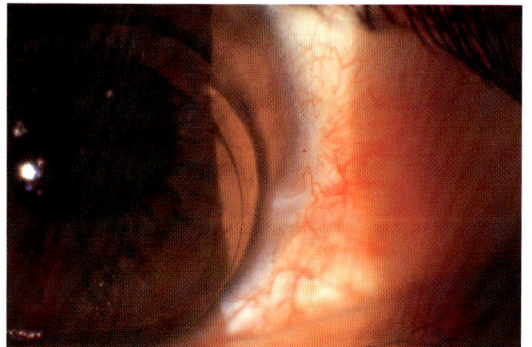

Figure 12.11 Pterygium-like lesion as a result of continued three and nine o'clock erosions

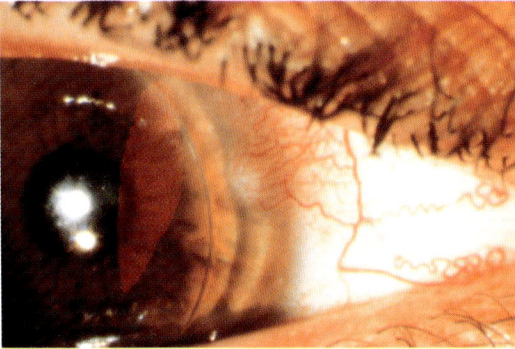

Figure 12.12 Nodular corneal infiltrate at the three o'clock position at the corneal periphery with a leash of feeding vessels

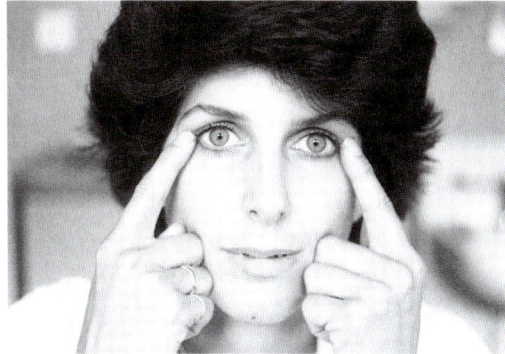

Figure 12.14 Exercises to promote normal blinking. The head is held erect and the eyes look straight forward. The tips of the forefingers are applied gently to the outer canthi. Blinking with full closure is performed every three seconds so that no orbicularis contractions are felt

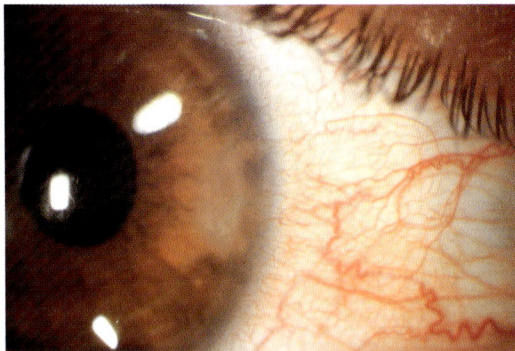

Figure 12.13 Large flat peripheral lightly vascularized corneal scar at the three o'clock position (Courtesy Dr Lali Moodaley)

type. The exercise should be done for five minutes in each hour while the patient is wearing the contact lenses.

The doctor should check that orbicularis contractions cannot be felt, by placing a forefinger at one of the patient's outer canthi (Figure 12.15). If there is any difficulty, the doctor should demonstrate the closure to the patient by asking the patient to place a forefinger at one of his or her outer canthi. Some patients have very spastic lids, especially when a contact lens is being worn, and it may be easier for them to start doing this exercise while the contact lenses are not worn.

Treatment

If three o'clock and nine o'clock localized corneal staining, perhaps with dellen formation, and associated ciliary injection are seen soon after a patient has been fitted with hard corneal lenses it is worth while trying to establish normal blinking by exercises – a sort of ocular physiotherapy. These exercises are performed as follows (Figure 12.14):

> The head is held erect and the eyes look straight ahead. The tips of the forefingers are applied gently at the outer canthi. Blinking with full closure is performed every three seconds so that no orbicularis contractions are felt. If orbicularis contractions are felt, it means that the blinking is abnormal and of sphincter

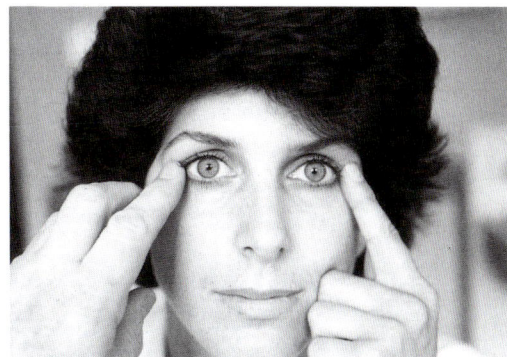

Figure 12.15 Exercises to promote normal blinking. The ophthalmologist should check that orbicularis contractions are not felt

These exercises are seldom effective in established contact lens wearers.

Many of these patients are determined to continue wearing contact lenses. Refitting with soft contact lenses should be considered. With soft contact lenses problems of blinking seldom arise and localized corneal drying never occurs.

Unfortunately, problems associated with withdrawal of the corneal contact lenses, as discussed in Chapter 10, become manifest. It may be expedient to refit these patients with hard gas permeable lenses for a period of six months to stabilize the refraction. Then they can be refitted with soft lenses which, of course, may have to be toric.

Removal of the pingueculae is often ineffective and there remains the probability of three and nine o'clock corneal infiltrates as well as further pinguecula formation if the lenses continue to be worn.

Vascularization

Vascularization is not common in wearers of hard corneal lenses and is not the important complication which is seen in soft contact lens wearers. It occurs in two forms.

The first is the peripheral form associated with the constant positioning of a corneal lens over one area of the limbus. This is often seen at the superior limbus in the case of a high riding immobile minus lens. Occasionally the vessels bleed and give rise to a subepithelial haemorrhage (Figure 12.16) which clears with time. The vascularization is not progressive, but when seen in association with giant papillary conjunctivitis it may lead to the erroneous diagnosis of trachoma. A high riding immobile minus lens is more prone to produce giant papillary conjunctivitis by a purely mechanical action on the superior tarsus.

The peripheral form of vascularization is also seen inferiorly in association with a dropping lens (Figure 12.17). In this situation the vessels are often deeply placed.

The second form of vascularization is the silent single leash of deep vessels which progressively grow towards the centre of the cornea, either to a pre-existing stromal opacity there or without any apparent reason. The stimulus is presumably hypoxia. The danger associated with these vessels is that they may silt out lipid into the corneal stroma and give rise to a lipid keratopathy out of all

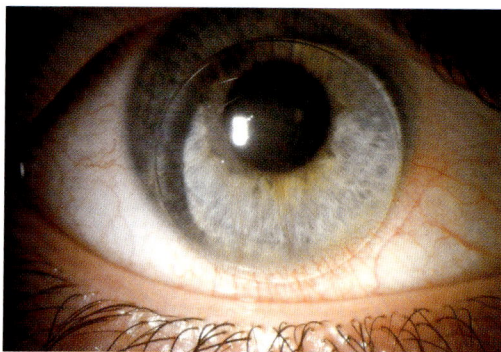

Figure 12.17 Gross, deep and superficial vascularization below in association with a dropping hard corneal lens worn over a period of two years. The other eye had the same type of lens fitting and did not show vascularization

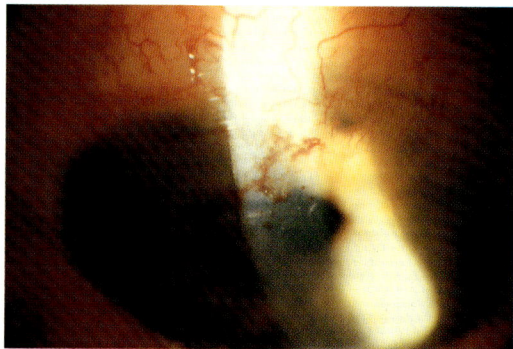

Figure 12.16 Subepithelial haemorrhage

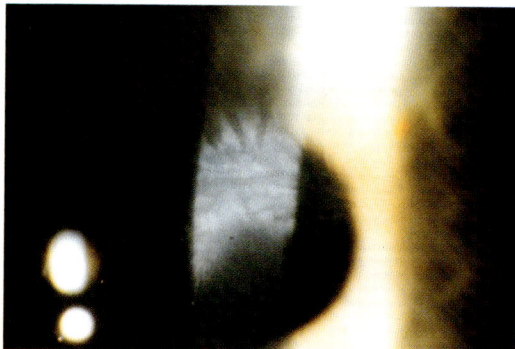

Figure 12.18 Lipid keratopathy in association with vascularization caused by a hard corneal lens

proportion in area to the size of the invading vessels (Figure 12.18). Lipid keratopathy looks unsightly and reduces the visual acuity.

Treatment

First form

This is directed, in the case of the high riding lens, to making it more mobile and perhaps of gas permeable material. Greater mobility may be achieved by flattening the posterior peripheral curve and introducing a front peripheral optic curve to diminish the bulk of the lens at its periphery. An attempt can be made to bring about centration of the lens. This will necessitate a marked reduction in its diameter.

In the case of a dropping lens an attempt should be made to convert it into a lens lid attachment fit and this can be achieved by introducing a front peripheral curve to the lens. Most dropping lenses are either of low minus power or of plus power.

Second form

The contact lens should be remade in gas permeable material and perhaps there may be a case for a very high Dk value (see Chapter 5). The cornea should be routinely inspected for progression of the vascularization. Nirankari *et al.* (1983) describe a case in which the deep stromal vascularization did not progress after the hard lenses were refitted in gas permeable material.

If there is a lipid keratopathy a blood lipid profile should be carried out since a dyslipoproteinaemia may be present. The lesion can be treated by argon laser application after anterior segment fluorescein angiography to identify the microvessels (Marsh and Marshall, 1982), but there is a danger of thinning of the cornea and even perforation after treating central lesions. Such therapy should probably only be considered when the lesion is cosmetically undesirable, or when the alternative, in view of the visual acuity, is a corneal graft. In mild lesions the lipid keratopathy is probably best left untreated. Many patients will wish to continue wearing their lenses, in which case the lens material should be changed to the gas permeable type and the cornea should be periodically inspected.

Corneal anaesthesia

Millodot (1978a) in a study of 91 subjects, who had worn hard corneal lenses for up to 22 years, found that corneal sensitivity diminished exponentially. However, in five subjects who abandoned their contact lenses after periods of between 12 and 16 years, recovery occurred within four months. Millodot suggests that loss of sensitivity, with hard corneal lens wear, ought to be heeded since the eye is thus put at a greater risk of infection. By this statement he means that subjects would be at greater risk of corneal infection occurring without their being aware of it. There is no clinical evidence whatever that this is the case. The problem in corneal infection is not that of patient awareness that something is wrong, but the long lapse of time that often ensues before an ophthalmologist is consulted.

It is certain that long-term wear of hard corneal lenses does not induce a condition similar to neuroparalytic keratitis (see Chapter 14) or the corneal condition similar to the latter disease which follows the continued use of topical local anaesthetics. Millodot (1978b) noted that some of his subjects who displayed a very high increase in corneal touch threshold (that is diminished sensitivity) believed that they had become more, and not less, sensitive. They reacted more sharply to a stimulus such as a piece of dust in the eye.

Preservative keratopathy

This includes thimerosal keratopathy and is seldom seen in wearers of hard corneal lenses, but is occasionally met in those patients who insert their lenses after instilling, into the concave surface, a drop of preserved wetting solution. Thimerosal keratopathy can be found, similar to that seen in soft contact lens wearers. It is very rare and it takes the form of an erosive punctate epitheliopathy, always maximal above and often showing tongue like processes of dysplastic opaque epithelium. Dendritiform figures are sometimes seen as part of the epithelial dysplasia, just as they are seen in soft lens wearers. These entities are discussed in Chapter 13.

Preservatives contained in preparations used with hard contact lenses are shown in Appendix 9.I.

Foreign bodies

Small foreign bodies are often trapped under hard corneal lenses, much to the discomfort of the patient. They leave tell-tale lines on the corneal epithelium which stain with fluorescein (Figure 12.19). These lines disappear after a few hours and the patient usually becomes asymptomatic as soon as the foreign body has been removed.

Crescentic erosions

Crescentic erosions are sometimes seen on a cornea after a hard corneal lens is removed (Figure 12.20). They are usually seen midway between the centre of the cornea and the periphery and consist of confluent small erosions. They are usually produced by a sharp transition between the curves on the back surface of the contact lens and can often be eradicated by blending the curves of the transition zone on the contact lens lathe.

Diffuse corneal erosions

Corneal erosions are sometimes seen after corneal lens removal. It is important that the hard corneal lens surface is carefully inspected, after washing, to exclude irregularities. In the absence of a special holder it is best to place the lens between the forefinger and thumb, steadying it by the edges. Look at it through the slit lamp microscope using

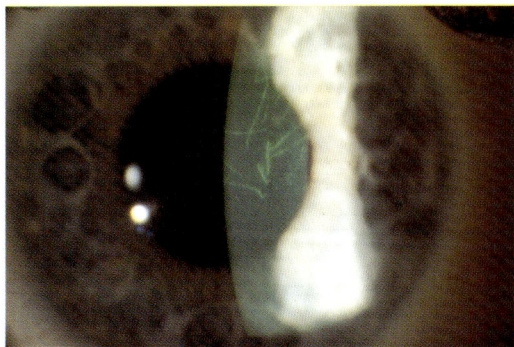

Figure 12.20 Crescentic corneal erosions caused by a hard corneal contact lens. These are usually related to a sharp transition between posterior curves or sediment on the posterior surface of the hard corneal lens

the third finger behind the lens as a retroilluminator (Figure 12.21). Deposit, which consists of magnesium and calcium carbonates or protein, may be seen on the surface of the lens. This lens coating is more common with gas permeable lenses. It acts as an abrasive. It occurs more frequently on the back surface of hard contact lenses. This deposit can also be seen at the junction between the front surface and the carrier of a reduced optic lens. If the coating is in this area it

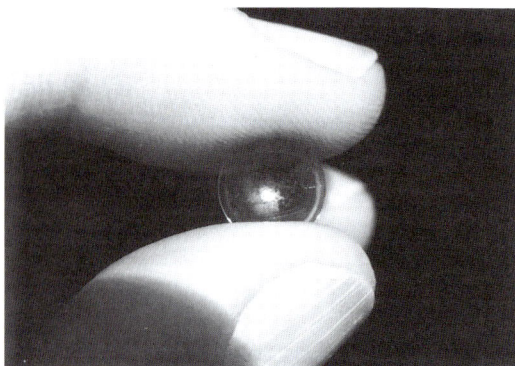

Figure 12.19 Foreign body erosions. These are usually linear and stain with fluorescein

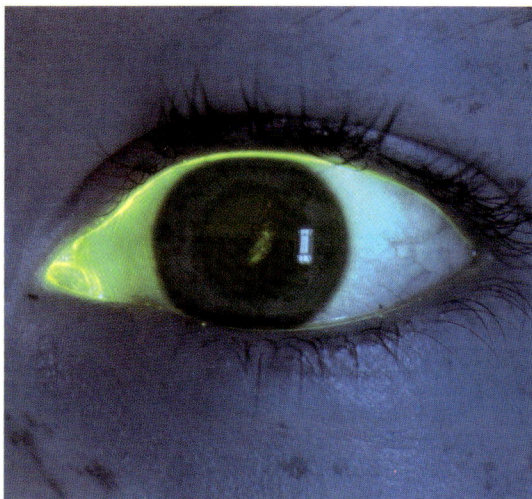

Figure 12.21 Method of inspecting a hard corneal lens for surface deposits and irregularities. The lens is placed between the forefinger and thumb and the third finger is used as a retroilluminator. The lens is viewed through the slit lamp microscope

acts as an abrasive on the palpebral conjunctiva and can be a factor in inducing giant papillary conjunctivitis.

Corneal endothelial polymegethism

Polymegethism means that there is much variation in cell size. Some of the early literature, mostly from Australia, refers to polymegathism, which implies many large cells. It has not been uncommon in the past to find both spellings in one paper, but now the truer term, polymegethism, is universally used.

This phenomenon (Figure 12.22) has been reported by Schoessler and Woloschak (1981) and Stocker and Schoessler (1985). Carlson, Bourne and Brubaker (1988) studied 40 long-term contact lens wearers (in excess of 23 years) and found that there was no difference between wearers of hard, soft, gas permeable and gas permeable plus prior lens usage, except that the gas permeable lens wearers had more hexagonal and less pentagonal cells. MacRae, Matsuda and Yee (1985) in a study of 12 patients (24 eyes) who had worn hard polymethylmethacrylate lenses for more than 10 years showed that the corneal endothelium of

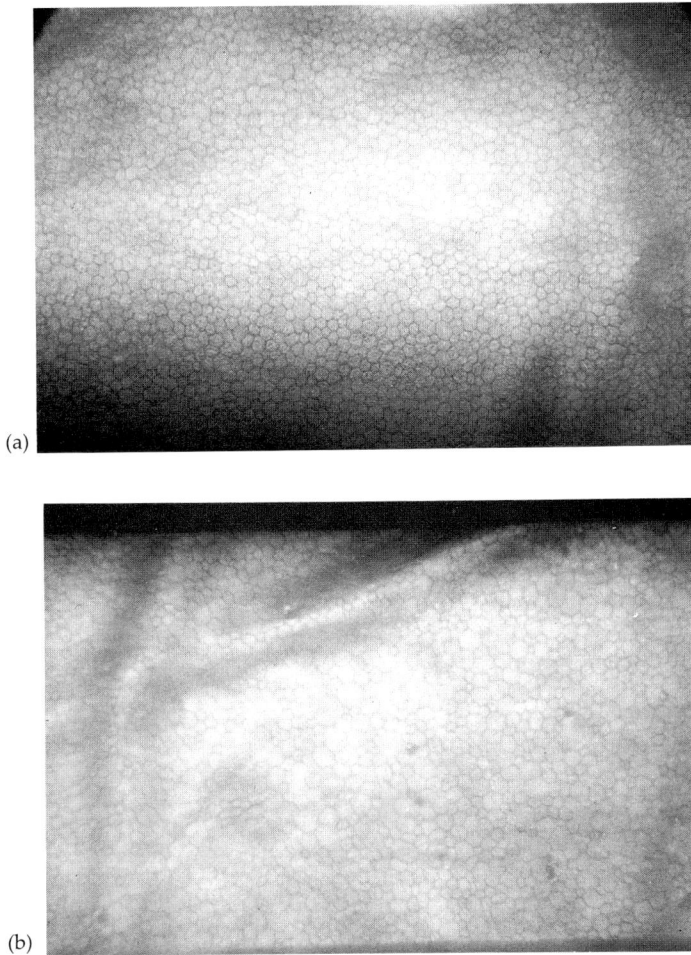

(a)

(b)

Figure 12.22 Endothelial polymegethism. (Courtesy of Mr Roger Buckley.) (a) Endothelium of a female aged 59 who had never worn contact lenses. (b) Endothelium of a female aged 56 who had worn hard PMMA lenses for 25 years. There is marked polymegethism but there was no evidence of corneal decompensation

these wearers (compared to non-wearers) had a higher coefficient of variation in cell area (polymegethism), lower number of hexagonal cells, higher number of other cell shapes (pleomorphism), and a lower figure coefficient (greater deviation from a lower hexagonal pattern). The cell density was within the limits of age matched controls.

The clinical significance of this finding is unclear. It has been shown that when preoperative cell densities are similar, polymegethic endothelium is more susceptible to surgical trauma than cells with more uniform areas (Bourne, Brubaker and O'Fallan, 1979; Rao *et al.*, 1979). In cataract surgery, patients with a greater preoperative polymegethism are more likely to develop corneal decompensation than those with uniform cell areas (Rao *et al.*, 1984). It is interesting that in this same study decreased cell density was not found to be associated with postoperative decompensation.

Endothelial polymegethism may be due to long-term corneal hypoxia (Schoessler, 1987), or it may be due to what Efron and Ang (1990) term hypercapnia, that is, the accumulation of carbon dioxide trapped under the lens which in turn leads to acidosis effects.

Suppurative keratopathy

Most of the published literature reports an equal incidence of this with hard and daily worn soft contact lenses. 'Catarrhal' ulcers do occur and must be distinguished. Fungal and acanthamoebic infections can both occur and the diagnosis and treatment is that outlined in Chapter 13. Infiltrates resulting from three and nine o'clock keratopathy are easily differentiated clinically from sterile ulcers (see Figure 12.13). They are often raised.

Nodular episcleritis

The author has noted the occurrence of this condition in association with hard corneal lens wear on a number of occasions. It occurs in the medial aspect of the episclera adjacent to the limbus in the three and nine o'clock zones (Figure 12.23). It occurs in the absence of pre-existing pingueculae.

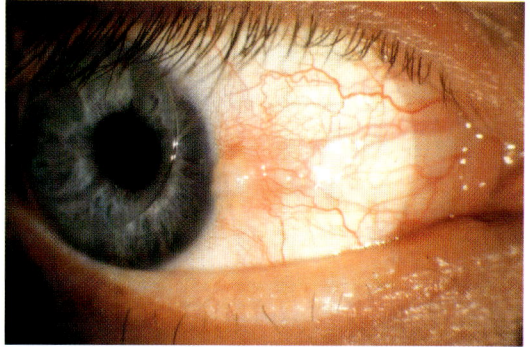

Figure 12.23 Nodular episcleritis associated with hard corneal lens wear

Treatment

The condition disappears in a day or two on the instillation of strong steroid drops such as dexamethasone 0.1%, three times daily.

Giant papillary conjunctivitis

This condition will be dealt with more fully in the section on soft contact lenses. The appearances are similar with hard and soft contact lenses. However, hard lens giant papillary conjunctivitis usually starts in the middle of the tarsal plate and moves to the zone adjacent to the lid margin (Zone 3) more rapidly than it moves to the zone adjacent to the tarsal fold (the junctional conjunctiva) (see Chapter 13).

Giant papillary conjunctivitis has been shown to occur in 10.5% of wearers of hard corneal lenses after a period of five years' wear (Korb *et al.*, 1980).

In the case of the hard corneal lens, trauma is probably the main causative factor. The condition can sometimes be resolved if a hard corneal contact lens is refitted to centralize rather than have lens lid attachment, but this is not always possible.

Stenson (1982) has reported three cases of focal giant papillary conjunctivitis from retained contact lenses (all rigid gas permeable). In all three patients the simple removal of the retained lens was sufficient to reverse the pathology. He pointed out that the focal nature of the changes observed in these patients as well as those cases occurring postoperatively, from exposed suture edges, would point towards an important direct mechanical aetiological factor in giant papillary conjunctivitis.

The plastic, contrary to accepted notions, has been shown to have antigenic potential (Heggers, Talmage and Barnes, 1978), but in order to have this potential it must be stressed. This stress may be produced by the continual movement of the upper lid against the surface of the lens, thus, in some way, changing the surface properties of the lens plastic. Allansmith and Ross (1988) have suggested that the lens, as a foreign body, grinds antigen against the conjunctiva, thus initiating the hypersensitivity response, and suggests a common immunological basis for giant papillary conjunctivitis and vernal conjunctivitis.

Giant papillary conjunctivitis may be localized or generalized as is the case in soft contact lenses and may induce a secondary ptosis. It is often asymptomatic in the hard corneal lens wearer, in contrast to giant papillary conjunctivitis associated with soft contact lens wear. Characteristic features of the soft lens disease are itch after removal and lens displacement, but these problems are seldom experienced in hard corneal lens disease. Discharge, however, is a feature.

Treatment

In attempting to eradicate hard lens disease an effort can be made to centralize the lens, but failing this the patient can be fitted with soft lenses, following an interim period in gas permeable lenses which help to stabilize the refraction. Where either the lens fit cannot be altered, or a soft lens cannot be introduced, as, for example, in keratoconus, topical medication may be helpful. Sodium cromoglycate has been shown to be effective (Matter, Rahi and Buckley, 1985), but is not curative while the lens continues to be worn. It will soon be superseded by other commercially available mast cell stabilizers of considerably greater potency. Clinical trials are already being carried out to assess the role of these agents in giant papillary conjunctivitis. The tetracycline group of drugs are helpful in diminishing the symptoms at this stage but they are not curative. They diminish the discharge and the hyperaemia of the conjunctiva. This can be helpful while the lens type is being changed. The mode of action of the tetracycline is not known, but it has been shown to have actions remote from its purely antibiotic function (Elewski *et al.*, 1983). It has also been shown to be concentrated in the goblet cells and the mucous coat of the external eye (Dilly and Mackie, 1981).

Tetracyclines can be given as oxytetracycline 250 mg twice daily or doxycycline 100 mg on alternate days over a course of many weeks. The latter drug has a much more convenient dosage schedule and does not have to be taken in the absence of milk or milk products. It is useful when there is gastrointestinal upset associated with tetracycline. It is, however, considerably more expensive.

Korb *et al.* (1983) found that when 15 keratoconic patients with this disease treated their hard lenses by soaking them for at least six hours in papain, after removal and cleaning at night, there was an increase in the wearing time in nine patients and diminished symptoms of mucus and itching in 12. In 13 control, lens-wearing keratoconic patients, three had a decrease, four had an increase and six had no change in wearing time. One had a diminution of symptoms.

Local steroids are seldom justified because of their hazards. The patient may become steroid dependent while he or she wears contact lenses.

It is important to realize that conjunctival scarring is seldom a feature of giant papillary conjunctivitis even after many years of hard contact lens wear. The author has repeatedly seen cases in which complete resolution of conjunctival signs has occurred, but such resolution may take one or two years. What scarring he has seen has been associated with ocular prostheses in the presence of anophthalmia. He does not consider the white heads of giant papillae to be scarring but rather hyaline degeneration and these white heads, in his experience, ultimately resolve.

Pseudochalazion

Sebag and Albert (1982) have supplied case reports and reviewed the literature on this phenomenon, where the hard contact lens imbeds itself into the upper lid and has to be removed sugically. The lens is usually one which has been deemed to have been lost and it is only when a swelling develops that its presence comes to light.

Ptosis

Unilateral ptosis occurs in some long-term wearers of hard corneal lenses in the absence of any other signs. The author has seen three referred patients who have undergone surgery without success while continuing to wear their hard corneal lenses. It does not appear that any new fitting philosophy with hard corneal lenses will eliminate the ptosis, but refitting with soft contact lenses has been very successful in the author's experience. Sometimes the ptosis is caused by a levator disinsertion, in which case a levator reatachment procedure is necessary. Epstein and Putterman (1981) have reported ptosis in hard and soft contact lens wearers and described bilateral cases. The bilateral ptosis, which develops in a number of long-term wearers of hard corneal lenses, often goes unnoticed by both the patient and his acquaintances. It is only when the patient is refitted with soft contact lenses that the previous heavy lidded appearance is noted to have disappeared.

Sheldon *et al.* (1979) have described both giant papillary conjunctivitis and ptosis in a contact lens wearer. In unilateral giant papillary conjunctivitis it is not uncommon to see some degree of ptosis on the affected side.

References

ALLANSMITH, M.R. and ROSS, R.N. (1988) Treatment of giant papillary conjunctivitis. *Transactions of the British Contact Lens Association International Conference*, 38–42. *BCLA Journal*, 1988, 5

BERGMANSON, J.P.G. and CHU, L.W.F (1982) Corneal response to rigid contact lens wear. *British Journal of Ophthalmology*, **66**, 667–675

BOURNE, W.M., BRUBAKER, R.F. and O'FALLAN, W.M. (1979) Use of air to decrease endothelial cell loss during intraocular lens implantation. *Archives of Ophthalmology*, **97**, 1473–1475

CARLSON, K.H., BOURNE, W.M. and BRUBAKER, R.F. (1988) Effect of long-term contact lens wear on corneal endothelial cell morphology and function. *Investigative Ophthalmology and Visual Science*, **29**, 2, 185–193

DILLY, P.N. and MACKIE, I.A. (1981) Surface changes in the anaesthetic conjunctiva in man, with special reference to the production of mucus from a non-goblet-cell source. *British Journal of Ophthalmology*, **65**, 12, 833–842

EFRON, N. and ANG, J.H.B. (1990) Corneal hypoxia and hypercapnia during contact lens wear. *Optometry and Visual Science*, **67**, 7, 512–521

ELEWSKI, B.E., LAMB, B.A.J., SAMS, W.M. and GAMMON, W.R. (1983) In vivo suppression of neutrophil chemotaxis by systemically and topically administered tetracycline. *Journal of the American Academy of Dermatology*, **8**, 807–812

EPSTEIN, G. and PUTTERMAN, A.M. (1981) Acquired blepharoptosis secondary to contact lens wear. *American Journal of Ophthalmology*, **91**, 634–639

HEGGERS, J.P., TALMAGE, J.P. and BARNES, S.T. (1978) Cellular immune response to methylmethacrylate in experimentally sensitized guinea pigs. *Military Medicine*, **143**, 192–195

HOLDEN, B.A., MERTZ, G.W. and GUILLON, M. (1980) Corneal swelling response of the aphakic eye. *Investigative Ophthalmology and Visual Science*, **19** (11), 1394–1397

KORB, D.R. (1962) Corneal transparency with emphasis on the phenomenon of central circular clouding. *Encyclopaedia of Contact Lens Practice* (Haynes, P.R., ed). Bernell Enterprises, South Bend, Indiana, USA, **4**, Appendix B, pp. 106–116

KORB, D.R., ALLENSMITH, M.R., GREINER, J., HENRIQUES, A.S., RICHMOND, P. and FINNEMORE, V. (1980) Prevalence of conjunctival changes in wearers of hard contact lenses. *American Journal of Ophthalmology*, **90**, 336–341

KORB, D.R. and EXFORD, J.M. (1968) The phenomenon of central circular clouding. *Journal of the American Optometric Association*, **39**, 3, 223–230

KORB, D.R., RICHMOND, P.R. and HERMAN, J.P. (1980) Physiological response of the cornea to hydrogel lenses before and after cataract extraction. *Journal of the American Optometric Association*, **51**, 3, 267–270

KORB, D.R., GREINER, J.V., FINNEMORE, V.M. and ALLANSMITH, M.R. (1983) Treatment of contact lenses with papain. *Archives of Ophthalmology*, **101**, 48–50

LANSCHE, R.F. and LEE, R.C. (1960a) Acute complications from corneal contact lenses. A recurring and serious problem in the command. *Medical Bulletin of the USA Army in Europe*, **17**, 236–544

LANSCHE, R.F. and LEE, R.C. (1960b) Acute complications from present day corneal contact lenses. *Archives of Ophthalmology*, **64**, 275–285

LEMP, M.A., HOLLY, F.J., IWATU, S. and DOHLMAN, C.H. (1971) The precorneal tear film. Factors in spreading and maintaining a continuous tear film over the corneal surface. *Archives of Ophthalmology*, **83**, 89–94

LITT, M., WOLF, D.P. and KHAN, M.A. (1977) Functional aspects of mucus rheology. In *Mucus in Health and Disease* (Elstin, M. and Parker, D.V., eds). Plenum Press, New York, pp. 191–201

MACKIE, I.A. (1966) Lesions at the corneal limbus at 3 o'clock and 9 o'clock in association with the wearing of contact lenses. In *Contact Lenses, Symposium in Munich – Feldafing*. 20th International Congress of Ophthalmology, Munich, 1966. S. Karger, Munich

MACKIE, I.A. (1971) Localized corneal drying in association with dellen, pterygia and related lesions. *Transactions of the Ophthalmological Society of the UK*, **91**, 129–145

MACRAE, S.M., MATSUDA, M. and YEE, R. (1985) The effect of long term hard contact lens wear on the corneal endothelium. *CLAO Journal*, **11**, 4, 322–326

MANDELL, R.B., POLSE, K.A. and FATT, I. (1970) Corneal swelling caused by contact lens wear. *Archives of Ophthalmology*, **83**, 3–9

MARSH, R.J. and MARSHALL, J. (1982) Treatment of lipid keratopathy with the argon laser. *British Journal of Ophthalmology*, **66** (2), 127–135

MATTER, M., RAHI, A.H.S. and BUCKLEY, R.J. (1985) Sodium cromoglycate in the treatment of contact lens-associated giant papillary conjunctivitis. *Proceedings of the 7th Congress of the European Society of Ophthalmology, 1984.* Yliopistopaino, Helsinki, 1985

MILLODOT, M. (1978a) Effect of long term wear of hard contact lenses on corneal sensitivity. *Archives of Ophthalmology*, **96**, 1225–1227

MILLODOT, M. (1978b) Long term wear of hard contact lenses and corneal integrity. *Contacto*, **22**, 7–12

NIRANKARI, V.S., KARESH, J., LAKHANPAL, V. and RICHARDS, R.D. (1983) Deep stromal vascularisation associated with cosmetic daily wear contact lenses. *Archives of Ophthalmology*, **101**, 46–47

PHILLIPS, C.I. (1990) Contact lenses and corneal deformation: cause, correlate or co-incidence? *Acta Ophthalmologica*, **68**, 661–668

PONDER, E. and KENNEDY, W.P. (1927) On the act of blinking. *Quarterly Journal of Experimental Physiology*, **18**, 89–110

RAO, G.N., SHAW, E.L., ARTHUR, E.J. *et al.* (1979) Endothelial cell morphology and corneal deturgescence. *Annals of Ophthalmology*, **11**, 885–899

RAO, G.N., AQUAVELLA, J.V., GOLDBERG, S.H. *et al.* (1984) Pseudophakia bullous keratopathy. Relationship to preoperative corneal endothelial status. *Ophthalmology*, **91**, 1135–1140

SCHOESSLER, J.P. (1987) The corneal endothelium after 20 years of PMMA contact lens wear. *CLAO Journal*, **13**, 3, 157–160

SCHOESSLER, J.P. and WOLOSCHAK, M.J. (1981) Corneal endothelium in veteran PMMA contact lens wearers. *International Contact Lens Clinic*, **8**, 19–25

SEBAG, J. and ALBERT, D.M. (1982) Pseudochalazion of the upper lid due to hard contact lens imbedding – case reports and a literature review. *Ophthalmic Surgery*, **13**, 634–636

SHELDON, L., BIEDNER, B., GELTMAN, C. *et al.* (1979) Giant papillary conjunctivitis and ptosis in a contact lens wearer. *Journal of Pediatric Ophthalmology and Strabismus*, **16**, 136–137

SMELSER, G.K. and CHEN, D.K. (1955) Physiological changes in the cornea induced by contact lenses. *Archives of Ophthalmology*, **53**, 676–679

STAINER, G.A., BRIGHTBILL, F.S., HOLM, P. and LAUX, D. (1981) The development of pseudo pterygia in hard contact lens wearers. *Contact Intraocular Lens Medical Journal*, **7**, 1, 1–4

STENSON, S. (1982) Focal giant papillary conjunctivitis from retained contact lenses. *Annals of Ophthalmology*, **14**, 9, 881–885

STOCKER, E.G. and SCHOESSLER, J.P. (1985) Corneal endothelial megathism induced by PMMA wear. *Investigative Ophthalmology and Visual Science*, **26**, 6, 857–863

13

Adverse reactions to soft contact lenses

Introduction

Adverse reactions to soft contact lenses are usually quite different from those of hard contact lenses. Soft contact lenses contain water and often solutes other than sodium chloride. They usually move very little on the eye and therefore do not interfere with blinking mechanisms. Unlike hard corneal lenses they bestride the limbus. All soft contact lenses interfere with the uptake of oxygen by the cornea. This results, to a lesser or greater extent, in swelling of the cornea which is related to corneal oedema.

Corneal oedema

The oxygen permeability of soft contact lenses is roughly linearly proportional to their water content (Refojo, 1979) (Figure 13.1). The oxygen transmission of these lenses is inversely proportional to their thickness and the latter relationship is not linear (Figures 13.2 and 13.3). The force that drives oxygen across contact lenses is the difference in partial pressures in front and at the back of the lens. Thus, the oxygen transmission of soft contact lenses will vary with the partial pressure in the ambient air. Thus, in cities like Denver or Mexico City, where the altitude is high, lenses which function well at sea level may give problems related to corneal oxygenation.

Furthermore, in closed eye conditions which are encountered in the use of therapeutic soft contact lenses and cosmetic extended wear soft contact lenses, the partial pressure of oxygen coming from the palpebral conjunctival vessels

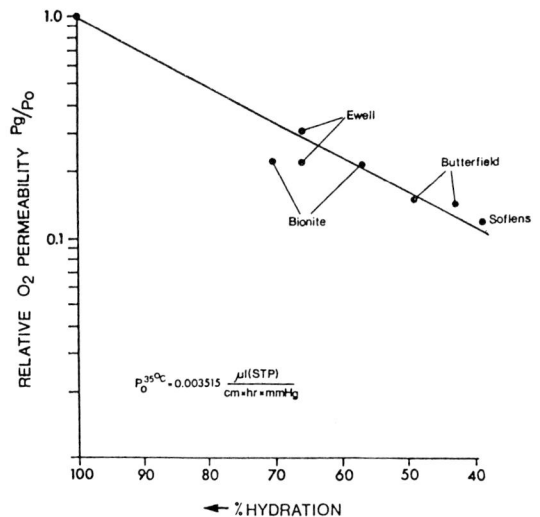

Figure 13.1 Linear relationship of relative permeability to oxygen and percentage hydration of hydrogel contact lenses at 35 °C. (Based on data from Fatt and St Helen) (Refojo, 1979)

will be much reduced. Refojo (1979) has graphically represented the oxygenation of the cornea, as a percentage of the minimum requirement before swelling starts, across hydrogel lenses of different hydration and thickness for open eye conditions (Figure 13.2) and closed eye conditions (Figure 13.3).

The volume increase in the cornea caused by oedema is proportional to the increase in corneal thickness and this increase in corneal thickness can be used as an index. Low levels of stromal oedema, say up to a 5% increase, can only be detected by a high resolution pachometer, but after a 5% increase striae begin to appear in

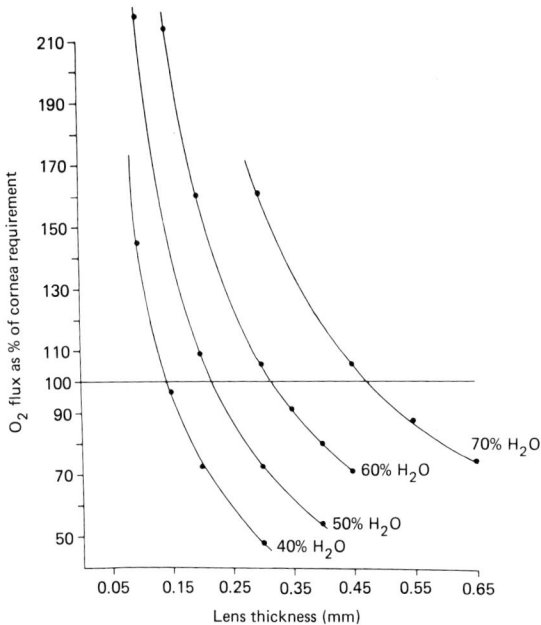

Figure 13.2 Open eye conditions. Oxygenation of the cornea across hydrogel lenses of diverse hydrations and thicknesses (Refojo, 1979)

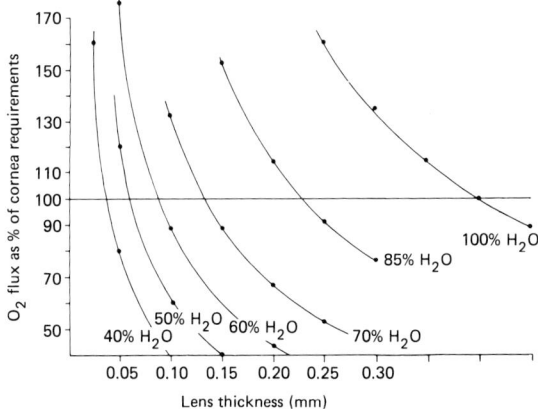

Figure 13.3 Closed eye conditions. Oxygenation of the cornea across hydrogel lenses of diverse hydrations and thicknesses. (Curve for 100% H_2O hydration represents hypothetical lenses made of a static layer of water.) (Refojo, 1979)

Descemet's membrane. These are fine greyish-white vertical lines which are easily missed unless a special search is made of the posterior cornea. Their presence is a source of concern, especially in patients with extended wear soft contact lenses.

Folds (or undulations) in Descemet's membrane appear when the degree of linear swelling of the cornea reaches 10 to 12%. These are an indication for cessation of wear and immediate removal and discontinuance of that particular lens. When the swelling exceeds 15% the cornea becomes hazy and there is a loss of visual acuity. Greater degrees of swelling result in bullous keratopathy.

In contradistinction to the case of scleral lens wearers, typical multicoloured haloes of the glaucomatous type are seldom reported in soft contact lens wearers. A few patients, however, volunteer this symptom, often with low levels of corneal oedema. They are usually middle-aged wearers of plus powered (and therefore centrally thick) soft contact lenses.

Klyce (1981) has explained the aetiology of contact lens induced stromal oedema in terms of alterations in epithelial metabolism. Oxygen availability to the cornea is restricted by contact lenses and in order to conserve energy the corneal epithelium begins to respire anaerobically. Lactate, which is a by-product of anaerobic metabolism, increases in concentration and moves posteriorly into the corneal stroma. This creates an osmotic load which is balanced by a movement of water into the stroma, resulting in oedema. There is also the factor of the accumulation of carbon dioxide under a contact lens and its potential toxic effect on the cornea (Bonanno and Polse, 1987).

The soft contact lens has a water content by weight of anything from 38% to 85% and it acts as a sponge which is applied to the eye on a long-term basis. This means that small amounts of chemicals, be they contaminants or contained in the solutions used for sterilization, can, because of their long time of application, have a significant effect on the cornea and conjunctiva, even when in great dilution. It is often difficult to identify contaminants in contact lenses and it is also difficult to aportion the blame to chemicals or to the soft contact lenses themselves.

There is also the factor of immunological reaction, in the cornea and conjunctiva, to lens material, lens contents such as chemicals and waste products. There is, in addition, trauma, and the latter can give a quasi-immunological reaction.

Finally, there is infection with microorganisms which may be related to the microtrauma which soft contact lenses produce and the fact that organisms actually adhere to soft lenses (see Chapter 9).

Corneal complications

Acute hypoxic keratopathy

Patients who sleep in soft contact lenses not intended for extended wear, or who sleep in extended wear lenses which do not satisfy the oxygen demands of their particular corneas, at that time, may awake with painful red eyes. Only one eye may be affected when both have been stressed in the same way. If the lens has been removed on awakening there may only be slight corneal epithelial oedema and slight stromal infiltration by the time the patient is seen. This condition soon clears without treatment.

In the case of a patient wearing an extended wear lens which has not been removed before being seen by the ophthalmologist the signs may be much more severe. The lens often appears to be adherent to the cornea. There is diffuse stromal oedema with folds in Descemet's membrane and often anterior chamber flare. In severe cases a sterile hypopyon may be present. This is the so-called 'tight lens syndrome'. Whether it is caused by a tight soft lens is a matter of debate.

Treatment

Dark glasses may be all that is necessary in the mild case. In the more severe case, where the lens is still in situ, some sterile saline should be instilled in the eye and the lens then removed. Epithelial loss will demand the instillation of a broad spectrum antibiotic ointment, such as gentamicin, or tobramycin and the application of an eye pad and firm two inch (5 cm) crepe bandage. Flare or a sterile hypopyon is an indication for the use of a mydriatic, such as cyclopentolate 1%, together with topical steroid drops such as prednisolone acetate 1% or dexamethasone 0.1% at two hourly intervals.

Acute toxic epitheliopathy

This can be seen after the enzyme treatment of soft contact lenses where the enzyme has not been washed off properly. It is, in this case, probably due to papain. There is pain when the lenses are inserted and examination reveals a punctate epitheliopathy. The pain and the kerato-pathy may last for two days. Another common cause is hydrogen peroxide.

Treatment

Dark glasses may be all that is necessary, but in severe cases a pad and bandage may be indicated. Topical antibiotic drops are usually prescribed.

Central focal epithelial necrosis

This complication is seen intermittently in wearers of soft contact lenses and usually after a number of hours of wear. The lens starts to become uncomfortable, much in the same way as a hard corneal lens which is producing anoxia. There may be related flushing of the face. Examination of the eye shows areas of corneal epithelial necrosis ('mush') (Figure 13.4) which may or may not be associated with gaps in the epithelium (mush and pits) (Figure 13.5). A tag of epithelium is often seen, reminiscent of operculae seen in association with retinal holes (Figure 13.6). This condition has not been reported in the literature. It would appear to be an anoxic phenomenon because removal of the soft contact lens produces immediate relief of symptoms although the signs remain for a number of hours. The complication seems to be associated with a particular lens. Changing to an identical soft lens of the same material may remedy the situation. It is more commonly seen with thick soft lenses and is sometimes a complication of aphakic soft lenses. The patient may have good days and bad days for this complication to occur.

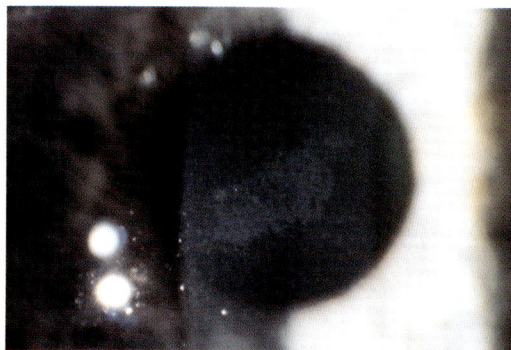

Figure 13.4 Central focal epithelial necrosis ('mush')

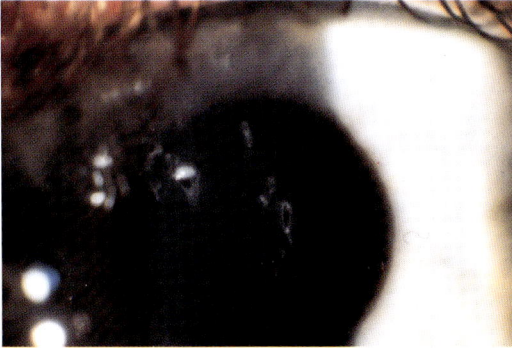

Figure 13.5 Central focal epithelial necrosis ('mush') with epithelial gaps (pits). This is the other eye of the patient in Figure 13.4

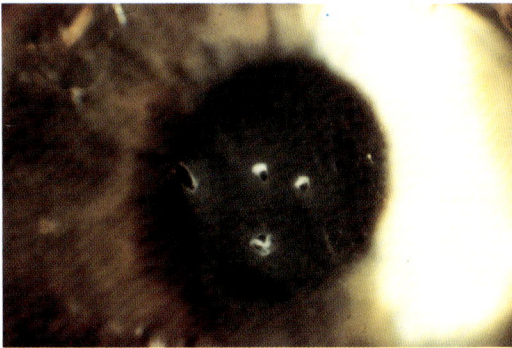

Figure 13.7 Peripheral focal epithelial necrosis. The lesion occurs superiorly in the cornea, is often arcuate and stains with fluorescein

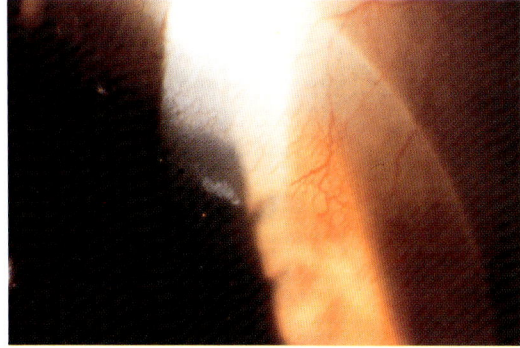

Figure 13.6 Central focal epithelial necrosis ('mush') with epithelial gaps (pits) and tags (operculae)

Treatment

A thinner, soft contact lens should be fitted, or, if the patient is hypermetropic, a lens of higher water content.

Peripheral focal arcuate epithelial necrosis

This complication, like the central form described above, may be due to corneal anoxia or perhaps the compression of the epithelium by the thicker edge of a minus lens. The symptoms experienced are less marked than that of the central form of epithelial necrosis and usually consist of only a slight irritation.

The lesion is white or greyish in colour and granular in appearance. It occurs near the limbus, is always above and is frequently arcuate in shape. It is often seen in association with the thickened peripheral area of a minus soft lens (Figure 13.7). It may occur on some days on which the lens is worn, and not on others. It may occur repeatedly with one lens. This lens may be changed and, after a period of time, the patient may revert to the lens which caused it without any problems. The danger of peripheral focal epithelial necrosis is that it may incite local superficial vascularization and scar formation.

Horowitz, Lin and Chew (1985) described this complication in 13 patients (10 women and three men, 16 to 39 years old) most of whom had tight eyelids. They assessed this by seeing how easy it was to evert the upper lid. In some cases the problem was unilateral and in others bilateral. No permanent keratopathy developed as a result of this complication, probably because of early detection and treatment of the problem. The condition is sometimes referred to as a superior epithelial arcuate lesion (SEAL), especially in the Australian literature.

Hine, Back and Holden (1987) found that 20 (14%) of 150 hyperopic and myopic presbyopes fitted with daily wear high water content lenses developed these lesions either unilaterally or bilaterally within one month. Fifty per cent of these arcuate lesions were resolvable by altering lens factors and/or care regimen.

Hine, Back and Holden (1987) put forward

three popular theories for their cause: (1) mechanical chafing of the limbal area; (2) hypoxia exacerbated by the position and pressure of the eyelid; and (3) the thickness of the lens edge. Their studies showed that the patient's age was an important factor, the presbyope suffering most.

Treatment

A thinner contact lens, front optic reduction, a back peripheral curve or a different make of soft lens may be tried in order to eradicate the condition. Hine, Back and Holden (1987) suggest that the patient be rested for seven days and then put back into the same lenses and followed. They found that there was then a 37% chance of the problem resolving without the need to do anything further. This is in accord with the author's observation that, just as in the case of the central form of epithelial necrosis, the penultimate contact lens which caused the peripheral arcuate lesion often does not cause it when its wear is resumed. Happily, patients are aware that something is wrong when these lesions occur and should be encouraged to seek advice.

Desiccation staining

Orsborn and Zantos (1988) performed several studies comparing very thin, high water content to very thin, low water content contact lenses. They also compared very thin, high water content lenses to thicker, high water content contact lenses. In addition, they explored the effects of ambient humidity and lens movements. They found that the incidence and severity of corneal staining and erosions was greatest with very thin, high water content lenses. The corneal staining did not correlate with patients' symptoms, nor the amount of movement or dehydration of the lens on the eye. Their results also showed that staining, which developed in a low relative humidity environment, disappeared when the patients were placed in a high relative humidity environment.

They concluded that thin (that is 0.05 Tc) high water (i.e. 70–75%) lenses cannot be used to increase the oxygen transmission to the eye.

Inferior closure staining

This stain can sometimes be seen on removing a soft lens and instilling fluorescein. It occurs in the intermediate zone of the cornea below. Its incidence in asymptomatic soft contact lens wearers has not been studied. It appears that it may be symptomatic in some.

Kline, DeLuca and Fishberg (1979) attribute this stain to incomplete closure of the upper lid on blinking. They state that lid pressure causes lens buckling which stagnates the tears, leading to corneal disruption.

Thimerosal keratopathy

This is a quite distinct clinical entity seen in association with the use of thimerosal in sterilizing, cleaning and soaking solutions (Wilson, Schlitzeer and Ahearn, 1981; Mondino, Salamon and Zaidman, 1982; Wright and Mackie, 1982). Thimerosal is commonly used because of its fungistatic action and because it does not react with the polymers used in contact lenses.

The reaction to thimerosal is one of hypersensitivity which may have been instituted by injected vaccines, such as those for diphtheria, tetanus and pertussis which commonly contain it.

The basis of this keratopathy is probably abnormal differentiation of limbal stem cells (Thoft, 1989). 'Stem cells', or progenitor cells for the corneal epithelial surface, is a concept introduced by Schermer, Galvin and Sun (1986).

The initial symptoms of the epitheliopathy are redness and burning of the eyes and progressive reduction of wearing time. Discharge from the eyes is uncommon at this time. The vision is not affected while the patient wears the soft lenses, since they restore the integrity of the front surface of the optical system, but the vision in spectacles is impaired. Many patients do not possess current spectacles and will be unaware of this important symptom.

The symptoms usually develop one to two years after exposure to thimerosal. Some sensitive patients present with very early disease while other stoical patients may have advanced corneal destructive changes when they are first seen. Exposure to thimerosal need only be intermittent – once a week while the patient wears his lenses to play football, or the housewife goes out for dinner with her husband. It is important to enquire what preparations are being used with the contact lenses. Thimerosal may be introduced to the eyes by a lens cleaner which is being used once a week, or even by an occasional drop of medication which is being used, for example, to whiten red eyes. The characteristic signs are discussed below.

1 Superior limbitis

A cellular, swollen, superior limbus which takes fluorescein and Bengal Rose stain is a valuable early sign (Figure 13.8). This sign may be present in association with what is only a mild and non-confluent erosive epitheliopathy.

2 Erosive corneal epitheliopathy

This epitheliopathy (Figure 13.9) consists of dense confluent erosions which are usually maximal in the upper half of the cornea unless the condition is of such severity that the whole cornea is evenly involved. The superior location is a valuable diagnostic sign and serves to differentiate the condition from other diseases which cause erosive epitheliopathy, such as staphylococcal disease and dry eyes, where the erosions are usually maximal in the lower half of the cornea.

In early cases, where the diagnosis of an epitheliopathy is in doubt, it is helpful to look for corneal staining subsequent to repeated fluorescein instillations (sequential staining) as described by Korb and Herman (1979) in another context.

This may show a much more extensive epitheliopathy than is visible in a cursory examination with fluorescein. The fluorescein is instilled at five minute intervals for up to 30 minutes. Normal corneas do not stain.

3 Corneal vascularization

The pannus is typically seen coming from above and may assume a florid appearance in advanced cases, even progressing so far as to form tufts at the end of vessels (Figure 13.10). Superficial vascularization may be seen entering the cornea from all areas (Figure 13.11). This superficial vascularization has been confused with that which appears as a result of corneal hypoxia.

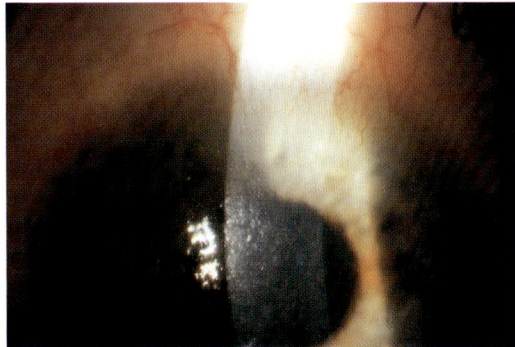

Figure 13.9 Thimerosal keratopathy. Dense, confluent epithelial erosions, maximal in the upper half of the cornea

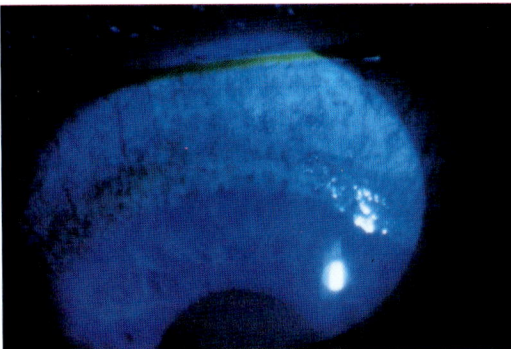

Figure 13.8 Thimerosal keratopathy. A cellular and staining limbus above (fluorescein with cobalt light)

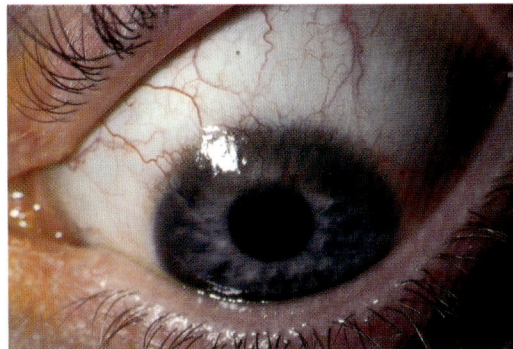

Figure 13.10 Thimerosal keratopathy. Florid pannus in an advanced case with tufting at the end of vessels

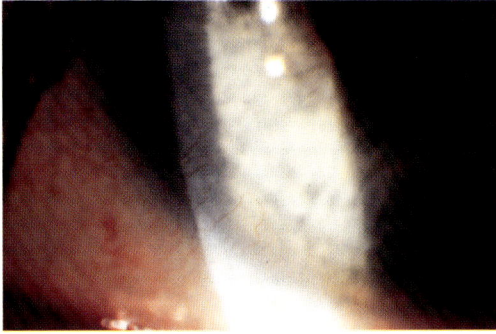

Figure 13.11 Thimerosal keratopathy. Superficial vascularization of the cornea in all areas

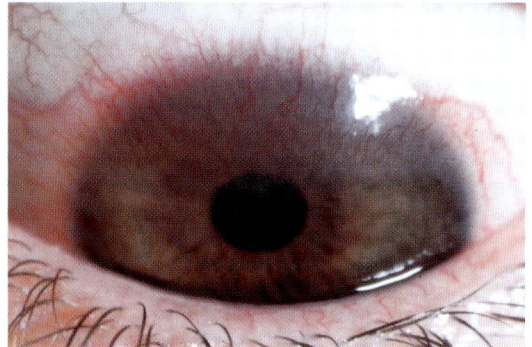

(a)

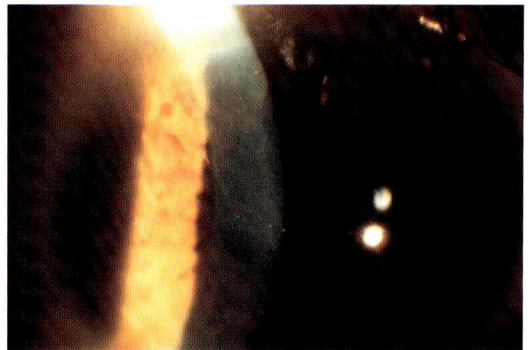

(b)

Figure 13.12 Thimerosal keratopathy. Aprons of dysplastic epithelium with blood vessels (a) and without blood vessels (b)

4 Corneal epithelial dysplasia

An apron of dysplastic epithelium may stretch down from the superior limbus, with blood vessels (Figure 13.12a), or without blood vessels (Figure 13.12b). This dysplasia does not totally resolve with time after the cessation of exposure to thimerosal. In mild disease, it may typically be seen after the episode as areas of opaque epithelium stretching down from the superior limbus in tongue-like processes (Figure 13.13). This sign is useful in making a retrospective diagnosis when the erosive epitheliopathy has resolved. It may be a few months after cessation of lens wear before the patient presents.

Occasionally, dendritic forms are seen on the cornea (Margulies and Mannis, 1983; Udell *et al.*, 1985) (Figure 13.14). These are peripheral, pigmented and flat and quite unlike those seen in herpes simplex or zoster.

On rare occasions the epithelial dysplasia progresses at an alarming rate so that the cornea is covered by a membrane of opaque tissue. When this happens there is no resolution. The stroma then slowly opacifies (Figure 13.15), confusing a retrospective diagnosis. The author has seen four patients, blinded in one eye, from this condition. Strangely, thimerosal corneal epitheliopathy is invariably asymmetrical.

5 Conjunctivitis

No special features are seen in the conjunctiva except hyperaemia and oedema. In particular, follicles, papillae and conjunctival infiltration are not seen. This is another important diagnostic feature. However, these signs may be present as part of another pathological entity related to contact lens wear and developing concurrently with the thimerosal hypersensitivity response.

Thimerosal would appear to initiate a Type 1 hypersensitivity reaction in the conjunctiva in some individuals, as evidenced by the findings of Wright and Mackie (1982). However, the corneal and limbal manifestations cannot be explained on this basis. These would appear to be a Type IV reaction. It is probable that Langerhans cells are involved in the corneal disease. These dendritic cells which lie between the corneal epithelial cells and which are analogous to those found in the skin and involved in contact dermatitis, have only recently been described in the cornea (Rodrigues, 1982). They are highly specialized in antigen presentation and may play an important role in inducing contact sensitivity dermatitis (Braathen and Thorsby, 1983). They are capable of inducing a strong proliferative T-cell response to a contact allergen (nickel sulphate) (Braathan, 1980). It has been shown that both the anatomical site where antigen is first encountered by the immune system and the nature of the cells which present the antigen, determine whether a contact sensitivity reaction will ensue and also whether is will be evanescent or long lasting (Ptak *et al.*, 1980).

As has already been stated, thimerosal can give rise to either a Type 1 (immediate) or Type IV (delayed) hypersensitivity reaction. These hypersensitivity reactions can be quite separate, according to an individual's particular response. In other words, if the eye becomes red and uncomfortable soon after thimerosal is inserted, that does not mean that continued exposure will necessarily result in a Type 4 reaction. Vice versa applies. The patients who have gross cellular changes with thimerosal and whose disease is well advanced before diagnosis, probably have no Type 1 response.

Objections may be raised that there is no real evidence of a Type I response in this keratopathy. However, Dr Murat Irkec, in a paper given at the 21st Anniversary Congress of the European Contact Lens Society of Ophthalmologists in London, 1991, showed the tear inflammatory mediator response was increased in patients using thimerosal disinfection techniques and was not increased in patients using either thermal or peroxide disinfection systems. There was a slight increase in leucotriene B_4 and an increase in both leucotriene C_4 and prostaglandin E_2 in the users of thimerosal preserved systems. It may be that those who suffer from thimerosal keratopathy, without much in the way of symptoms, do not get these increases in inflammatory mediator levels.

It would also appear that in some patients the erosive epitheliopathy predominates (see Figure 13.9) while in others it may be the pannus (see Figure 13.10). In a further group it may be the dysplasia which is the main feature (see Figure 13.12). The epithelial erosions disappear and the pannus regresses some months after withdrawal of thimerosal, but the epithelial dysplasia may remain and it is this that is the real danger. The dysplastic opacified epithelium is followed by an opacified stroma (see Figure 13.15), presumably because the epithelium controls the biosynthesis of stromal proteins (Cremer-Bartels, 1977).

The author has observed a few patients who have developed thimerosal hypersensitivity, ceased lens wear or the use of thimerosal and

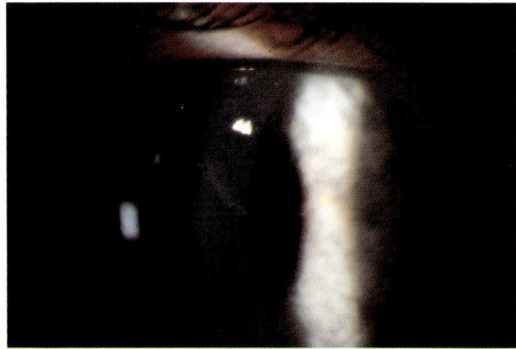

Figure 13.14 Thimerosal keratopathy. Dendritic figures. These are pigmented and flat and quite unlike those seen in herpetic disease

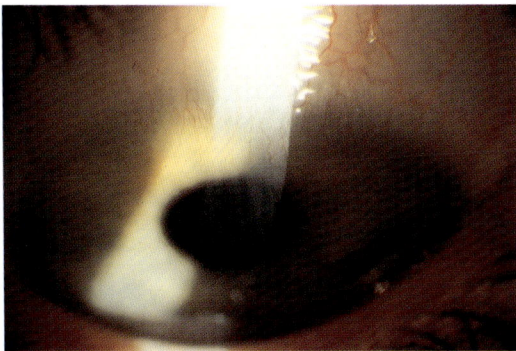

Figure 13.13 Thimerosal keratopathy. Tongue-like processes of opaque epithelium. This is a late feature and may allow a retrospective diagnosis when the erosive epitheliopathy has cleared

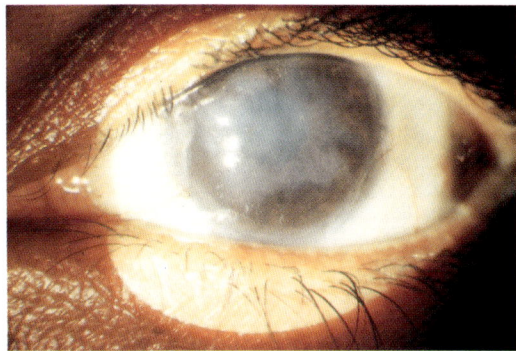

Figure 13.15 Thimerosal keratopathy. The corneal epithelium and stroma are opaque and the eye is blind with a visual acuity of less than 6/60. (Photographed in June, 1991)

then have had one repeated exposure to the preservative after a long period. One such case is illustrated (Figure 13.16). The reaction is intense and fulminating and patients should be warned of this danger.

Treatment

The management of thimerosal epitheliopathy demands the complete withdrawal of thimerosal from any therapeutic or lens care regimen. A search should be made for this ubiquitous preservative in everything which may go into the eye. In the late 1970s when this distinctive keratopathy was not recognized to be due to thimerosal, the author was using prednisolone preserved with thimerosal as treatment. Some symptomatic relief was produced, but the keratopathy continued, leading to stromal thinning and opacification.

The soft lens disinfection method can be changed so that a heat method is used or it can be carried out by a solution system which does not contain thimerosal. In early disease it is not usually necessary to wait for the complete resolution of the physical signs before reinserting the lens. This may take many months. However, florid disease should be allowed to quieten first.

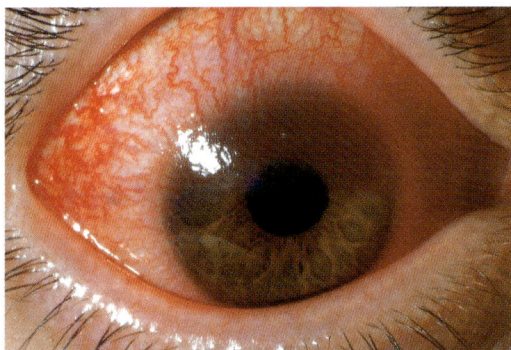

Figure 13.16 Reactivation of thimerosal hypersensitivity after two years. This patient had worn soft contact lenses for four years and had been advised to discontinue their use because of signs of thimerosal hypersensitivity. He was then refitted with rigid gas permeable contact lenses and wore these mainly for sport for two years. He lost one lens before an important football match and went into an optician's shop and purchased a pair of soft lenses. He wore the lenses, which had been soaked in thimerosal solution, once to play the game, and appeared at a hospital casualty department five days later with both eyes in the condition illustrated

Thimerosal does not fix to soft contact lenses and can be removed by, say, ten soakings in fresh normal saline for half an hour each time. So far as medication is concerned, local steroids with the ever present problem of a fresh sensitivity developing to their preservatives have little to offer. If the eyes are particularly hyperaemic and uncomfortable, oxytetracycline 250 mg twice daily or doxycycline 100 mg on alternate days, by mouth, may be used for their anti-inflammatory effect on the conjunctiva.

If there is a total epithelial dysplasia and consequent blindness, the operative procedure advocated by Kenyon and Tseng (1989) can be performed. Their operative technique involves the transfer of two free grafts of limbal tissue (epithelial 'stem cells') from the uninjured or less injured donor eye of the patient, to the severely injured recipient eye, the latter having been prepared by limited conjunctival resection and superficial dissection of fibrovascular pannus without keratectomy (Figure 13.17).

Impression cytology in a selection of the cases, described by Kenyon and Tseng, showed restoration of the corneal epithelial phenotype and regression of goblet cells from the recipient cornea. Three of the 26 consecutive cases they described were of contact lens induced keratopathy. Their results were impressive. The procedure is a modification of the operation of keratoepithelioplasty described by Thoft (1984) and Turgeon *et al.* (1990), whereby healthy limbal epithelium is obtained from fresh donor eyes in which the epithelium is intact and clear.

Preservatives contained in ophthalmic preparations are listed in Appendix 9.III.

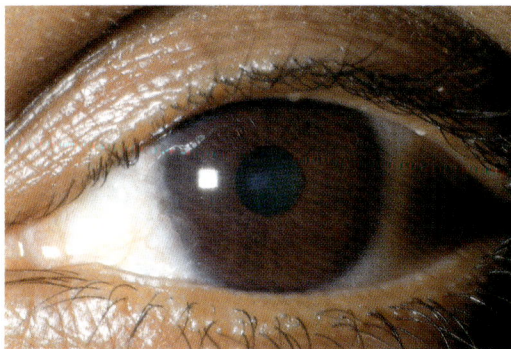

Figure 13.17 The same eye as in Figure 13.15 some months after limbal autograft transplantation and now with a visual acuity of 6/9. (Photographed in May, 1992)

Chronic chemical epitheliopathy

Quite apart from thimerosal, other chemicals used as preservatives or stabilizers in cleaning, wetting and sterilizing solutions may cause an erosive epitheliopathy. This, in turn, can lead to the appearance of peripheral vascularization of the cornea. The end result is seldom the picture described above as seen with thimerosal. The epitheliopathy lasts for a few weeks rather than months. It tends to be generalized rather than maximal above. Limbitis and pannus are rare.

Treatment

The offending chemicals must not be instilled in the eye. It is important to realize that solutions which are said to contain no preservatives may contain stabilizers. This is particularly true of peroxide sterilization systems (see Chapter 9). An alternative method of sterilization is called for, as outlined in Chapter 9.

Preservatives contained in preparations used with soft contact lenses are listed in Appendix 9.II.

Granular epithelial keratopathy

Rosenfeld *et al.* (1990) have described four patients who, using extended wear soft contact lenses for myopia, abruptly developed ocular irritation and injection associated with elevated granular opacities initially confined to the central corneal epithelium (Figure 13.18). Cultures of the granular epithelial lesions were positive for *Pseudomonas aeruginosa* in all patients. Cultures of the contact lenses and lens case solutions grew Pseudomonas species and other Gram-negative organisms. All patients responded to discontinuation of lens wear and frequent topical antibiotics. All recovered baseline visual acuity and three have successfully resumed contact lens wear.

Acute corneal distortion

In this condition the patient usually presents complaining of diminished vision in one eye and it is found that the vision, which has deteriorated to perhaps halfway down the Snellen chart, cannot be improved by over-refraction. There is no discomfort. Removal of the soft contact lens reveals that the vision still cannot be improved to normal with a spectacle refraction. The keratometry is found to be regular and unchanged.

Examination of the red reflex with the ophthalmoscope held at a distance of 25 cm (10 inches) from the eye shows a 'bleb' within the red reflex, something like that seen in keratoconus, but translucent. Slit lamp examination shows no abnormality.

Schanzer *et al.* (1989) have reported the development of irregular corneal astigmatism in three patients who wore annular tinted soft contact lenses on a daily basis for 1.5 to 3 years. There was severe keratometer mire distortion and midperipheral corneal topographical irregularities in four of six eyes. Scanning electron microscopy of four contact lenses revealed physical deformations in three of the lenses, worn on affected eyes. They propose the latent stress vectors were created when the affected contact lenses were tinted and that with usage these matured into physical deformations which induced irregular astigmatism.

Treatment

The condition can be related to an abnormality of the centre of an old, thin soft contact lens and is seen in myopes where the centre is thin. With

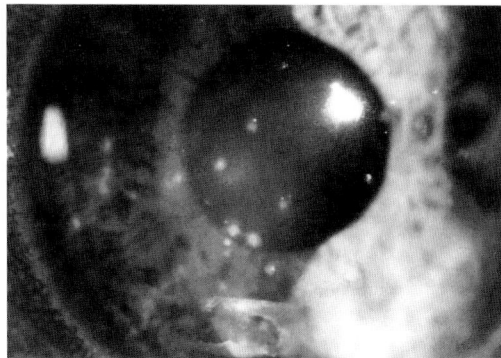

Figure 13.18 Granular epithelial keratopathy. The elevated granular epithelial opacities, on culture, were positive for *Pseudomonas aeruginosa*. (From Rosenfeld, S.I. *et al.* (1990) *American Journal of Ophthalmology*, **109**, 17–22. Published with permission of the *American Journal of Ophthalmology*. Copyright by the Ophthalmic Publishing Company)

discontinuation of lens wear the cornea clears and vision is restored within a few days. The lens should be replaced. Schanzer *et al.* (1989) found that the condition they reported resolved upon discontinuation of the offending contact lens.

Delayed response keratopathy

In this condition the patient who usually wears soft contact lenses without difficulty finds one morning that his vision in contact lenses is slightly smoky, misty or foggy. He either removes the lenses and substitutes spectacles, in which case his vision is still blurred, or continues to wear the lenses for part of the day, in which case the vision becomes more blurred. He has no discomfort at all on this day. On the following day he experiences excruciating pain, usually bilaterally, but occasionally unilaterally. Examination at this time may reveal an oedematous corneal epithelium and stroma, with perhaps epithelial loss (Figure 13.19), but more often than not the epithelium and stroma show little change. There may be faint staining with fluorescein. If the cornea is inspected with the thin beam of the slit lamp the stroma may be seen to be oedematous, but examination is difficult, even with a local anaesthetic. The lids are not oedematous and there is no discharge as there would be in an adenoviral infection. This agonizing condition, coupled with extreme photophobia, usually lasts

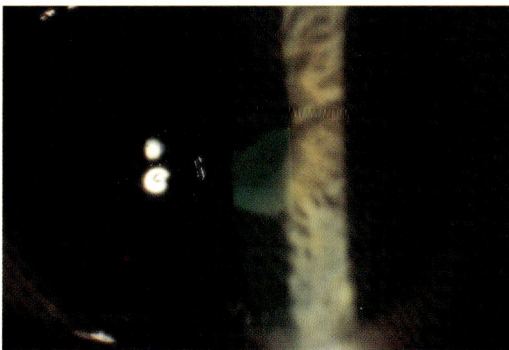

Figure 13.19 Delayed response keratopathy. There is corneal oedema and a circumscribed area of epithelial loss shown with fluorescein staining

for as long as a week and has, in the author's experience, always resolved without any detectable corneal sequelae. The author has seen 26 such patients over a period of 13 years.

The long latent period, during which the only symptom is slight mistiness of vision, together with the stromal oedema and the long period of subsequent severe distress, distinguishes this condition from the syndrome of Lansche and Lee already described as a complication of hard corneal lens wear (Chapter 12). It is unlikely to be caused by anoxia and is probably a toxicity reaction caused by a subtle chemical contamination of the lens. Nevertheless, gas chromatography analysis of the fluid in the contact lens containers of a number of the author's patients has revealed no impurities. In the author's experience it has occurred in members of the same family living together. The condition can recur if the same lens is used again, but does not do so immediately. It is conceivable that some environmental compound in everyday use can contaminate the lens in minute quantities and is active because it is held in contact with the cornea for a long time.

Wright (1982) has described a similar delayed toxic keratopathy in scuba divers which he attributed to the improper use of commercial defogging agents on the divers' masks. The mechanism of delayed keratopathy in response to chemical agents has not been established, but it has been suggested that it is related to changes in nucleic acid function within epithelial cells (Grant, 1974). This would explain the characteristic delay.

Williams (1986) has described such a condition to which he has given the name Soft Contact Lens Toxic Occlusion Phenomenon. Williams described two types of the condition. Type I was like that which has been described here, and type II was of lesser severity. In this type II, the initial subjective symptom was not foggy vision but moderate discomfort and photophobia. Initial punctate staining with oedema limited to the epithelium could be seen and the resulting discomfort severity was much less than with type I.

Williams saw a total of 18 patients with type I from 1979 until he wrote his paper. They ranged in age from 16 to 62 years. Eleven were female and seven were males. Six patients lived in the same house as another of the patients. Some patients had multiple episodes even when the soft lens type was changed. Of 18 patients, 8 had unilateral episodes and 10 had bilateral episodes.

The age of their contact lenses was two weeks to two years.

Williams (1986) had the opportunity to see a few patients on the day when the vision was blurred and the eye was not painful. He saw central corneal oedema. He pointed out that the vision was not so much 'foggy' as 'steam bath' in nature and that no ocular redness or discomfort accompanied this state. This was followed after about 12 hours by a central de-epithelialization in some patients. (The author has observed this in only one patient.) He did not find patching helpful.

Treatment

Atropine 1% drops, double padding and bandaging afford some relief. The reaction does not appear to be influenced in any way by strong topical steroid, for example, dexamethasone 0.1% drops every two hours, but seems to run its course relentlessly over the period of a week. During this time the patient needs reassurance and, perhaps, sedation.

Corneal epithelial microcysts

Brown and Lobascher (1975) first drew attention to the occurrence of corneal epithelial microcysts in wearers of soft contact lenses. These cysts were identified by retroillumination and were commonly present in small numbers. Observed punctate staining spots in their patients were accounted for by microcysts, punctate epithelial erosions and punctate epithelial keratitis.

These signs increased with lens spoilage and were at their greatest with extended wear of the lenses. In these extended wear patients a coarse, subepithelial punctate epithelial keratitis was seen.

Brown and Lobascher were studying aphakic patients wearing Permalens (Pilkington Barnes Hind) high water content lenses worn on an extended basis. Humphreys, Larke and Parrish (1980) also observed microcysts in extended contact lens wearing patients and noted that it took an average of 10 weeks after cessation of lens wear for the microcysts to disappear. In only one of their cases were the microcysts associated with symptoms of discomfort.

Holden (1989) believes that epithelial microcysts are one of the best indicators of chronic extended wear-induced hypoxia and Madigan *et al.* (1990) think that microcysts are dead or ageing cells that are trapped in the epithelium and brought to the surface at a slower rate than normal epithelial cells. Microcysts can also occur with daily wear of hydrogel lenses (Holden *et al.*, 1987).

Grant, Terry and Holden (1990) advocate refitting the patient with higher Dk lenses or even high Dk rigid gas permeable lenses.

Treatment

On occasion the author has been presented with an area in a cornea of a daily wear patient with brightly staining cystic change in the epithelium (Figure 13.20). It has not been his policy to forbid wear, but to change the lens. Ultimately, after a period measured in months, the cystic area has resolved.

Subepithelial haemorrhages

These haemorrhages, which were described in Chapter 12 (see Figure 12.16) as an adverse reaction to hard corneal lenses, also occur in wearers of soft contact lenses. They are usually found where there are pre-existing vessels in association with a cataract wound and the aphakic soft lens is, of necessity, thick.

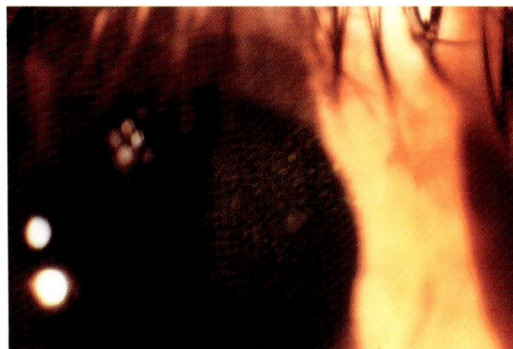

Figure 13.20 Area of gross microcystic epitheliopathy in a soft contact lens wearer. Many of the cysts stain brightly with fluorescein

Treatment

No treatment is necessary.

Limbitis and limbal follicles

Circumcorneal injection is seen from time to time in soft contact lens wearers. It may be localized (Figure 13.21) or involve the whole circumference of the cornea (Figure 13.22). This limbitis is often painful and at least causes discomfort. It would appear to be a short step from this injection to the development of limbal follicles (Figure 13.23) and Trantas' spots. These features in a contact lens wearer have been shown by Meisler, Zaret and Stock (1980) to be an allergic phenomenon. They scraped the corneoscleral limbus and the inferior fornix in one patient. Cytological examination with Giemsa stain revealed epithelial and mono-nuclear cells and eosinophils in the limbal and inferior fornix smears. Additionally, polymorpho-nuclear leucocytes were noted in the smear from the inferior fornix. They compared their observations with limbal disease found in vernal conjunctivitis and concluded that these findings, in relation to giant papillary conjunctivitis, make up a total picture of contact lens induced disease very similar to vernal conjunctivitis. Nevertheless, the author has not seen limbal follicles associated with giant papillary conjunctivitis, has not seen the occurrence of limbal follicles precede the development of giant papillary conjunctivitis and has not known limbal follicles to be a progressive disease such as giant papillary conjunctivitis.

The condition tends to appear for no good reason. It resolves over a week or so, when contact lenses are discontinued, and tends to recur from time to time as the contact lenses are worn. It is cosmetically embarrassing and the eye is somewhat uncomfortable. It is probable that cells with immunological potential are lodged at the limbus and activated by trauma, but chemicals in solutions may play a part. The condition ultimately resolves over a period of months while the lenses continue to be worn.

Treatment

Topical sodium cromoglycate should be of use in the prophylaxis of this condition, but, in fact, the author has not found it to be effective. It may be that new more potent mast cell stabilizers which will be commercially available will be effective.

When the lesion occurs, contact lens wear should be discontinued. The follicles clear rapidly within two days if fluorometholone 0.1% drops are used four times daily. This steroid is chosen because of its minimum effect on intraocular

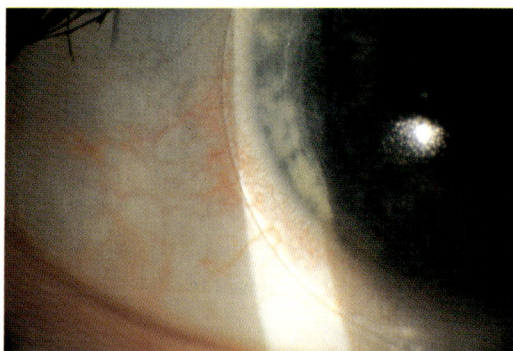

Figure 13.21 Localized circumcorneal injection

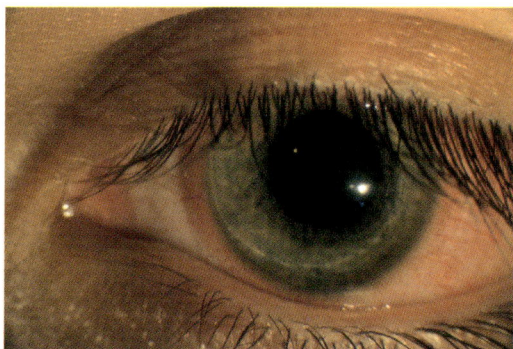

Figure 13.22 Generalized circumcorneal injection

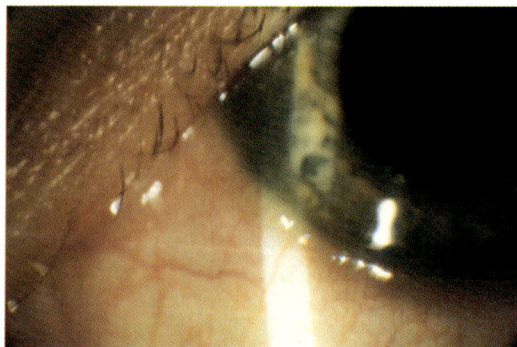

Figure 13.23 Limbal follicles

pressure. When the lesions have resolved contact lens wear can be resumed. To prevent recurrence one drop of fluoromethalone is used each night after the lens is removed. This can be continued for a few weeks. Then the patient is weaned off the drops gradually, first by using them on alternate nights and then, perhaps, once or twice weekly until they are discontinued.

Nummular keratitis

A nummular keratitis (Figure 13.24) is sometimes seen to develop in wearers of soft contact lenses. It usually presents as a red eye. The appearance of the lesions is reminiscent of that seen in herpes zoster ophthalmicus. They are fluffy, round and intrastromal. This is probably a further example of a hypersensitivity reaction in association with soft contact lens wear. The role which chemicals in solutions play in the pathogenesis of this condition has not been assessed.

Nummular keratitis is rare in non-contact lens clinical practice, except in cases of herpes zoster ophthalmicus where a clear history of the attack is usually obtainable and there is dermatological evidence of a past episode. However, the Epstein–Barr virus can cause nummular keratitis (Pinnolis, McCulley and Urman, 1980) and this may not be associated in time with an episode of glandular fever.

Harrer and Rubey (1981) reported a disease resembling nummular keratitis which developed in patients wearing HEMA lenses. The large, disc-shaped, subepithelial opacities were accompanied by pathological changes in the endothe-lium of the peripheral parts of the cornea. They believe that there is an immunological process acting on components of the lenses and the solutions they are cleaned with and kept in. They discuss the differential diagnosis between this disease, Dimmer's nummular keratitis and herpetic corneal disease.

Eggink, Pinckers and Aandekerk (1991) report the appearance of nummular stromal opacities in three patients, associated with the wearing of soft contact lenses of a copolymer of polymethacrylate and polyvinylpyrrolidone and manufactured by Lunelle, France. In all three cases the opacities disappeared – first with a change to gas permeable lenses, secondly with cessation of wear and thirdly with exclusion of thimerosal from the disinfecting regimen. All three patients used a peroxide disinfecting system and stored their lenses in thimerosal and EDTA preserved solutions. They considered the clinical picture to be most consistent with a delayed hypersensitivity reaction.

Treatment

The condition responds quickly to a moderately potent steroid such as gutt. fluoromethalone 0.1% four times daily. However, the residual opacities take many months to disappear and may persist in the long term. There does not seem to be a tendency for the nummular keratitis to recur.

Catarrhal ulcer

Catarrhal ulcers have been shown to be a hypersensitivity phenomenon to staphylococci and may be in this sense related to nummular keratitis. Their diagnosis in non-contact lens wearers is easy. In the contact lens wearer there is always the possibility that one is dealing with a peripheral corneal abscess caused by a potent bacterium or fungus.

Treatment

Since the condition may be a peripheral corneal abscess it should be treated aggressively. Topical steroid, which is adequate for the non-contact lens wearer, is not sufficient when contact lenses are worn. The treatment should anticipate that it

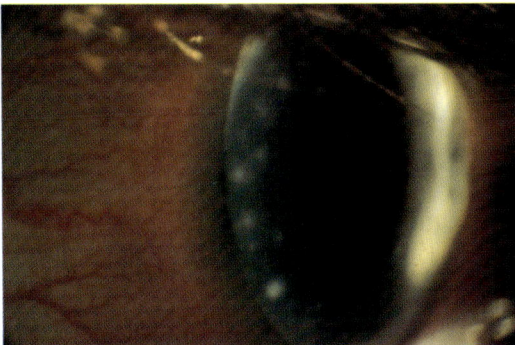

Figure 13.24 Nummular keratitis. There are discrete, fluffy infiltrates in the stroma

is a corneal abscess and broad spectrum antibiotics should be used hourly. If, after six hours, there is no progression of the disease, topical steroid can be used. If there is progression of the disease a corneal scrape should be performed for microscopy and culture and the lesion should be treated as a suppurative keratopathy.

Sterile corneal infiltrates

These stromal infiltrates, which may be more centrally located lesions of the catarrhal ulcer type, or intense expressions of nummular keratitis, are referred to as sterile because corneal cultures prove negative. Stein *et al.* (1988) examined 50 patients to determine whether differences exist between the initial clinical signs and symptoms associated with infected versus sterile corneal infiltrates. Ocular findings were correlated with the results of corneal cultures. Increased pain, discharge, epithelial staining and anterior chamber reaction were associated with infected ulcers. Sterile infiltrates were usually smaller, multiple or arcuate and without significant pain, epithelial staining or anterior chamber reaction.

Treatment

Sterile infiltrates are, by definition, not associated with microbial invasion of the cornea. Nevertheless, every stromal infiltrate should be treated as a suppurative keratitis until proved otherwise by the rapidity of its resolution. Peripheral, focal, arcuate epithelial necrosis (SEALS) and the infiltrates resulting from three and nine o'clock staining are easily identifiable (see Chapter 12) and should not be confused with sterile infiltrates. Sterile infiltrates respond to topical steroid.

Suppurative keratitis

Bacterial keratitis

Over the past several years there have been reports of an alarming increase in serious contact lens related infectious ulcerative keratitis (Krachmer and Purcell, 1978; Galentine *et al.*, 1984; Alfonso *et al.*, 1986). The danger is greatly increased when extended wear soft lenses are used. Mondino *et al.* (1986) have estimated that

there is a 4.6 times greater risk with extended wear compared with daily wear. Graham *et al.* (1986) have reported that in two years of follow up, suppurative keratitis occurred in 3% of their group of elderly patients with aphakia wearing soft contact lenses continuously, but in none of those which removed their lenses daily.

Galentine *et al.* (1984) reviewed their experience with ulcerative keratitis associated with contact lens wear at Wills Eye Hospital, Philadelphia, from 1 January, 1978, to 1 July, 1983 – a period of five and half years. There were 322 cases of ulcerative keratitis recorded. Fifty-six cases (17%) were associated with the use of contact lenses. Twenty-nine (52%) of the 56 cases of contact lens associated ulcers were culture positive. Pseudomonas was the most common isolate occurring in 13 (23%) of the 56 cases. Staphylococcus species were the second most common, occurring in 11 (20%) of the 56 cases. In this series contact lens associated ulcers were seen frequently in those wearing soft lenses (40 out of 56 cases, 86%) and in those wearing aphakic lenses (32 out of 56 cases, 57%). They stressed the importance of prompt, appropriate and intensive treatment to prevent visual loss.

Poggio *et al.* (1989) have carried out a prospective study of the epidemiology of ulcerative keratitis in contact lens wearers. They estimate the risk of wearing lenses on a daily wear basis to be 0.02 to 0.03% per annum and on an extended wear basis to be 0.22 to 0.32% per annum. The risk for overnight wear is ten to fifteen times as great as daily wear.

Treatment   In the author's experience, eyes are lost not just because contact lenses may facilitate the entry of bacteria into the cornea, but because of the considerable delay which is experienced by most patients before adequate treatment can be obtained. This delay is particularly noticeable when the patient is aphakic, old and infirm and is thus, by necessity, wearing an extended wear soft lens.

Lustbader, Stark and Kracher (1986) have reported the relationship between delay in treatment and the resultant loss in vision. They suggest that if the lens is removed and treatment is sought within 12 hours of a problem arising, the likelihood of vision loss is small. If lens removal and treatment is delayed 48 hours or more, substantial loss of vision is almost certain.

The management entails the identification of the organism and the institution of the correct therapy and is in the domain of the medical specialist. Too often time is wasted in waiting to see a non-medical contact lens practitioner and then further time is lost in arranging for a medical consultation. Except at large centres, appropriate treatment is often not immediately at hand because the indicated antibiotics are not commercially available in a topical form. All contact lens wearing patients should be told:

1. There is some danger in most human activities and contact lens wearing is no exception.
2. If an eye is painful, comparable to toothache, it is probably something more serious than conjunctivitis, that is, a corneal infection. This is especially true if there is a white spot on the cornea of the affected eye. Conjunctivitis is seldom painful.
3. The lens should then be removed and help sought without delay.
4. Never go to bed with a red or painful eye.
5. You may waste valuable time in waiting to consult or in consulting a general medical practitioner, a contact lens practitioner or a chemist.
6. You must be seen by an ophthalmologist or an ophthalmic surgeon, for example, at the casualty department of a hospital. He is in the best position to assess the gravity or otherwise of the condition and to institute the proper treatment, which is not that usually given for conjunctivitis. It is a good thing to know where such help is available before it is needed.
7. The longer you delay, the more chance there is of losing the vision in the eye.

When a corneal ulcer or abscess is present the first requirement is to identify the organism. This involves scraping the ulcer site to obtain material for microscopy (see Appendices 13.I and 13.II) and culture and sensitivity testing to antibiotics. The ideal is to plate the material directly (see Appendix 13.III), perhaps by getting a bacteriology technician to come from the laboratory to the consulting room. Initial examination of the microscope slides will indicate whether the organism is a Gram-positive coccus or a Gram-negative bacillus. Frequently no organisms are seen, or cultured, even in ideal situations. In this case it is

possible that the basis of these suppurative lesions is an initial allergic response which releases inflammatory mediators and sets off the activation of complement by the alternative pathway (Mondino, Brown and Rabin, 1978). Perhaps the soft lens prevents the dispersal of inflammatory substances and products of metabolism.

It has been pointed out by Maske, Hill and Oliver (1986) and Baum (1986) that microscopy of corneal scrapings may be misleading and that treatment should be started with antibiotics having a broad spectrum of activity. The unreliability of the microscopy is probably due to the fact that not all organisms stain with Gram stain. Dr David Seal at Moorfields Eye Hospital, London, has evolved a method of staining with various stains, using the same microscopy slide. It is given in Appendix 13.II.

So far as immediate treatment is concerned an excellent selection is a cephalosporin – cefuroxime or ceftazidime – together with gentamicin. This selection is based on the premise that the worst possible Gram-positive coccus is a penicillinase-producing *Staphylococcus aureus* and the most difficult Gram-negative bacillus to treat is *Pseudomonas aeruginosa* (Coster, 1985).

Cefuroxime 5% has a superior effect on Gram-positive bacteria to ceftazidime 5%, but the latter is effective against *Pseudomonas* which may be resistant to the gentamicin. Gentamicin resistant staphylococci are more likely to be seen in infections acquired in hospital.

Cefuroxime drops 5% can be prepared by injecting 5 ml water for injection from an ampoule into a 250 mg vial of cefuroxine powder (Zinocef, Glaxo Labs Ltd) and transferring the solution to a sterile dropper bottle. It has a refrigerator shelf life of three days. Ceftazidime 5% can be prepared by injecting 10 ml sterile water from an ampoule into a 500 mg vial of ceftazidime powder (Fortum, Glaxo Labs Ltd) and transferring the solution to a sterile dropper bottle. It has a refrigerator shelf life of seven days. As already stated, it is active against *Pseudomonas aeruginosa*. It is, furthermore, the drug of choice for *Pseudomonas* when the patient is allergic to gentamicin and it, and therefore other aminoglycosides, cannot be used. Hypersensitivity to one aminoglycoside usually involves hypersensitivity to others.

Methicillin 2%, if buffered with sodium citrate 0.5%, has a refrigerator shelf life of 12 weeks, so it may be practical to stock it in anticipation of use, instead of a cephalosporin. It is effective against penicillinase-producing staphylococci, but methicillin resistance by staphylococci has been reported (Khan, Hoover and Ide, 1984).

Vancomycin 5% solution, which has an effective refrigerator shelf life of two weeks, may be an effective alternative to ceftazidime. It is effective against both methicillin-resistant *Staphylococcus epidermidis* (Lowy and Hammer, 1983) and methicillin-resistant *Staphylococcus aureus* (Boyce *et al.*, 1981).

Further information on the preparation of these eye drops can be obtained from the Chief Pharmacist, Moorfields Eye Hospital, London, EC1V 2PD.

Fortified gentamicin drops (1.5%) should be used. They can be made up by adding 80 mg (2 ml) of intravenous gentamicin solution to a 5 ml bottle of commercial gentamicin (Genticin 0.3%). Resistance has been documented to gentamicin when used at a concentration of 1.5% (the commercial preparation is 0.3%) and this is especially true in the USA where it has become the standard, all-purpose, topical antibiotic for eye infections, displacing topical chloramphenicol, to which fatal adverse reactions have been reported. It may be expedient instead to use tobramycin (1.5%) which has the same spectrum. Both these antibiotics have a shelf life of one year when in drop form.

When only common proprietary preparations are available Polytrim (Wellcome Medical Division), which contains trimethoprim and polymixin B, or Neosporin (Calmic), which contains polymixin B, neomycin and gramicidin, can be used. Both are effective against Gram-positive and Gram-negative organisms.

Drops should be instilled every 15 minutes or at one minute intervals for the first five minutes of each hour.

In the latter part of the 1980s new fluoroquinolone antibiotics began to be used. These kill bacteria as well as inhibit their growth. Those organisms not killed initially do not begin to grow again for two to six hours after exposure to a fluoroquinolone. This is called the post antibiotic effect and may have importance in topical administration to the eye where peak antibiotic levels are not maintained because of the intermittent instillation of antibiotic and subsequent run-off into the lacrimal drainage system.

In the USA one of these antibiotics has been made commercially available as an eye drop (Ciloxan, Alcon Laboratories Inc., Fort Worth). This is ciprofloxacin HCl 0.3%. Experience so far has indicated that this antibiotic has an exceedingly low incidence of resistance. It has a wide spectrum of antibiotic effect, being effective against both Gram-positive and Gram-negative bacteria. In particular, it is effective against *Staph. aureus, Ps. aeruginosa, Serratia marcescens, Strep. pneumoniae* and *Mycobacteria*.

Leibowitz (1991) has reported a multicentre, prospective study of 148 culture proven cases of bacterial keratitis treated with ciprofloxacin 0.3% ophthalmic solution compared with a group of patients treated conventionally with fortified cefazolin and fortified gentamicin or tobramycin and a further group treated during the year before the initiation of the ciprofloxacin study. Treatment with ciprofloxacin yielded a 91.9% success rate. Standard therapy yielded an 88.2% success rate and the success rate in the previous year was 88.3%. These differences are not statistically significant.

Ciprofloxacin has excellent penetration into the aqueous. The most frequently observed event associated with topical ciprofloxacin therapy is a white crystalline precipitate of the antibiotic, commonly located in the superficial position of the corneal epithelial defect. This precipitate does not appear to interfere with epithelial healing and can be irrigated or scraped from the ulcer bed.

Borrman and Leopold (1988) have reported that between 8% and 10% of ulcerative keratitis caused by *Ps. aeruginosa* are resistant to aminoglycosides.

The manufacturers recommend a dosage regimen for Ciloxan in bacterial keratitis of two drops in the affected eye every 15 minutes for the first six hours and then two drops every 30 minutes for the remainder of the day. On the second day two drops are instilled hourly and on the third to the 14th day two drops are instilled four hourly.

This new antibiotic would appear to be a big step forward in the management of bacterial keratitis. Fortified aminoglycosides can rapidly become toxic to the cornea and prolong ulceration. It is interesting to note that the quinolones achieve high concentrations in lacrimal secretions when taken systemically.

In the UK, norfloxacin, another fluoroquinolone antibiotic with a comparable wide spectrum of activity to ciprofloxacin, has become available in eye drop form (Noroxin, Merck Sharp and Dohme).

The role of topical steroids is a controversial issue. Recent work by Badenoch *et al.* (1985), in a rat model, has shown that it is probably safe and desirable to suppress corneal inflammation with steroid after the effectiveness of antimicrobial therapy has been confirmed by a non-progressive course.

Huang *et al.* reported on the clinical features of six cases of atypical (i.e. non-tuberculous) mycobacterial keratitis at the meeting of the American Academy of Ophthalmology in 1988. Two of their cases were associated with corneal trauma, three with contact lens usage, and one with penetrating keratoplasty. Of the six cases, five were caused by *M. chelonae* and one by *M. fortuitum*. They found the organisms sensitive to amikacin and tobramycin. Malcolm Kerr Muir (personal communication) has treated a case in which the organism was not sensitive to either of these antibiotics, but sensitive to imipenem. Mycobacteria are sensitive to ciprofloxacin.

This keratitis is mentioned here because its presenting clinical features are quite atypical (Figure 13.25). The suppuration is chronic and presents as a slowly spreading stromal infiltrate without an epithelial break. The definitive diagnosis usually demands a corneal biopsy. This can be done with a 1 or 2 mm Elliott trephine and a sharp blade in peripheral affected cornea. Microscopy can be performed, as indicated in Appendices 13.I and 13.II. Culture and sensitivity should be performed using Lowenstein-Jensen medium if mycobacteria are suspected.

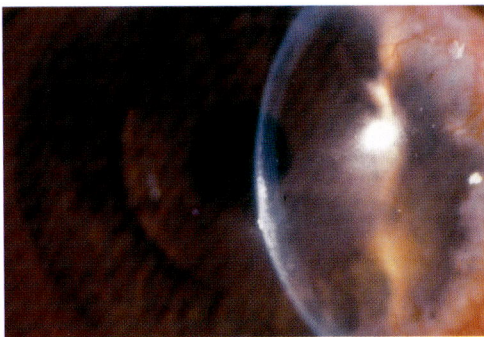

Figure 13.25 Atypical mycobacteria keratitis. There is a spreading stromal infiltrate without an epithelial break. (Courtesy Dr Andrew Huang *et al.*)

Jackson *et al.* (1989) suggest the use of fluorescein-conjugated lectins for visualizing atypical mycobacteria.

Fungal keratitis

Suppurative keratitis may be due to fungi, although this cause is rare when compared with bacterial keratitis. Fungi are also capable of directly invading soft contact lens material (Wilson and Ahearn, 1986). Fungal keratitis usually progresses more slowly than is the case with bacterial infection and most cases are associated with therapeutic soft contact lens wear. The fungi may be yeasts or filamentous forms.

Wilhelmus *et al.* (1988) found in a retrospective review of cases of microbial keratitis that fungal infection occurred in four (4%) of 90 cosmetic or aphakic contact lens wearers and in four (27%) of 15 patients using a therapeutic soft lens. Predisposing factors included improper lens care by the refractive lens wearers and a chronic epithelial defect with topical corticosteroid use among the therapeutic lens wearers. Filamentous fungi were more likely to be associated with cosmetic or aphakic lens wear, whereas yeasts were more frequently found with therapeutic lens use.

The diagnosis is made from corneal scrapings. These should always be performed when there is a suppurative corneal lesion. Giemsa stain (Appendix 13.I) is especially useful for the identification of fungi as also is Calcofluor white stain (Appendix 13.I). The latter is also useful for the identification of amoebae (Wilhelmus *et al.*, 1986).

Treatment The initial drug of choice in the USA for either filamentous fungal or yeast keratitis is 5% natamycin suspension (Jones, 1980). It is a relatively stable suspension at room temperature and is non-irritating to the cornea following topical application which should be once every quarter hour or five times at minute intervals each hour. In the UK the commonest fungus would appear to be Candida, although this has not been documented. Fusarium, common in the USA, is rare here. Accordingly, the first choice in the UK is probably miconazole 1%, but a new oral fungicide, itraconazole, is particularly active against Candida. It remains to be seen whether it is effective against ocular candidiasis. The possibility of a mixed bacterial and fungal infection should be borne in mind.

Thereafter, the drug therapy should be based on the results of culture and on advice from a microbiologist. Three review articles, in addition to the one quoted above (Jones, 1980) are helpful. They are by Jones (1975), Lemp, Blackman and Koffler (1980) and O'Day (1987).

Acanthamoeba keratitis

Infection of the cornea with Acanthamoeba was first described by Nagington *et al.* (1974). There followed a series of reports of such corneal infection and one was associateded with fatal meningoencephalitis (Jones, Visvesvara and Robinson, 1975) and another with both anterior and posterior scleritis (Mannis *et al.*, 1986). Harwood *et al.* (1988) have described the isolation of Acanthamoeba from a cerebral abscess.

A review of the literature (Mannis *et al.*, 1986) showed an association with contact lens wear in 39% of reported cases. Of these 11 reported cases, two were wearers of hard corneal lenses and nine were wearers of soft contact lenses, one of whom wore them on an extended basis.

Moore, McCulley and Newton (1987) described their experience with 11 cases. Eight were culture and/or stain positive for Acanthamoeba and three were presumed to have Acanthamoeba based on the history and clinical findings. Six wore soft contact lenses. Two wore extended wear soft contact lenses, one wore a PMMA hard lens, one wore a gas permeable contact lens and one wore a Saturn lens.

Acanthamoeba is a non-flagellate protozoon and produces fine tapered cytoplasmic projections called acanthapodea. Its cyst is double walled and stellate. Both are uninucleate and contain a large centrally located nucleolus (Figure 13.26).

The disease is often confused initially with ocular herpes simplex and dendritic figures may appear on the cornea.

Early features of acanthamoebic infection are:

1. A central punctate corneal epitheliopathy which often breaks down to an erosion. This is seen in the absence of a stromal infiltrate in the central area.
2. A perineural infiltration of the corneal nerves proceeding from the centre to the periphery (Figure 13.27).
3. A superficial nummular keratitis.

Severe ocular pain, out of proportion to the inflammatory process, is a hallmark of the keratitis.

A later feature of diagnostic value is a ring infiltrate of the cornea (Theodore *et al.*, 1985)

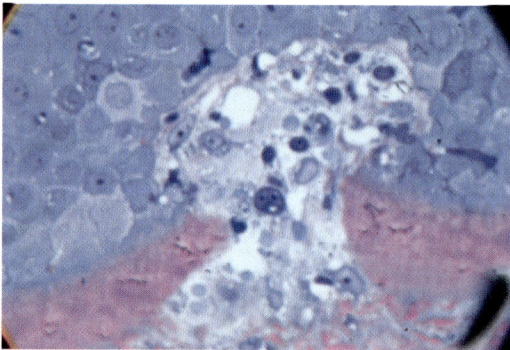

Figure 13.26 Acanthamoeba keratitis. Light micrograph of corneal epithelium and anterior stromal infiltrates. Note break in Bowman's membrane with cysts and trophozoites migrating into the stroma (same case as Figure 13.22.) (Haematoxylin – eosin, original magnification × 40.) (Courtesy Dr Michael S. Insler *et al.*, Louisiana State University Eye Center, USA and *Archives of Ophthalmology* (**106**, 883, 1988); Copyright 1988 American Medical Association)

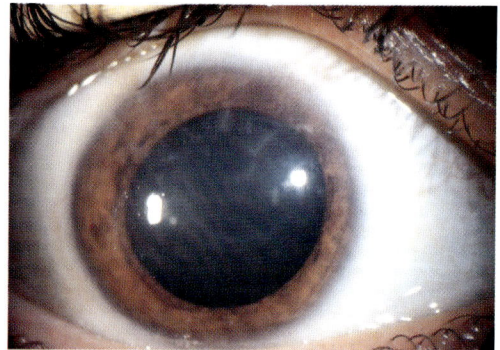

Figure 13.27 Acanthamoeba keratitis. Right eye of 32-year-old soft contact lens wearer with three-week history of red painful eye. The cornea showed numerous radial linear and branching anterior stromal infiltrates extending to the limbus and resembling 'highlighted' corneal nerves. Radial instrastromal lines are probably the result of migrating trophozoites with minimal inflammation. (Courtesy of Dr Michael S. Insler *et al.*, Louisiana State University Eye Center, USA and *Archives of Ophthalmology* (**106**, 883, 1988); Copyright American Medical Association)

(Figure 13.28). Hypopyon which waxes and wanes is found and secondary glaucoma is common.

Wilhelmus, McCulloch and Osato (1988) have reported seeing small refractile opacities within the corneal stroma in patients subsequently confirmed to have Acanthamoeba keratitis (Figure 13.29a and b). They documented these multiple intrastromal crystalline-like refractile granules by specular microscopy. The opacities are most easily identified just central to a ring infiltrate and vary in shape from spherical to ellipsoid. Wilhelmus, McCulloch and Osato suggest that there is a reduction in these opacities following successful treatment and that specular microscopy provides a non-invasive photographic biopsy that can assist in the clinical evaluation of Acanthamoeba keratititis.

Florakis *et al.* (1988) have described elevated epithelial lines as another clinical sign in Acanthamoeba corneal infection (Figure 13.30). Histopathological examination of these lines revealed trophozoites and cysts. In one patient these lines appeared in the cornea one month after the initial symptoms.

A culture technique has been described for the diagnosis of Acanthamoeba by Wright, Warhurst and Jones (1985). The rapid diagnosis using calcofluor white has been reported by Wilhelmus *et al.* (1986). The diagnosis can also be made by direct immunofluorescence with fluorescein labelled antibody against Acanthamoeba in corneal scrapings or, preferably, a corneal biopsy (Epstein *et al.*, 1986). Silvany, Luckenbach and

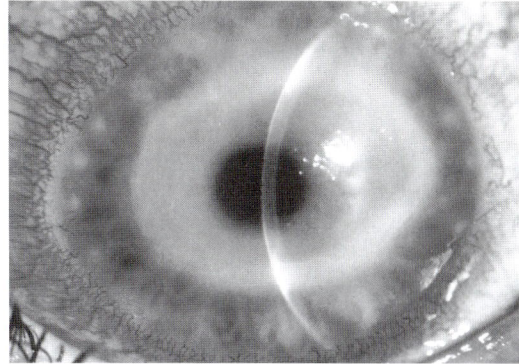

(a)

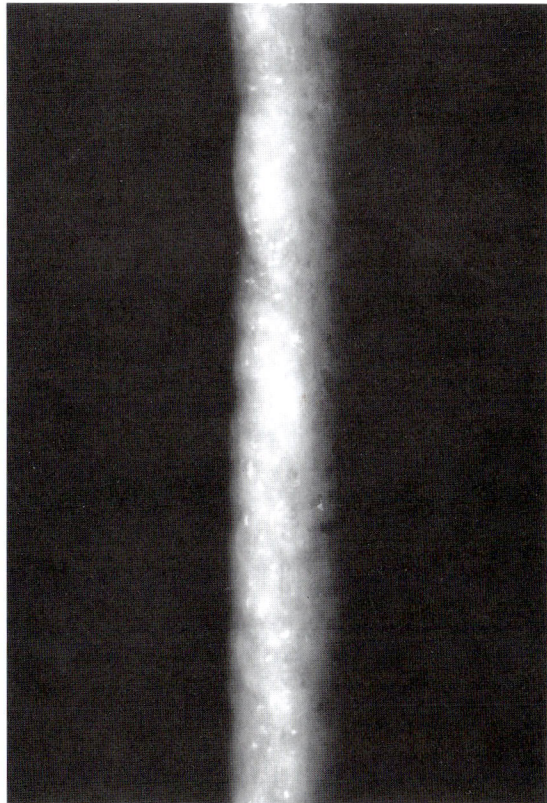

(b)

Figure 13.29 Acanthamboeba keratitis. (a) A ring infiltrate in a soft contact lens wearer. (b) Specular microscopy of the same case showing multiple intrastromal refractile opacities. (Courtesy Dr Kirk R. Wilhelmus *et al*. Dept. of Ophthalmology, Cullen Eye Institute, Baylor College of Medicine and the Editor of the *American Journal of Ophthalmology*, 1988, **106**, 5, 626–630)

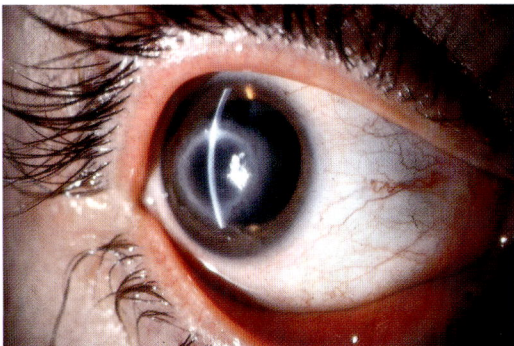

Figure 13.28 Acanthamoeba keratitis. Ring infiltrate of the cornea. (Courtesy of F.H. Theodore and the Editor of *Ophthalmology*, 1985, **92**, 1471–1479)

Moore (1987) have described the rapid detection of Acanthamoeba in paraffin embedded sections of corneal tissue with calcofluor white.

Johns *et al.* (1989) have drawn attention to the fact that the identification of amoebic cysts on the surface of a patient's hydrophilic contact lens, by direct examination with light microscopy, can provide rapid confirmation of the diagnosis of Acanthamoeba keratitis. Lenses can be examined, unstained, or after the application of calcofluor white.

Treatment   There is general agreement that the earlier the diagnosis is made the more successful treatment is likely to be.

There was a debate as to whether early keratoplasty or medical treatment is the best management of the disease. Keratoplasty, unfortunately, often does not always remove all the infected tissue and recurrences of the infection have been described (Jones, McGill and Steele, 1975).

The successful treatment of Acanthamoeba keratitis has been reported using propamidine drops, together with neomycin drops and dibromopropamidine ointment (Wright, Warhurst and Jones, 1985). It is now apparent that these drops and ointments must not be used with the same aggressiveness as is indicated by a bacterial keratitis, as otherwise the eye will become severely inflamed despite the improvement in corneal signs. Initially the drops are used hourly and the ointment four hourly during the night. This treatment must be continued on a long-term basis.

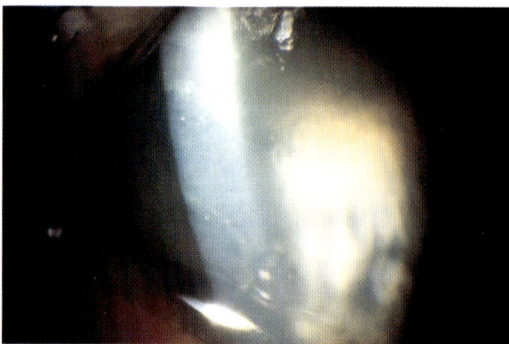

Figure 13.30 Coarsely elevated corneal epithelial line in Acanthamoeba keratitis. The elevated line is that seen at the junction of the middle and inferior thirds of the illuminated slit. By kind permission of George Florakis *et al.* and the Editor of *Archives of Ophthalmology*, 1988, **106**, 1202–1206

Propamidine drops are available commercially, in the UK, over the counter, without prescription, as Brolene eye drops (May and Baker) and dibromopropamidine cream as Brolene cream (May and Baker).

Moore and McCulley (1989) have reported the successful management of six consecutive cases of Acanthamoeba keratitis. Five patients were treated with topical neomycin, polymyxin B, gramicidin (Neosporin, Wellcome) and propamidine drops. Two patients required keratoplasty. All six patients required keratoplasty. All six patients achieved 6/6 vision. The authors state that early diagnosis and medical treatment alone can result in resolution of corneal infiltrates due to Acanthamoeba.

The effects of cryotherapy and antibiotics (paromycin, neomycin or propamidine isothionate) on the viability of *Acanthamoeba polyphaga* and *A. castellani* cysts were studied in vitro by Matoba *et al.* (1989). Either cryotherapy or exposure to antibiotic led to a decrease in the number of viable *A. castellani* detected. *Acanthamoeba polyphaga* showed variable response to the antibiotics tested. The combination of cryotherapy and antibiotic therapy was more cysticidal than either modality alone and eliminated detectable visible organisms in five of six experiments. Of the antibiotic solutions tested, paromycin (15 mg/ml) was the most effective.

At a meeting of the Ocular Microbiology and Immunology Group in Las Vegas on 7th October, 1988, it was the consensus of opinion of ophthalmologists familiar with the disease that steroids were almost totally contraindicated in Acanthamoeba keratitis. Their use leads to a temporary improvement and relief of pain which is then followed by exacerbation of the disease. Sometimes, however, their use is necessary to suppress inflammation.

Driebe *et al.* (1988) have drawn attention to the potential role for topical clotrimazole in combination therapy for Acanthamoeba keratitis. This antifungal agent has been shown to have excellent in vitro activity against most strains of Acanthamoeba. They reported successful use in four patients.

Ishibashi *et al.* (1990) have reported good results in three patients treated orally with a new antifungal agent, itraconazole. This was used in association with topical miconazole and surgical debridement. Oral itraconazole is said to have fewer side effects compared with oral ketoconazole.

A review and account of experience in the management of Acanthamoeba keratitis at Moorfields Eye Hospital, London, is given by Ficker (1988).

Larkin, Kilvington and Dart (1992) have described the successful use of polyhexamethylene biguanide (PHMB) in the management of Acanthamoeba keratitis at Moorfields Eye Hospital. It is a polymeric biguanide disinfectant which is effective against trophozoite forms and is cysticidal at low concentrations. Toxicity to the ocular surface was not evident with PHMB, unlike propamidine or neomycin. It is used in conjunction with propamidine.

Koenig *et al.* (1987) have reported that sulindac, a non-steroidal anti-inflammatory agent, has proven to be an effective analgesic in their patients who had Acanthamoeba keratitis. It produced more symptomatic relief than other non-steroidal agents or mild narcotic–analgesic combinations.

Acanthamoeba keratitis should be treated in specialist centres or, at least, with specialist advice. Referral should be very early in the course of the disease, even at the stage of suspicion. Only specialist centres have the necessary microbiological facilities.

Corneal vascularization

Corneal vascularization in wearers of soft contact lenses may be due to anoxia or may be secondary to changes in the corneal epithelium. These changes can be brought about by hypersensitivity or toxic reactions to chemicals or by trauma. A further possible cause is the exacerbation of potential or subclinical ocular rosacea caused by the wearing of contact lenses.

If the changes are due to anoxia the vessels may be superficial or deep and they may progress from the limbus in all areas. The superficial vascularization from the periphery usually recedes without trace if the soft contact lens is withdrawn or replaced with one with a higher oxygen transmissibility. The danger with deep penetration is that the cornea may lose its regular shape if the vascularization is marked. In much the same way as visual acuity is reduced, after an attack of interstitial keratitis, because of irregular thickness

and irregular contour, so may a cornea be left after deep vascularization has been induced by a soft contact lens. Occasionally a silent, single leash of vessels will penetrate to the centre of the cornea without involvement of the peripheral cornea. This leash of vessels may silt out lipid as has been illustrated in the case of the hard corneal lens (see Figure 12.18).

Vascularization secondary to hypersensitivity or toxic reactions of the cornea to chemicals is almost invariably superficial. In contrast to superficial vascularization caused by anoxia, there are often accompanying dysplastic changes in the corneal epithelium. Such changes usually remain when the stimulus is stopped and the accompanying vessels are slow to recede if, in fact, they ever do.

If superficial vascularization is seen it is important to stain the cornea with fluorescein for evidence of epitheliopathy. In its early stages such an epitheliopathy may only manifest as sequential staining (Korb and Herman, 1979). Sequential staining is fluorescein staining of the cornea which develops some time after fluorescein has been instilled. It is not a feature of normal corneas and in the opinion of the author is an early sign of preservative hypersensitivity or toxicity.

Trauma, even with a soft contact lens, can cause disruption of the corneal epithelium and subsequent superficial vascularization. It may be the cause of peripheral epithelial necrosis (mush) (see Figure 13.7).

Treatment

The treatment of vascularization entails identifying the cause and removing it. Lipid keratopathy can be dealt with as described in Chapter 12 in the paragraph on vascularization.

Corneal thinning

Holden *et al.* (1988), using an electronic digital pachometer, examined 27 patients who had worn high water content hydrogel contact lenses in one eye only for an average of 62 plus or minus 29 months (mean plus or minus SD). The stroma of the lens wearing eye was found to be significantly thinner ($P < 0.05$) than that of the contralateral eye after lens-induced oedema was allowed to subside. Recovery had not occurred after 33 days.

They concluded that contact lenses can induce stromal thinning.

Intracorneal haemorrhage

Yeoh, Cox and Falcon (1989) have described the unusual complication of spontaneous intracorneal haemorrhage in an aphakic patient who used an extended wear contact lens. This was severe enough to cause corneal blood staining and ulceration which required a pre-Descemet's lamellar graft.

Posterior corneal complications

Polse, Sarver and Harris (1973) observed vertical striae at the level of Descemet's membrane in association with soft contact lens wear. These are now taken to be one manifestation of corneal hypoxia. The striae develop with time and are associated with an oedematous stroma.

Transient endothelial changes occurring within minutes of insertion of soft contact lenses were described by Zantos and Holden (1977). These changes consist of blebs in the endothelium which can start within five minutes of insertion of a soft contact lens. Their number and size increase with time and after about half an hour they start to disappear. A thicker lens gives more blebs sooner and corneas vary in their proneness to produce blebs. The blebs appear to be on the stromal side of the endothelium.

Endothelial bedewing as a localized phenomenon in the cornea at the level of the inferior papillary margin and associated with poor soft contact lens tolerance has been reported by McMonnies and Zantos (1979).

Total endothelial bedewing

This has been observed by the author as an acute phenomenon in soft contact lens wearers (Figure 13.31). It is presumably due to endothelial oedema and resolves within two days. The cause is unknown and in the author's experience it has not recurred on resumption of lens wear. The patient presents with blurred vision.

Posterior annular keratopathy

This is a condition which has much in common with the posterior annular keratopathy described by Payrau and Raynaud (1965). These authors described a condition occurring after blast injuries of the cornea in five cases. They assumed penetration of the cornea by foreign bodies without a clinically perceptible track. They also described transient annular configurations on the posterior face of the cornea which disappeared without a trace. Vogt (1930) produced drawings of such lesions in his *Atlas of Slit Lamp Microscopy*. The notion of minute foreign bodies penetrating the cornea is hard to believe. The annular lesions may be initiated by metabolic changes.

Stulting, Rodrigues and Nay (1986) have examined the ultrastructure of traumatic corneal endothelial rings in a four-year-old boy after a fatal gunshot wound to the forehead. Electron microscopy showed the injury to consist of an annular area of endothelial loss and disruption with adherent macrophages. Endothelial cell disruption was localized to the circular area where mechanical distortion of endothelium and Descemet's membrane caused by the inpact of a projectile would be maximal.

Such lesions have been observed by the author in association with soft contact lens wear. The patient presents with an uncomfortable but not painful eye, and a slight central epithelial irregularity may be observed. Diffuse stromal cellular infiltration is also discernible on using a fine beam at the slit lamp. On the following day the patient

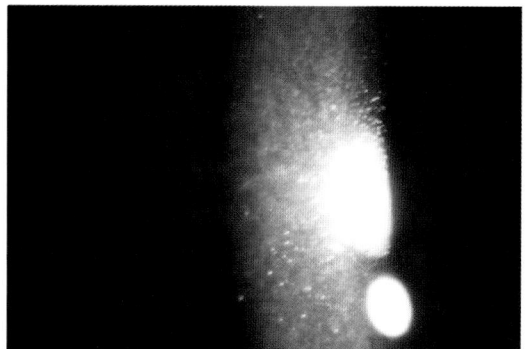

Figure 13.31 Total endothelial bedewing. This was observed by the author as an acute phenomenon which resolved without sequel

may return with a comfortable eye, but the endothelium is totally bedewed, apart from a central area in which it appears to be missing (Figure 13.32). The endothelium seems to end in a fringe ('franges') around this central zone just as in the Payrau and Raynaud description. There is a fusiform swelling of the cornea in the region of the apparently absent endothelium, mainly projecting posteriorly. Resolution occurs within a few days and subsequent endothelial specular microscopy shows no abnormality. If there is a great deal of stromal infiltration, normality may only be achieved over a longer time.

The author has seen five such cases and the last one was associated with a hypopyon which cleared rapidly in a day, leaving a flare on the second day. Although there was no focal stromal infiltration amounting to a corneal abscess, a diagnosis of suppurative keratopathy had been made on the previous day and *Pseudomonas aeruginosa* was cultured from the corneal scrape. The patient had also had a subconjunctival injection of gentamicin. Here there may have been a double pathology of posterior annular keratopathy and sterile hypopyon. Sterile hypopyon is sometimes seen in the management of corneal conditions with therapeutic soft lenses and is dealt with in Chapter 14.

The precise nature of posterior annular keratopathy in contact lens wearers is unclear. Some light is thrown on the situation by Bergmanson and Chu (1982). These authors studied the corneal response to extended rigid contact lens wear in three Rhesus monkeys by electron microscopy. They described changes among keratocytes which were evident, mainly posteriorly, and which were frequently severe. In these monkeys there was an apparent loosening of the endothelial adhesion to the posterior limiting lamina (Descemet's membrane).

In view of the work of McCulley, Maurice and Schwartz (1980) and Maurice, McCulley and Schwartz (1981), on the behaviour of corneal endothelial cells, it is probable that endothelial cells are missing from the posterior corneal surface and are suspended as spherical cells in the aqueous. They then become reattached to the posterior corneal surface and assume their hexagonal shape in order to pack together.

In the case of traumatic posterior annular keratopathy, Maloney *et al.* (1979) have shown by specular microscopic studies in two patients that the rings consist of disrupted and swollen endothelial cells. The damaged cells were evident many days after the rings had disappeared. Despite lengthy searches with the specular microscope in two patients, examination of the area of injured endothelium four and a half months after the injury did not disclose either localized abnormal cell structure or a decrease in cell density compared with unaffected areas of the same cornea, or with normal corneas of the same age. In a further two patients with more severe injuries, a substantial decrease in endothelial cell density was found, compared with normal corneas of the same age.

Treatment

A topical steroid such as prednisolone acetate 1.0%, or dexamethasone 0.1%, should be used four times daily in an attempt to control the stromal infiltration. The condition is self-limiting.

Posterior stromal opacification

The author has seen opacification develop in the deep stroma in the central area in three cases. In all three cases one eye had much more advanced changes than the other. The presenting complaint was that the vision had deteriorated in one eye. In one case (Figure 13.33a) the visual acuity was

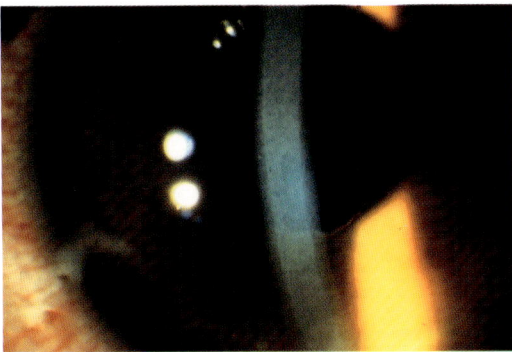

Figure 13.32 Posterior annular keratopathy. There is total endothelial bedewing apart from a central area in which the endothelium appears to be missing. A fringe of endothelium appears to surround this central zone. There is fusiform swelling of the cornea in the area where the endothelium is absent. This was associated with soft contact lens wear

less than 6/60 in the more severely affected eye. In this eye the opacification extended forwards at least two-thirds of the thickness of the stroma and there was concurrent corneal flattening in the central area. The other eye (Figure 13.33b) showed much less opacification and the visual acuity was normal. The condition developed after a few years of soft contact lens wear. Specular endothelial microscopy in this case revealed a normal endothelium. The condition did not resolve.

Twelve such cases of posterior stromal opacification (including those of the author) were seen at the Endothelial Specular Photography Clinic at Moorfields Eye Hospital, City Road, London. In all cases there were deep opacities, that is just anterior to Descemet's membrane. The opacities ranged from small spots, through discoid forms, to scattered discs and wispy central areas. One

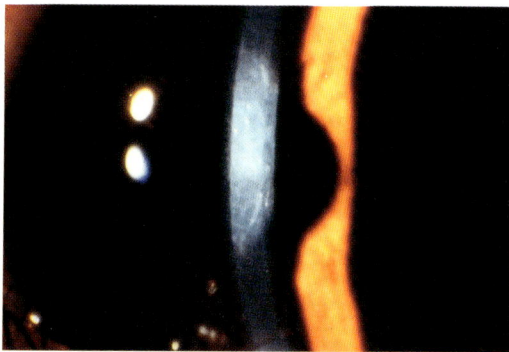

(a)

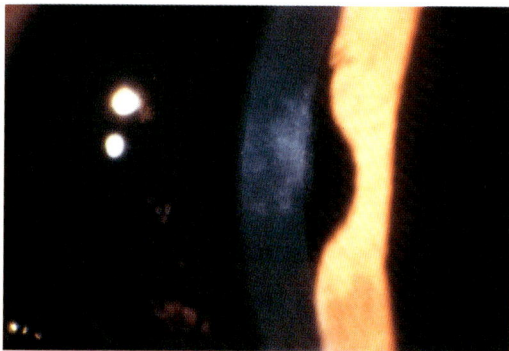

(b)

Figure 13.33 (a) Dense posterior stromal opacification. The deep stroma is opacified over a wide central area with concurrent corneal flattening and gross reduction in visual acuity. (b) The other eye showing early deep stromal change

case showed a distinct green coloration and the opacities were located at the superior and inferior limbus. Other cases showed a polychromatic coloration. The age range of the patients was 23 to 45 years. Six cases were male and six female. They had worn contact lenses from 3 to 13 years.

In its early stages, the condition resembles the central cloudy dystrophy of Francois (Francois, 1956; Strachan, 1969). The cloudy dystrophy of Francois, in contrast to the adverse reaction to contact lenses, is non-progressive and does not affect vision, although the patient may be photophobic.

Eight of the Moorfields cases showed abnormal posterior corneal rings (described by Sherrard and Buckley (1981a, b) as a feature of normal corneas). They were weak or incomplete or absent. One case showed endothelial polymegethism (see below) outside the normal range and two patients had low endothelial cell counts.

Two patients with deep stromal opacities after prolonged contact lens wear have recently been described by Brooks *et al.* (1986).

Remeijer *et al.* (1990) described whitish corneal opacities which they had seen between 1981 and 1988 in the deep layers of the corneas of 32 patients with long-term contact lens wear. These opacities were seen in 29 patients wearing soft HEMA contact lenses and three patients wearing rigid PMMA lenses. All the patients used a chemical care regimen in which thimerosal was the only common preservative. Endothelial specular microscopy showed a higher coefficient of cell size. Two cases were illustrated. Case no. 1 showed a slow reduction in the opacities after a seven-month period when the soft lenses were replaced by rigid gas permeable lenses. Case no. 2 (Figure 13.34a and b) had normal visual acuity and the lesions disappeared after nine months. In five cases permanent scarring persisted.

Pinckers *et al.* (1987) have described four of these cases which they tentatively label 'Contact lens induced pseudo-dystrophy of the cornea'. They saw whitish dots in the stroma of the cornea resembling the cloudy dystrophy in four patients wearing HEMA contact lenses. They saw a lattice-like corneal pattern in another patient wearing HEMA contact lenses. There were no complaints. Visual acuity was normal. Corneal sensitivity was normal or reduced. The pseudo-dystrophies vanished after replacement of the HEMA lenses by Boston IV material.

Gobbels, Wahning and Spitznas (1989) studied the corneal endothelial permeability of 21 patients with a more than ten-year-old history of contact lens wear (HEMA 38%), compared with that of an age-matched group of eight healthy individuals without ocular disease. They used a computerized automatic fluorometer. The corneal endothelial permeability of contact lens wearers with deep corneal opacities was found to be significantly increased when compared with contact lens wearers without corneal opacities. Contact lens wearers without corneal opacities showed no significant increase of their endothelial permeability in comparison with the control group.

Treatment

In the light of our present knowledge contact lens wear should be discontinued if the opacities are at all marked. In mild disease, contact lenses of

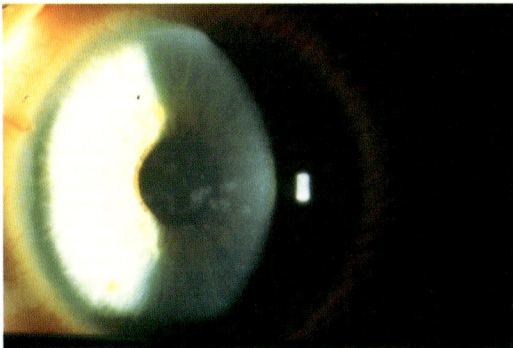

(a)

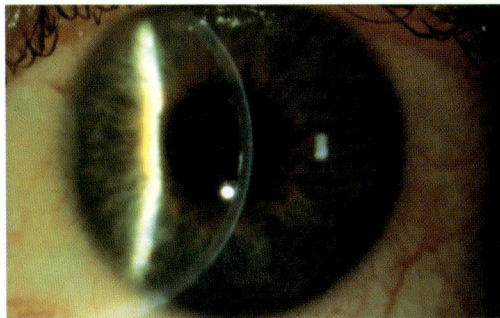

(b)

Figure 13.34 Posterior stromal opacification. (a) Early disease shown by general illumination. (b) Seen by slit illumination showing the depth of the disease in the cornea. (Courtesy Dr G. van Rij *et al.*, Oogziekenhuis, Rotterdam)

higher oxygen transmissibility may be fitted and the condition carefully watched. Penetrating, or deep lamellar keratoplasty may be indicated if the visual acuity is severely diminished after a suitable length of time has elapsed to ensure that the process does not resolve.

Prolonged bullous keratopathy

The author has seen one case of bilateral bullous keratopathy which rapidly developed and persisted for three weeks in a women aged 24 years. She had worn soft contact lenses successfully for two years. One day, after removing the lenses, her vision quickly deteriorated to counting fingers. After one week it was still counting fingers. After a further week the vision was still counting fingers but tended to improve as the day progressed. Within a further week the vision had returned to normal and the bullous keratopathy had disappeared. Subsequent endothelial specular microscopy was normal.

Treatment

In the absence of the cause of this condition, no rational treatment can be given, but no harm and some benefit may be achieved by using a topical steroid such as prednisolone acetate 1.0%, or dexamethasone 0.1% two hourly.

Corneal endothelial polymegethism

Variation in endothelial size has been found as a feature of the ageing process, but recently attention has been drawn to its occurrence in wearers of hard, soft daily and soft extended wear lenses (Hirst *et al.* 1984; Holden *et al.*, 1985; Carlson, Bourne and Brubaker, 1986; MacRae *et al.*, 1986). The condition has been found in one eye where only that eye had been wearing a contact lens (Woloschak, 1983).

Endothelial polymegethism (see Figure 12.22) may be caused by chronic corneal hypoxia (Schoessler, 1987). It may be caused by what Efron and Ang (1990) refer to as hypercapnia, that is, the accumulation of carbon dioxide under a contact lens which leads to acidosis effects. Holden *et al.* (1985) demonstrated a slight trend towards recovery after ceasing lens wear, but this could not be statistically verified over a six-month period. They suggest that if polymegethism does recover, it is a very slow process that occurs over many months or years.

Carlson and Bourne (1988) performed anterior segment fluorophotometry and endothelial cell photography on 11 subjects who had used extended wear contact lenses for at least two years. Forty subjects of similar age who did not wear contact lenses served as a control group. The coefficient of variation of cell size was increased in the contact lens group compared with the control group; no significant difference in mean endothelial cell size was found. No difference in corneal clarity, central corneal thickness, endothelial permeability to fluorescein, or rate of flow of aqueous humour, was found between the groups. There was a significant correlation between duration of lens wear and mean endothelial size. They detected no functional impairment, despite the morphological changes in the corneal endothelium.

Connor and Zagrod (1986) suggest that these changes may compromise the ability of the cornea to withstand added stresses such as surgery.

Treatment

In the light of our present knowledge chronic corneal oxygen deprivation should be avoided by fitting thin, gas permeable hard corneal lenses, thin soft contact lenses or, when this is not practicable because of the refraction, high water content lenses.

Conjunctival complications

Acute bacterial conjunctivitis

This is not a significant problem in wearers of soft contact lenses. Many wearers can abandon all daily sterilization procedures and apparently have no problem with infection. Quite apart from this, the conjunctiva can become hyperaemic and oedematous in response to corneal pathology and this should always be borne in mind. The cornea should always be stained with fluorescein. It must be emphasized that conjunctivitis, in contradistinction to keratitis, is not normally a painful disorder.

Treatment

In the absence of corneal involvement, chloramphenicol 0.5% drops should be used hourly. Alternatively, fusidic acid 1% drops (Fucithalmic, Leo Labs. Ltd) can be used twice daily. These preparations are highly effective against staphylococci which are the commonest cause of acute conjunctivitis. A broader spectrum is provided by gentamicin 0.3% or tobramycin 0.3% in drop form.

Allergic conjunctivitis

Hyperaemia and oedema of the conjunctiva can be seen as a type 1 allergic reaction to the constituents of contact lens cleaning and soaking solutions. It was reported as a reaction to thimerosal by Wright and Mackie (1982) and it can be seen quite independently as a type 1 reaction to this substance in the absence of corneal lesions. Occasionally a conjunctivitis is seen as part of an allergic dermatoconjunctivitis where the skin of the lids is involved in an eczematous reaction.

Treatment

The offending chemical should be removed from the sterilization regimen. In the case of an allergic dermatoconjunctivitis it is helpful to use a topical steroid such as fluocinolone acetonide 0.025% (Synalar cream, ICI) to the skin.

Giant papillary conjunctivitis

This condition was first described by Spring (1974) and one of the reasons why an Australian was first to describe it was that soft contact lenses were dispensed as a practicable proposition for myopes some two years earlier in Australia than in America or the UK. Spring correctly diagnosed the condition as an allergic manifestation and described papillae and not follicles. Previously, contact lens literature had referred to follicular conjunctivitis, or folliculosis. It must be remembered that this condition had, from time to time, been seen as a complication of wearing all types of contact lenses and prostheses, but it became much commoner because of the advent of the soft contact lens.

The disease bears a considerable resemblance to juvenile vernal conjunctivitis, but the slit lamp appearances are quite distinctive. In giant papillary conjunctivitis the giant papillae are more regular in size (Figure 13.35) and never assume the large, irregular, often pedunculated form which is frequently seen in vernal conjunctivitis. Furthermore, in vernal conjunctivitis the whole upper lid conjunctiva is involved, if not with giant papillae, at least with gross cellular infiltration. This is in contradistinction to the localized form of giant papillary conjunctivitis (Figure 13.36) where the adjacent conjunctiva may be normal.

Biopsy shows giant papillae with irregular hyperplastic epithelium with many downgrowths into the stroma and occasional inclusion cysts. The epithelium is infiltrated with a large number

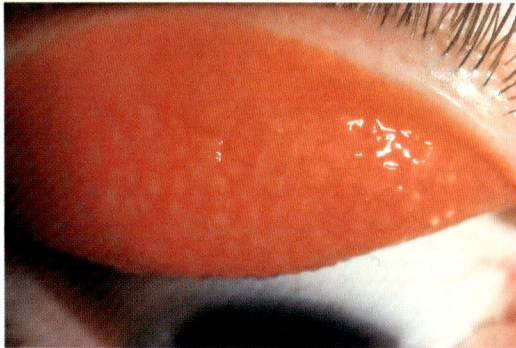

Figure 13.35 Giant papillary conjunctivitis. Regular giant papillae

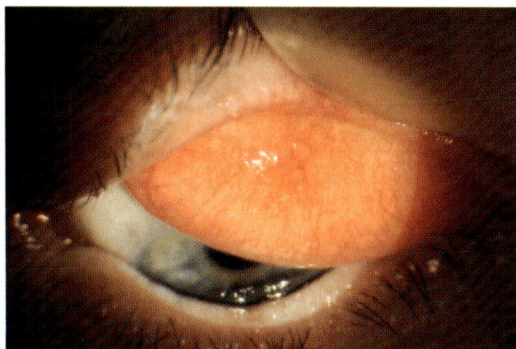

Figure 13.36 Giant papillary conjunctivitis. Localized giant papillae. The adjacent conjunctiva is normal

of eosinophils and there is an increase in the goblet cell population. The stroma is diffusely infiltrated with eosinophils.

Trocme *et al.* (1989) have investigated the role of the eosinophil in vernal keratoconjunctivitis and contact lens associated giant papillary conjunctivitis, by assessing the presence of eosinophil granule major basic protein in conjunctival tissues by immunofluorescence. Vernal keratoconjunctivitis and giant papillary conjunctivitis groups had significantly more major basic protein deposition than controls. No significant correlation between severity of disease and degree of major basic protein deposition was found. Thus, they explain, eosinophil degranulation commonly occurs in vernal keratoconjunctivitis and giant papillary conjunctivitis with release of eosinophil granule major basic protein and presumably other toxic granule proteins on to affected tissues. These cationic proteins are potent cytotoxins and are able to stimulate mast cell degranulation.

Tagawa and Matsuda (1988) have demonstrated that Langerhans cells are markedly increased in patients with giant papillary conjunctivitis and with vernal conjunctivitis. In giant papillary conjunctivitis the increase is in the substantia propria, whereas in vernal conjunctivitis it is in both epithelium and substantia propria. In allergic conjunctivitis the increase is in the epithelium only.

Allansmith, Baird and Greiner (1979) have compared and contrasted vernal conjunctivitis and contact lens associated giant papillary conjunctivitis. Biopsies were subjected to sophisticated cell counting and this was statistically evaluated. They found that vernal conjunctivitis and contact lens associated giant papillary conjunctivitis had abnormalities of mast cells in the epithelium and eosinophils and basophils, both in the epithelium and substantia propria. They concluded that vernal conjunctivitis and contact lens associated giant papillary conjunctivitis may represent different subtypes of a general category of conjunctival abnormality characterized by giant papillae.

Using light microscopy, Allansmith and Baird (1981) determined the percentage of degranulated mast cells in sections of tissue from 10 persons with vernal conjunctivitis, 10 with giant papillary conjunctivitis associated with contact lens wear and 10 normal subjects. Tissues from both groups of patients had a significantly higher percentage of mast cells (80%) than did normal tissue (25%). The fully granulated mast cells in the three groups did not appear morphologically different, nor did the degranulated mast cells in the three groups. The percentage of degranulated mast cells in vernal conjunctivitis did not differ significantly from that in giant papillary conjunctivitis associated with contact lens wear. They concluded that the histamine level in the tears of patients with vernal conjunctivitis, which is four times higher than that of normal subjects (Abelson, Baird and Allansmith, 1980), and that of patients with giant papillary conjunctivitis associated with contact lens wear, cannot be explained by a difference in the percentage of degranulated mast cells detected by light microscopy.

Henriques, Kenyon and Allansmith (1981) studied the mast cell ultrastructure in contact lens associated giant papillary conjunctivitis and vernal conjunctivitis. Most mast cells from normal subjects were fully granulated and showed granule forms previously reported for the conjunctiva. All mast cells from patients with giant papillary conjunctivitis had some degree of degranulation. The number of granules in approximately 30% of mast cells from patients with giant papillary conjunctivitis was sufficiently reduced that the cells probably would not have been recognized as mast cells using light microscopy. Mast cells from vernal conjunctivitis patients had the most extensive degranulation. The vast majority of these cells, at least 80%, had so few granules that it is unlikely they would have been recognized if light microscopy alone had been used.

In a previous paper Allansmith *et al.* (1977) assessed the atopic status of patients with giant papillary conjunctivitis by means of a detailed questionnaire. They found that there was no significant difference between patients and controls. Mackie and Wright (1979) did not find any significant elevation of IgE in 11 patients whom they surveyed. The level was raised in only one patient (320 units/ml compared with an upper limit of normal of 150 units/ml; the levels in nine of the other patients were below 10 units/ml). Donshik and Ballow (1983) found elevated levels of IgE and IgG in the tears of patients with giant papillary conjunctivitis in comparison with normal controls and contact lens wearers without symptoms. Apart from atopic status there would appear to be a definite susceptibility to the disease. At one time in the mid 1970s the author was involved in a study of an American prototype soft

lens which produced giant papillary conjunctivitis in one-third of wearers in the course of one year. This was a very high incidence which suggests that different soft contact lenses have different potentials for causing the disease. It is interesting to record that the author, who stocked these lenses in quantity, still had some patients wearing them after ten years without conjunctival abnormality. The disease affects mainly the upper palpebral conjunctiva, but occasionally the lower palpebral conjunctiva may be involved.

Many normal asymptomatic individuals exhibit giant papillae in the junctional zone between the fornix and the tarsal conjunctiva, especially at the lateral extremities. These papillae can be stained with fluorescein and the excess mucus, which takes the fluorescein stain, can be wiped away. Allansmith *et al.* (1977) regard it as a sign of active disease if the apices of the papillae take the fluorescein stain, as viewed with the cobalt light of the slit lamp. This is an important sign when measures are being taken to eradicate the disease while maintaining the patient's status as a contact lens wearer. However, the concomitant presence, or absence, of typical symptoms is also an impressive indication. The papillae in giant papillary conjunctivitis do not extend into the superior fornix as follicles do in chlamydial infection. The disease has been confused with this infection (Kaufman, Gasset and Votila, 1972).

Korb *et al.* (1983) pointed out that in the disease associated with soft contact lenses giant papillae are seldom found in the zone adjacent to the eyelid margin (zone 3) without also occurring in the intervening zones. Involvement of zone 3 without involvement of the intervening zones is often seen in the disease associated with hard corneal lens wear. The zones of the conjunctiva are illustrated in Figure 13.37.

Some patients have giant papillae with white heads (Figure 13.38) which seem to be the result of a hyaline change with persistence of the stimulus. The white head develops some time after the papilla appears and disappears after the papilla matures. This appearance has been taken by some to be evidence of conjunctival scarring, but the author has repeatedly seen these white heads disappear and such resolution is not a feature of conjunctival scarring.

Some patients, in the early stage of the disease, develop a cellular infiltration of the conjunctiva without the formation of giant papillae. The normal architecture of the deep conjunctival vessels is obscured and a network of fine dilated vessels is seen. In the early stages of such infiltration one is aware of a space (packed with inflammatory cells) between the large branching conjunctival vessels and the conjunctival surface. The conjunctival vessels are, in fact, buried. The conjunctiva is three dimensional instead of having its normal two dimensional appearance. It must be borne in mind that a number of patients who have worn hard corneal lenses for many years show this cellular infiltration in the absence of symptoms. Before assessing this sign it is prudent to ask whether the patient wore hard lenses before the change was made to soft, as is often the case.

This type of infiltration is seen in diseased

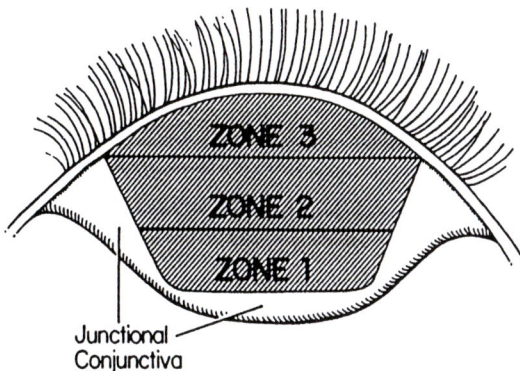

Figure 13.37 Zones of the upper palpebral conjunctiva

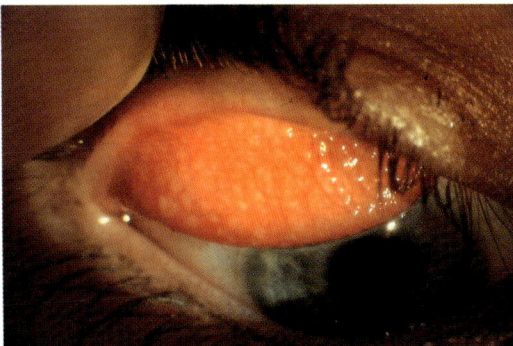

Figure 13.38 Giant papillary conjunctivitis. Giant papillae with white heads. White heads are a late feature

states unassociated with contact lens wear, notably in atopic conjunctival disease and in chlamydial infection. Atopic conjunctival disease is not necessarily associated with general atopy, but is often associated with high IgE serum values (Jay, 1981). A negative serological test for microimmunofluorescent antibodies will rule out chlamydia.

Some patients seem to develop only a localized form of the disease in an otherwise avascular, uninfiltrated lid (see Figure 13.30) and in many cases only one eye is affected.

Patients characteristically complain of:

1. *Discharge* – at first excess 'sleep' in the morning and then during wear. Non-goblet cell mucus was originally described by Srinivasan *et al.* (1977) and in the context of giant papillary conjunctivitis by Greiner *et al.* (1980). This mucus is contained in membrane-bound bodies which lie just under the conjunctival microvillae within the superficial epithelial cells and contributes to the excess seen in giant papillary conjunctivitis (Greiner *et al.*, 1980). Allansmith, Baird and Greiner (1981) have established that the density of goblet cells in this disease is not significantly different from that of normal subjects. However, the conjunctiva in giant papillary conjunctivitis is thicker and has a greater surface area.
2. *Itch or pain* – at first on *removing* the lenses and then during wear. Clinically, vernal conjunctivitis causes far more itching than giant papillary conjunctivitis and this is perhaps a reflection of the tear histamine levels which have already been noted in the two diseases.
3. *Blurred vision* – this is due to two factors. First a coating of mucus on the lens itself and second the eventual displacement of the lens upwards as it is pulled up by the top lid. The adhesion is produced by tackiness of both lid and lens.

Fowler, Greiner and Allansmith (1979) studied soft contact lenses from patients with giant papillary conjunctivitis. They pointed out that deposits on lenses do not invariably lead to disease. They found that the surfaces of all worn lenses are strikingly different from those of unworn lenses. It is commonly observed that replacing a patient's lenses will relieve the symptoms for up to two weeks before they start again. This may indicate that some change has to take place in the plastic or the lens for antigenicity to appear. Alternatively it could mean that some change has to take place in the mucous coat to produce antigenicity. Perhaps this change is brought about by the plastic of the lens itself.

Fowler, Greiner and Allansmith (1979) also found that there was no sigificant difference between the morphological appearance of lenses from subjects with giant papillary conjunctivitis and those lenses from asymptomatic wearers. They concluded that the capacity to develop giant papillary conjunctivitis was influenced more by individual differences than by differences in lens deposits.

Mackie and Wright (1978) cultured the lids and conjunctivae in 18 patients. In 16 there was a moderate or heavy growth of coagulase-negative *Staphylococcus epidermidis*. In one patient pneumococcus was isolated and in another *Staph. aureus*. It has been suggested that giant papillary conjunctivitis is a staphylococcal allergic phenomenon. These results are what one would expect in a normal population and therefore do not support this idea.

Mackie and Wright (1978) also studied conjunctival scrapings in 15 cases. Eosinophils were seen in only one case. This finding is contrary to that of true vernal conjunctivitis. It is significant that eosinophil granule major basic protein which is a marker for hypersensitivity disease in the tears was found to occur in vernal conjunctivitis but not in giant papillary conjunctivitis (Udell *et al.*, 1981).

There may be three factors causing giant papillary conjunctivitis:

1 *Mechanical factors*

Lid problems associated with protruding sutures are well known to ophthalmologists who look under the top lid. They are seen after cataract extraction and keratoplasty. The influence of the mechanical factors can sometimes be seen in high riding hard corneal lenses where there is a prism base out construction at the periphery of the lens. Refitting to centralize the lens and lose lid attachment can cure the disease and allow the patient to continue wearing hard corneal lenses.

It it is interesting that Rahi (1982, personal communication) is of the opinion that the rubbing action of a hard or soft corneal lens on the conjunctiva is a sufficient stimulus to degranulate surface mast cells and thus initiate an allergic type reaction.

This concept of a mechanical cause, however, is not supported by the observations of Tagawa and Matsuda (1988). As already noted, they found a marked increase in Langerhans cells in the substantia propria of patients with contact lens induced papillary conjunctivitis. However, in patients with giant papillary conjunctivitis associated with interrupted prolene sutures, used in cataract surgery, no such increase was found compared with normal subjects. They concluded that giant papillary conjunctivitis associated with prolene sutures was not immunogenic in origin.

Elgebaly *et al.* (1991) designed a study to determine the presence of neutrophil chemotactic factors in the tears of patients with giant papillary conjunctivitis. Elevated levels of chemotactic activity were found in the tears of symptomatic contact lens wearers compared with control tears of asymptomatic contact lens wearers and non-contact lens wearers. Using radioimmunoassay, C5a, leucotriene B_4 and interleukin-1 were not detected in the tears of symptomatic patients. These authors determined whether injured conjunctival cells participate in this process by releasing neutrophil chemotactic factors. Isolated rabbit bulbar conjunctiva incubated with culture medium for four and six hours released high levels of neutrophil chemotactic factors. The release of these factors from injured conjunctiva supports the premise that physical trauma of conjunctival cells, induced by contact lenses, may be an important component of the pathophysiology of giant papillary conjunctivitis.

2 *Protein on the lens*

Using amino acid analysis Karageozian (1976) found that deposits on lenses are almost entirely lysozyme and that the spectophotometric curves of the lens protein and lysozyme were almost identical.

Refojo and Holly (1977) have drawn attention to the fact that a substantial amount of research has been carried out on the blood compatibility of synthetic materials for use in heart valves and other devices. Foreign surfaces immersed in plasma adsorb rapidly at least a monomolecular layer of protein. This has been identified as the initial step that triggers the blood coagulation process. Tears, like plasma, contain dissolved protein. Refojo and Holly suggested that denaturation may take place to a different extent with different materials. If the allergy is to a product of denatured protein then one plastic may cause it more than another.

However, whether protein on the contact lens is the cause of giant papillary conjunctivitis or not, its removal by various enzymatic agents does not appear either to prevent the onset or to cure the disease.

Ballow *et al.* (1989) suggest that the syndrome is the result of a complex immunological process, an idea supported by the presence of elevated tear concentrations of IgG and IgE in giant papillary conjunctivitis. They took two soft contact lenses from patients with giant papillary conjunctivitis (GPC), two from asymptomatic contact lens wearers, and two clean unused lenses, and placed them in one eye of each of a group of cynomolgus monkeys. The lenses were held in place with a partial tarsorrhaphy. Tears from the two monkeys with GPC lenses showed increased levels of IgG, IgA and IgE, 35 to 75 days post lens placement. The tears from the two monkeys with clean lenses and the two lenses from asymptomatic contact lens wearers had elevated levels of IgG compared to the contralateral control eye without a lens, but the tear IgE levels remained normal. Histopathology studies of tarsal conjunctival biopsy material from the monkeys with GPC lenses showed an intense round cell infiltrate at the epithelial–stromal junction. Mast cells were seen in the epithelial layers. These authors suggest that some factor (or factors) in the lens coating from GPC patients was able to induce a local IgE response and histopathological changes in monkeys.

3 The plastic itself

It has been shown that plastic has immunogenic potential (Heggers, Talmage and Barnes, 1978). However, the mere implantation of plastic into tissue is not enough. The plastic must be stressed. In a contact lens, this stress may be produced by its continual movement with the eye against the upper lid.

Free monomer does not appear to be the problem since the chemistry has to be of a very high order in the contact lens industry in order to maintain the physical characteristics of the plastic and thus the parameters of the lens.

The surface characteristics of the plastic may be important, or perhaps its electrical charge. The walls of arteries and platelets have been shown to have a negative charge (Williams and Roaf, 1973) and a plastic may have a positive, neutral, or a different negative charge. This electrical charge may be important in the causation of giant papillary conjunctivitis.

Studies have been carried out (Kennedy *et al.*, 1978), comparing the infrared spectroscopy of plastics used in heart valves with the platelet morphology in the blood in which they are immersed using a scanning electron microscope. Similar work could be carried out to compare the infrared spectroscopy of contact lens plastics with the morphology of conjunctival cell cultures.

Treatment

Giant papillary conjunctivitis usually resolves within three months to two years if lens wear is discontinued. The disease usually becomes asymptomatic as soon as contact lens wear is discontinued and it is not necessary to prescribe topical steroids except perhaps in the rare case in which symptoms continue.

However, most patients wish to go on wearing their contact lenses and this may be necessary for visual reasons in patients with corneal pathology. The first objective should be to change the lens plastic, if possible to a different polymer, and if that is not possible, to a lens produced by a different manufacturer. The edge thickness, form and finish of a soft lens are critical to the development of giant papillary conjunctivitis. Changing these features while using the same plastic can reverse the ability of the lens to produce the disease.

Donshik *et al.* (1984) treated 45 patients with symptomatic giant papillary conjunctivitis by one of the following methods: (1) changing to a new lens of the same type; (2) changing to a different type of contact lens; or (3) changing the lens and adding 2% cromolyn sodium eye drops (sodium cromoglycate). Sixty-five per cent of the patients who were treated by changing to a new lens of the same type were able to continue wearing their lenses satisfactorily (for an average of 15.2 months). Seventy-five per cent of patients who were changed to a different type of contact lens were able to wear their lenses without any significant problems (for an average of 11.9 months). Seventy-eight per cent of the patients who had a return of symptoms after their contact lenses were changed were able, when treated with a new lens and cromolyn eye drops, to maintain contact lens wear (for an average of 7.7 months). By utilizing all three modalities they were able to keep 82% of their giant papillary conjunctivitis patients wearing contact lenses.

Reports are appearing in the literature that disposable lenses are useful in the management of giant papillary conjunctivitis (Cho, Norden and Chang, 1988; Coursaux *et al.*, 1989). The supposition is that, since these lenses are replaced frequently, deposit formation is less likely. However, proper evaluative studies will have to be performed to establish whether this modality is superior to merely changing the type of contact lens.

The giant papillary conjunctivitis which took many months to develop will take a long time to resolve and an interim period occurs when the new lens may be associated with a continuing inflammatory response. Gutt. sodium cromoglycate (Opticrom in the UK, Cromolyn in the USA) has been shown to be effective (Matter, Rahi and Buckley, 1985). Donshik *et al.* (1984) stated that cromolyn eye drops appeared to help in the treatment of their cases of refractory giant papillary conjunctivitis.

In the author's opinion it is useful, but is in no way curative. If the antigenic or mechanical factor is still present the disease will pursue a relentlessly progressive course despite the use of sodium cromoglycate. More potent mast cell stabilizers will soon be commercially available and it remains to be seen what effect these will have on the disease. The manufacturers of sodium cromoglycate in the UK insert a warning in their package to the effect that their drops must not be used in the presence of soft contact lenses. This warning was issued some six years after the drops were first introduced, despite the fact that there had been no reports of adverse reaction (Fisons, 1985, personal communication). It was introduced because the drops are preserved with benzylkonium chloride. This preservative has been shown to be toxic to corneal epithelial cells if in sufficient concentration.

Iwasaki *et al.* (1988) have studied the absorption of topical disodium cromoglycate and its preservative by soft contact lenses. The drug was administered to patients wearing both extended wear and daily wear soft contact lenses. The contact lenses and their soaking solutions were analysed for disodium cromoglycate, benzalkonium chloride, 2-phenylethanol and EDTA. During the study no side effects of disodium cromoglycate were observed in any of the patients. They concluded that commercial disodium cromoglycate, applied topically to contact lenses, does not result in the accumulation of either the drug or its preservatives in lenses and that disodium cromoglycate can be safely applied directly on to a worn contact lens.

Unit dose Opticrom (Fisons), without preservative, is available in some countries and here on a named patient basis.

Wood *et al.* (1988) have conducted a multicentre study of patients with contact lens associated giant papillary conjunctivitis treated with suprofen. This is a recently developed non-steroidal, anti-inflammatory agent, which inhibits prostaglandin synthesis through its inhibition of the cyclooxygenase system. The study was a randomized, double-masked comparison of 1.0% suprofen solution versus the suprofen vehicle solution (placebo). The patients were given two drops of medication four times daily for up to 28 days. Treatment with suprofen led to a greater overall reduction in ocular signs and symptoms than with placebo. Strong trends approaching statistically significant levels were found for reductions in the principal ocular sign, papillae, and in mucous strands which also favoured suprofen.

The tetracycline groups of drugs is helpful in reducing discharge and quietening the eye in this interim period. They are used at half the normal daily dose over a period of weeks, or even months, for example, Tabs. oxytetracycline 250 mg twice daily or Caps. doxycycline 100 mg on alternate days. Tetracycline has been shown to have anti-inflammatory as well as antibiotic activity (Elewski *et al.*, 1983) and given systemically finds its way to the goblet cells of the conjunctiva and thus the mucous coat of the eye (Dilly and Mackie, 1985). Doxycycline, although more expensive, may be useful where there is a compliance problem or where the twice daily tablet produces gastrointestinal problems. Because of its high lipid solubility doxycycline achieves high levels of concentration in tears in contrast to the low levels found with tetracycline and oxytetracycline (Hoeprich and Warshauer, 1974).

Topical steroids are rarely indicated. There may be a place for them when the contact lenses are the only means by which the patient can obtain adequate vision.

Finally, just as vernal conjunctivitis in children and young adults tends to run a course of about five years and then clear up, so may contact lens associated giant papillary conjunctivitis. The author has had a number of patients, for whom contact lens wearing was mandatory, who put up with the disease while using sodium cromoglycate and occasional systemic tetracycline group antibiotics. After a number of years the symptoms and signs have decreased. In no case has conjunctival scarring developed.

Visual complications

Insler, Hendricks and George (1988) have drawn attention to visual constriction caused by coloured contact lenses. They performed Goldmann visual field testing on 10 patients while they were wearing Durasoft 3 coloured soft contact lenses. All patients but one had visual field constriction ranging from 5° to 20°. When the areas inside the three tested isopters were averaged, the amount of field loss ranged from 21% to 47%.

References

ABELSON, M.B., BAIRD, R.S. and ALLANSMITH, M.R. (1980) Tear histamine levels in vernal conjunctivitis and other ocular inflammations. *Ophthalmology*, **87**, 812–815

ALFONSO, E., MANDELBAUM, S., FOX, M.J. *et al.* (1986) Ulcerative keratitis associated with contact lens wear. *American Journal of Ophthalmology*, **101**, 429–433

ALLANSMITH, M.R. and BAIRD, R.S. (1981) Percentage of degranulated mast cells in vernal conjunctivitis and giant papillary conjunctivitis associated with contact lens wear. *American Journal of Ophthalmology*, **9**, 1, 71–75

ALLANSMITH, M.R., BAIRD, R.S. and GREINER, J.V. (1979) Vernal conjunctivitis and contact lens associated giant papillary conjunctivitis compared and contrasted. *American Journal of Ophthalmology*, **87**, 544–555

ALLANSMITH, M.R., BAIRD, R.S. and GREINER, J.V. (1981) Density of goblet cells in vernal conjunctivitis and contact lens associated giant papillary conjunctivitis. *Archives of Ophthalmology*, **99**, 884–885

ALLANSMITH, M.R., KORB, D.R., GREINER, J.V., HENRIQUEZ, A.S., SIMON, M.A. and FINNEMORE, V. (1977) Giant papillary conjunctivitis in contact lens wearers. *American Journal of Ophthalmology*, **83**, 697

BADENOCH, P.R., HAY, G.J., MCDONALD, P.J. and COSTER, D.J. (1985) A rat model of bacterial keratitis. Effects of antibiotics and corticosteroid. *Archives of Ophthalmology*, **103**, 718–722

BALLOW, M., DONSHIK, P.C., RAPACY, P., MAENZA, R., YAMASE, H. and MUNCY, L. (1989) Immune responses in monkeys to lenses from patients with contact lens induced giant papillary conjunctivitis. *CLAO Journal*, **15**, 1, 64–70

BAUM, J. (1986) Therapy for ocular bacterial infection. *Transactions of the Ophthalmological Society of the UK*, **105**, part 1, 69–77

BERGMANSON, J.P.G. and CHU, L. (1982) Corneal response to rigid contact lens wear. *British Journal of Ophthalmology*, **66**, 667–675

BONANNO, J.A. and POLSE, K.A. (1987) Corneal acidosis during contact lens wear: effects of hypoxia and CO_2. *Investigative Ophthalmology and Visual Science*, **28**, 9, 1514–1520

BORRMAN, L.R. and LEOPOLD, I.H. (1988) The potential use of quinolones in future ocular antimicrobial therapy. *American Journal of Ophthalmology*, **106**, 227–229

BOYCE, J.M., LANDRY, M., DEETZ, T.R. and DU PONT, H.L. (1981) Epidemiology of methicillin resistant *Staphylococcus aureus* infections. In *Current Chemotherapy and Infectious Disease. Proceedings of the 11th International Congress of Chemotherapy and the 19th Interscience Conference on Antimicrobial Agents and Chemotherapy* (Nelson, J.D. and Grassi, C. eds). American Society for Microbiology, Washington DC, pp. 503–504

BRAATHEN, L.R. (1980) Studies on human epidermal Langerhans cells III. Induction of T lymphocyte response to nickel sulphate in sensitised individuals. *British Journal of Dermatology*, **103**, 517–526

BRAATHEN, L.R. and THORSBY, E. (1983) Human epidermal Langerhans cells are more potent than blood monocytes in inducing antigen-specific T cell responses. *British Journal of Dermatology*, **108**, 139–146

BROOKS, A.H., GRANT, C., WESTMORE, R. and ROBERTSON, I.F. (1986) Deep corneal stromal opacities with contact lenses. *Australian and New Zealand Journal of Ophthalmology*, **14**, 3, 243–247

BROWN, N. and LOBASCHER, D. (1975) Complications of soft contact lens use in the correction of simple refractive errors. *Proceedings of the Royal Society of Medicine*, **68**, 52–53

CARLSON, K.H. and BOURNE, W.M. (1988) Endothelial morphological features and function after long term extended wear of contact lenses. *Archives of Ophthalmology*, **106**, 1677–1679

CARLSON, K.H., BOURNE, W.M. and BRUBAKER, R.F. (1986) Effect of long term contact lens wear on corneal endothelial cell morphology and function. *Investigative Ophthalmology and Visual Science*, **27**, 2, 185–193

CHO, M.H., NORDEN, L.C. and CHANG, F.W. (1988) Disposable extended wear soft contact lenses for the treatment of giant papillary conjunctivitis. *Southern Journal of Optometry*, 6, 1, 9–12

CONNOR, C.G. and ZAGROD, M.E. (1986) Contact lens induced corneal endothelial polymegethism: functional significance and possible mechanisms. *American Journal of Optometry and Physiological Optics*, 63, 539–544

COSTER, D.J. (1985) Bacterial corneal ulcers. In *Current Ocular Therapy* (Fraunfelder, F.T. and Roy, F.H., eds). W.B. Saunders, Philadelphia and London

COURSAUX, G., BLOCH-MICHEL, E., FELLOUS, J.C. and MASSIN, M. (1989) Refitting of giant papillary conjunctivitis patients with Acuvue disposable contact lenses. *Contactologia* (English edition), 12, 1, 26–28

CREMER-BARTELS, G. (1977) The effect of the corneal epithelium on the biosynthesis of keratan sulphate in the stroma with regard to curvature variations important for wearing contact lenses. *Klinische Monatsblatter fur Augenheilkunde*, 171, 6, 981–986

DILLY, P.N. and MACKIE, I.A. (1985) Distribution of tetracycline in the conjunctiva of patients on long term systemic doses. *British Journal of Ophthalmology*, 69, 1, 25–28

DONSHIK, P.C. and BALLOW, M. (1983) Tear immunoglobulins in giant papillary conjunctivitis induced by contact lenses. *American Journal of Ophthalmology*, 96, 460–466

DONSHIK, P.C., BALLOW, M., LUISTRO, A. and SAMARTINO, L. (1984) Treatment of contact lens-induced giant papillary conjunctivitis. *CLAO Journal*, 10, 4, 346–349

DRIEBE, W.T., STERN, G.A., EPSTEIN, R.J., VISVESVARA, G.S., ADI, M. and KOMADINA, T. (1988) Acanthamoeba keratitis. Potential role for topical clotrimazole in combination chemotherapy. *Archives of Ophthalmology*, 106, 1196–1201

EFRON, N. and ANG, I.H.B. (1990) Corneal hypoxia and hypercapnia during contact lens wear. *Optometry and Visual Science*, 67, 7, 512–521

EGGINK, F.A.G.J., PINCKERS, A.J.L.G. and AANDEKERK, A.L. (1991) Subepithelial opacities in daily wear high water content soft contact lenses. *Contactologia*, 13, 4, 173–176

ELEWSKI, B.E., LAMB, B.A.J., SAMS, W.M. and GAMMON, W.R. (1983) In vivo suppression of neutrophil chemotaxis by systemically and topically administered tetracycline. *Journal of the American Academy of Dermatology*, 8, 807–812

ELGEBALY, S.A., DONSHIK, P.C., RAHHAL, F. and WILLIAMS, W. (1991) Neutrophil chemotactic factors in the tears of giant papillary conjunctivitis patients. *Investigative Ophthalmology and Visual Science*, 32, 1, 208–213

EPSTEIN, R.J., WILSON, L.A., VISVESVARA, G.S. and PLOURDE, E.G. (1986) Rapid diagnosis of acanthamoeba keratitis from corneal scrapings using indirect fluorescent antibody staining. *Archives of Ophthalmology*, 104, 1318–1321

FICKER, L. (1988) Acanthamoeba keratitis – the quest for a better prognosis. *Eye*, 2, (Suppl.), 537–545

FLORAKIS, G.T., FOLBERG, R., KRACHMER, J.H., TSE, D.T., ROUSSEL, T.J. and VRABEC, M.P. (1988) Elevated corneal epithelial lines in Acanthamoeba keratitis. *Archives of Ophthalmology*, 106, 1202–1206

FOWLER, S.A., GREINER, J.V. and ALLANSMITH, M.A. (1979) Soft contact lenses from patients with giant papillary conjunctivitis. *American Journal of Ophthalmology*, 88, 1056–1061

FRANCOIS, M.J. (1956) Une nouvelle dystrophie heredofamiliale de la cornée. *Journal de Genetique Humaine*, 5, 189–196

GALENTINE, P.G., COHEN, E.J., LAIBSON, P.R. et al. (1984) Corneal ulcers associated with contact lens wear. *Archives of Ophthalmology*, 102, 891–894

GOBBELS, M., WAHNING, A. and SPITZNAS, M. (1989) Endothelial function in contact lens-induced deep corneal opacities. *Fortschritte der Ophthalmologie*, 86, 5, 448–450

GRAHAM, C.M., DART, J.K.G., WILSON-HOLT, N.W. and BUCKLEY, R.J. (1986) Prospects for contact lens wear in aphakia. *Eye*, 2, 48–55

GRANT, T., TERRY, R. and HOLDEN, B.A. (1990) Extended wear of hydrogel lenses. Clinical problems and their management. *Problems in Optometry*, 2, 4, 599–622

GRANT, W.M. (1974) Survey of types of toxic effects involving the eyes or vision. In *Toxicology of the Eye*, 2nd edn. Charles C. Thomas, Springfield, pp 5–18

GREINER, J.V., KENYON, K.R., HENRIQUEZ, A.S., KORB, D.R., WEIDMAN, T.A. and ALLANSMITH, M.R. (1980) Mucus secretory vesicles in conjunctival epithelial cells of wearers of contact lenses. *Archives of Ophthalmology*, 98, 1843–1846

HARRER, S. and RUBEY, F. (1981) Differentialdiagnose von Hornhautveranderungen bei Tragern von Hema-Linsen. *Klinische Monatsblatter fur Augenheilkunde*, 179, 445–447

HARWOOD, C.R., RICH, G.E., MCALEER, R. and CHERIAN, G. (1988) Isolation of acanthamoeba from a cerebral abscess. *Medical Journal of Australia*, 148, 1, 47–49

HEGGERS, J.P., TALMAGE, J.B. and BARNES, S.T. (1978) Cellular immune response to methylmethacrylate in experimentally sensitized guinea pigs. *Military Medicine*, 143, 192–195

HENRIQUEZ, A.S., KENYON, K.R. and ALLANSMITH, M.R. (1981) Mast cell ultrastructure comparison in contact lens-associated giant papillary conjunctivitis. *Archives of Ophthalmology*, 99, 7, 1266–1272

HINE, N., BACK, A. and HOLDEN, B. (1987) Aetiology of arcuate epithelial lesions induced by hydrogels. *Transactions of BCLA Conference*, 1987. British Contact Lens Association, London, pp. 48–50

HIRST, L., AUER, C., COHN, J., TSENG, S. and KHODADOUST, A. (1984) Specular microscopy of hard contact lens wearers. *Ophthalmology*, 91, 1147–1153

HOEPRICH, P.D. and WARSHAUER, D.M. (1974) Entry of four tetracyclines into saliva and tears. *Antimicrobial Agents and Chemotherapy*, **5**, 330–336

HOLDEN, B.A. (1989) The Glenn A. Fry Award Lecture, 1988. The ocular response to contact lens wear. *Optometry and Visual Sicence*, **66**, 717–733

HOLDEN, B.A., GRANT, T., KOTOW, M., SCHNIDER, C. and SWEENEY, D.F. (1987) Epithelial microcysts with daily wear and extended wear of hydrogel and rigid gas-permeable contact lenses. *Investigative Ophthalmology and Visual Science*, **28** (Suupl.), 372

HOLDEN, B.A., SWEENEY, D.F., EFRON, N., VANNAS, A. and NILSSON, K.T. (1988) Contact lenses can induce stromal thinning. *Clinical and Experimental Optometry*, **71**, 4, 109–113

HOLDEN, B.A., SWEENEY, D., VANNAS, A., NILSSON, K. and EFRON, N. (1985) Effects of long term extended contact lens wear on the human cornea. *Investigative Ophthalmology and Visual Science*, **26**, 1489–1501

HOROWITZ, G., LIN, J. and CHEW, H.C. (1985) An unusual corneal complication of soft contact lens. *American Journal of Ophthalmology*, **100**, 794–797

HUMPHREYS, J.A., LARKE, J.R. and PARRISH, S.T. (1980) Microepithelial cysts observed in extended contact-lens wearing subjects. *British Journal of Ophthalmology*, **64**, 888–889

INSLER, M.S., HENDRICKS, C. and GEORGE, D.M. (1988) Visual field constriction caused by coloured contact lenses. *Archives of Ophthalmology*, **106**, 1680–1682

ISHIBASHI, Y., MATSUMOTO, Y., KABATA, T. *et al.* (1990) Oral itraconazole and topical miconazole with debridement for Acanthamoeba keratitis. *American Journal of Ophthalmology*, **109**, 2, 121–126

IWASAKI, W., KOSAKA, Y., MOMOSE, T. and YASUDA, T. (1988) Absorption of topical disodium cromoglycate and its preservatives by soft contact lenses. *CLAO Journal*, **14**, 3, 155–158

JACKSON, M., CHAN, R., MATOBA, A.Y. and ROBIN, J.B. (1989) The use of fluorescein-conjugated lectins for visualizing atypical Mycobacteria. *Archives of Ophthalmology*, **107**, 1206–1209

JAY, J.L. (1981) Clinical features and diagnosis of adult atopic keratoconjunctivitis and the effect of treatment with sodium cromoglycate. *British Journal of Ophthalmology*, **65**, 335–340

JOHNS, K.J., HEAD, W.S., PARRISH, C.M., WILLIAMS, T.E., ROBINSON, R.D. and O'DAY, D.M. (1989) Examination of hydrophilic contact lenses with light microscopy to aid in the diagnosis of Acanthamoeba keratitis. *American Journal of Ophthalmology*, **108**, 3, 329–331

JONES, B.R. (1975) Principles in the management of oculomycosis. XXXI Edward Jackson Memorial Lecture. *American Journal of Ophthalmology*, **79** (5), 719–751

JONES, B.R., MCGILL, J.I. and STEELE, A.D.MCG. (1975) Recurrent suppurative keratouveitis with loss of eye due to infection by *Acanthamoeba castellani*. *Transactions of the Opthalmological Society of the UK*, **95**, 211–213

JONES, D.B. (1980) Strategy for the initial management of suspected microbial keratitis. In *Symposium on Medical and Surgical Diseases of the Cornea. Transactions of New Orleans Academy of Ophthalmology*. C.V. Mosby Co., St Louis

JONES, D.B., VISVESVARA, G.S. and ROBINSON, H.M. (1975) *Acanthamoeba polyphaga*, keratitis and acanthamoeba uveitis associated with fatal meningoencephalitis. *Transactions of the Ophthalmological Society of the UK*, **95**, 221–232

KARAGEOZIAN, H.L. (1976) Use of amino acid analyser to illustrate the efficacy of an enzyme preparation for cleaning hydrophilic lenses. *Contacto*, **20**, 5–10

KAUFMAN, H.E., GASSET, A.R. and UOTILA, M.H. (1972) Treatment of corneal disease with soft contact lenses. In *Transactions of New Orleans Academy of Ophthalmology. Symposium on Contact Lenses* (Black, C.J., ed). CV Mosby Co., St Louis, Chapter 17, pp 174–180

KENNEDY, J.K., ISHIDA, H., STAIKOFF, L.S. and LEWIS, C.W. (1978) Correlation of infrared spectroscopy and platelet morphology in blood compatibility studies of polydimethylsiloxane membranes. *Medical Devices and Artifical Organs*, **6**, 3–8

KENYON, K.R. and TSENG, S.C.G. (1989) Limbal autograft transplantation for ocular surface disorders. *Ophthalmology*, **96**, 5, 709–723

KHAN, J.A., HOOVER, D. and IDE, C.H. (1984) Methicillin-resistant *Staphylococcus epidermidis*. *American Journal of Ophthalmology*, **98**, 562–565

KLINE, L.N., DELUCA, T.J. and FISHBERG, G.M. (1979) Corneal staining relating to contact lens wear. *Journal of the American Optometric Association*, **50**, 3, 353–357

KLYCE, S.D. (1981) Stromal lactate accumulation can account for corneal oedema osmotically following epithelial hypoxia in the rabbit. *Journal of Physiology*, **321**, 49

KOENIG, S.B., SOLOMON, J.M., HYNDIUK, R.A., SUCHER, R.A and GRADUS, M.S. (1987) Acanthamoeba keratitis associated with gas permeable contact lens wear. *American Journal of Ophthalmology*, **103**, 832

KORB, D.R. and HERMAN, J.P. (1979) Corneal staining subsequent to sequential fluorescein instillation. *Journal of the American Optometric Association*, **50**, 3, 361–367

KORB, D.R., GREINER, J.V., FINNEMORE, V.M. and ALLAN-SMITH, M.R. (1983) Biomicroscopy of papillae associated with wearing of soft contact lenses. *British Journal of Ophthalmology*, **67**, 733–736

KRATCHMER, J.H. and PURCELL, J.J. JR (1978) Bacterial corneal ulcers in cosmetic soft contact lens wearers. *Archives of Ophthalmology*, **96**, 57–61

LARKIN, D.F.P., KILVINGTON, S. and DART, J.K.G. (1992) Treatment of Acanthamoeba keratitis with polyhexamethylene biguanide. *Ophthalmology*, **99**, 2, 185–191

LEIBOWITZ, H.M. (1991) Clinical evaluation of ciprofloxacin 0.3% ophthalmic solution for treatment of bacterial keratitis. *American Journal of Ophthalmology*, **112**, 34S–47S

LEMP, M.A., BLACKMAN, H.J. and KOFFLER, B.H. (1980) Therapy for bacterial and fungal infections. *International Ophthalmology Clinic*, **20** (3), 135–147

LOWY, F.D. and HAMMER, S.M. (1983) *Staphylococcus epidermidis* infections. *Annals of Internal Medicine*, **99**, 834

LUSTBADER, J.M., STARK, W.J. and KRACHER, G.P. (1986) Corneal ulcers in extended contact lens wearers. *Investigative Ophthalmology and Visual Science*, **27** (Suppl.), 139

MCCULLEY, J.P., MAURICE, D.M. and SCHWARTZ, B.D. (1980) Corneal endothelial transplantation. *Ophthalmology (Rochester)*, **87**, 3, 194–201

MCMONNIES, C.W. and ZANTOS, S.G. (1979) Endothelial bedewing of the cornea in association with contact lens wear. *British Journal of Ophthalmology*, **63**, 7, 478–481

MACKIE, I.A. and WRIGHT, P. (1978) Giant papillary conjunctivitis (secondary vernal) in association with contact lens wear. *Transactions of the Ophthalmological Society of the UK*, **98**, 3–9

MACKIE, I.A. and WRIGHT, P. (1979) Giant papillary conjunctivitis – an iatrogenic disease resembling vernal conjunctivitis. In *The Mast Cell* (Pepys, J., Edwards, A.M., eds). Pitman Medical Publishing Co. Ltd, Tunbridge Wells, Kent

MACRAE, S.M., MATSUDA, M. and SHELLANS, S. (1989) Corneal endothelial changes associated with contact lens wear. *CLAO Journal*, **15**, 1, 82–87

MACRAE, S.M., MATSUDA, M., SHELLANS, S. and RICH, L.F. (1986) The effects of hard and soft contact lenses on the corneal epithelium. *American Journal of Opthalmology*, **102**, 50–57

MADIGAN, M.C., PENFOLD, P.L., HOLDEN, B.A. and BILLSON, F.A. (1990) Ultrastructural features of contact lens-induced deep corneal neovascularisations and associated stromal leucocytes. *Cornea*, **9**, 2, 144–151

MALONEY, W.F. COLVARD, M., BOURNE, W.M. and GARDON, R. (1979) Specular microscopy od traumatic posterior annular keratopathy. *Archives of Ophthalmology*, **97**, 1647–1650

MANNIS, M.J., TAMARU, R., ROTH, A.N., BURNS, M. and THIRKILL, C. (1986) Acanthamoeba sclerokeratitis. *Archives of Ophthalmology*, **104**, 1313–1317

MARGULIES, L.J. and MANNIS, M.J. (1983) Dendritic corneal lesions associated with soft contact lens wear. *Archives of Ophthalmology*, **101**, 1551–1553

MASKE, R., HILL, J.C. and OLIVER, S.P. (1986) Management of bacterial corneal ulcers. *British Journal of Ophthalmology*, **70**, 199–201

MATOBA, A.Y., PARE, P.D., TRANG, D. LE and OSATO, M.S. (1989) The effects of freezing and antibiotics on the viability of Acanthamoeba cysts. *Archives of Ophthalmology*, **107**, 439–440

MATTER, M., RAHI, A.H.S. and BUCKLEY, R.J. (1985) Sodium cromoglycate in the treatment of contact lens associated giant papillary conjunctivitis. *Proceedings of the 7th Congress of the European Society of Ophthalmology, 1984*. Yliopistopaino, Helsinki

MAURICE, D.M., MCCULLEY, J.P. and SCHWARTZ, B.D. (1981) The use of cultured endothelium in keratoplasty. *Vision Research*, **21** (1), 173–174

MEISLER, D.M., ZARET, C.R. and STOCK, E.L. (1980) Trantas' dots and limbal inflammation associated with soft contact lens wear. *American Journal of Ophthalmology*, **89**, 66–69

MONDINO, B.J., BROWN, S.I. and RABIN, B.S. (1978) Role of complement in corneal inflammation. *Transactions of the Ophthalmological Society of the UK*, **98** (3), 363–366

MONDINO, B.J., SALAMON, S.M. and ZAIDMAN, G.W. (1982) Allergic and toxic reactions in soft contact lens wearers. *Survey of Ophthalmology*, **26**, 337–343

MONDINO, B.J., BARRY, A., WEISSMAN, O.D., FARB, M.D. and PETTIT, T.H. (1986) Corneal ulcers associated with daily-wear and extended-wear contact lenses. *American Journal of Ophthalmology*, **102**, 58–65

MOORE, M.B. and MCCULLEY, J.P. (1989) Acanthamoeba keratitis associated with contact lenses: six consecutive cases of successful management. *British Journal of Ophthalmology*, **73**, 271–275

MOORE, M.B., MCCULLEY, J.P. and NEWTON, C. (1987) Acanthamoeba keratitis. A growing problem in soft and hard contact lens wearers. *Ophthalmology*, **94**, 12, 1654–1661

NAGINGTON, J., WATSON, P.G., PLAYFAIR, T.J., MCGILL, J.I., JONES, B.R. and STEELE, A.D.MCG. (1974) Amoebic infection of the eye. *Lancet*, ii, 1537–1540

O'DAY, D.M. (1987) Selection of appropriate antifungal therapy. *Cornea*, **6** (4), 238–245

ORSBORN, G.N. and ZANTOS, S.G. (1988) Corneal desiccation staining with thin high water content contact lenses. *CLAO Journal*, **14**, 2, 81–85

PAYRAU, P. and RAYNAUD, G. (1965) Lesions de la cornea par souffle; corps etranger perforantes microscopiques: anneaux veloutes posterieurs. *Annales D'Oculistique*, 2nd edn. 198, 1057–1074

PINCKERS, A., EGGINK, F., AANDERKERK, A.L. and VAN 'T PAD BOSCH, A. (1987) Contact lens-induced pseudo-dystrophy of the cornea? *Documenta Ophthalmologica*, **65**, 433–437

PINNOLIS, M., MCCULLEY, J.P. and URMAN, J.D. (1980) Nummular keratitis associated with infectious mononucleosis. *American Journal of Ophthalmology*, **89**, 791–794

POGGIO, E.C., GLYNN, R.J., SCHEIN, O.D. *et al.* (1989) The incidence of ulcerative keratitis among users of daily wear and extended wear soft contact lenses. *New England Journal of Medicine*, **321**, 12, 779–783

POLSE, K.A., SARVER, D. and HARRIS, M.G. (1973) Corneal oedema and vertical striae accompanying the wearing of hydrogel lenses. *American Journal of Optometry and Physiological Optics*, **52**, 183–191

PTAK, W., TOZYCKA, D., ASKENASE, P.W. and GERSHON, R.K. (1980) The role of antigen presenting cells in the development and persistence of contact hypersensitivity. *Journal of Experimental Medicine*, **151**, 362–375

REFOJO, M.F. (1979) Materials in bandage lenses. *Contact and Intraocular Lens Medical Journal*, 5, 1, 34–44

REFOJO, M.F. and HOLLY, F.J. (1977) Tear protein adsorption on hydrogels: A possible cause of contact allergy.

Contact and Intraocular Lens Medical Journal, **3** (1), 23–35

REMEIJER, L., VAN RIJ, G., BEEKHUIS, H., POLAK, B.C.P. and NES, J. (1990) Deep corneal stromal opacities in long term contact lens wear. *Ophthalmology*, **97**, 3, 281–285

RODRIGUES, M.M. (1982) Langerhans cells in the normal conjunctiva and peripheral cornea of selected species. *Investigative Ophthalmology and Visual Science*, **21**, (5), 759–765

ROSENFELD, S.I., MANDELBAUM, S., CORRENT, G.F., PFLUGFELDER, S.C. and CULBERTSON, W.W. (1990) Granular epithelial keratopathy as an unusual manifestation of Pseudomonas keratitis associated with extended-wear soft contact lenses. *American Journal of Ophthalmology*, **109**, 17–22

SCHANZER, M.C., MEHTA, R.S., ARNOLD, T.P., ZUCHERBROD, S.L. and KOCH, D.D. (1989) Irregular astigmatism induced by annular tinted contact lenses. *CLAO Journal*, **15**, 3, 207–211

SCHERMER, A., GALVIN, S. and SUN, T-T. (1986) Differentiation related expression of a major 64K corneal keratin in vivo and in culture suggests limbal location of corneal epithelial stem cells. *Journal of Cell Biology*, **103**, 49–62

SCHOESSLER, J.P. (1987) The corneal endothelium after 20 years of PMMA contact lens wear. *CLAO Journal*, **13**, 157–160

SHERRARD, E.S. and BUCKLEY, R.J. (1981a) Cliniccal specular microscopy of the corneal epithelium. *Transactions of the Ophthalmological Society of the UK*, **101**, 156–162

SHERRARD, E.S. and BUCKLEY, R.J. (1981b) Endothelial wrinkling – a complication of clinical specular microscopy. In *The Cornea in Health and Disease. Transactions of the VIth Congress of the European Society of Ophthalmology, 1981* (Trevor Roper, P.D. ed.). Academic Press and Royal Society of Medicine, London, Series 40, pp. 69–74

SILVANY, R.E., LUCKENBACH, M.W. and MOORE, B. (1987) The rapid detection of acanthamoeba in paraffin-embedded sections of corneal tissue with calcofluor white. *Archives of Ophthalmology*, **105**, 10, 1366–1367

SPRING, T.F. (1974) Reaction to hydrophilic lenses. *Medical Journal of Australia*, **1**, 449–450

SRINIVASAN, B.D., WORGUL, B.V., IWAMOTO, T. and MERRIAM, G.R. (1977) The conjunctival epithelium. Histochemical and ultrastructural studies on human and rat conjunctivae. *Ophthalmic Research*, **9**, 65–79

STEIN, R.M., CLINCH, T.E., COHEN, E.J., GENVERT, G.I., ARENTSEN, J.J. and LAIBSON, P.R. (1988) Infected vs sterile corneal infiltrates in contact lens wearers. *American Journal of Ophthalmology*, **105**, 6, 632–636

STRACHAN, I.M (1969) Cloudy central corneal dystrophy of Francois. *British Journal of Ophthalmology*, **53**, 192–194

STULTING, R.D., RODRIGUES, M.M. and NAY, R.E. (1986) Ultrastructure of traumatic corneal endothelial rings. *American Journal of Ophthalmology*, **101**, 156–159

TAGAWA, Y. and MATSUDA, H. (1988) Langerhans cells in

allergic conjunctival diseases. *Proceedings of the XXVth International Congress of Ophthalmology, Rome, 1986*, pp. 82–84. Kugler Publications, Berkeley, and Ghedini Editore, Milan

THEODORE, F.H., JACOBIEC, F.A., JUECHTER, K.B. *et al.* (1985) The diagnostic value of a ring infiltrate in acanthamoebic keratitis. *Ophthalmology*, **92**, 1471–1479

THOFT, R.A. (1984) Keratoepithelioplasty. *American Journal of Ophthalmology*, **97**, 1–6

THOFT, R.A. (1989) The role of the limbus in ocular surface maintenance and repair. *Acta Ophthalmologica*, **67** (Suppl. 192), 91–94

TROCME, S.D., KEPHART, G.M., ALLANSMITH, M.R., BOURNE, W.M. and GLEICH, G.J. (1989) Conjunctival deposition of eosinophil granule major basic protein in vernal keratoconjunctivitis and contact lens-associated giant papillary conjunctivitis. *American Journal of Ophthalmology*, **108**, 57–63

TURGEON, P.W., NAUHEIM, R.C., ROAT, M.I., STOPAK, S.S. and THOFT, R.A. (1990) Indications for keratoepithelioplasty. *Archives of Ophthalmology*, **108**, 233–236

UDELL, I.J., GLEICH, G.J., ALLANSMITH, M.R., ACKERMAN, S.J. and ABELSON, M.B. (1981) Eosinophil granule major basic protein and Charcot-leyden crystal protein in human tears. *American Journal of Ophthalmology*, **92**, 824–828

UDELL, I.J., MANNIS, M.J., MEISLER, D.M. and LANGSTON, R.H.S (1985) Pseudodendrites in soft contact lens wearers. *CLAO Journal*, **11**, 1, 51–53

VOGT, A. (1930) *Lehrbuch und atlas der spaltenlampe mikroskopie des lebenden auges*, **1**, 238–241. Springer, Berlin

WILHELMUS, K.R., OSATO, M.S., FONT, R.L., ROBINSON, N.M. and JONES, D.B. (1986) Rapid diagnosis of acanthamoeba keratitis using Calcofluor White. *Archives of Ophthalmology*, **104**, 1309–1312

WILHELMUS, K.R., MCCULLOCH, R.R. and OSATO, M.S. (1988) Photomicrography of Acanthamoeba cysts in human cornea. *American Journal of Ophthalmology*, **106**, 5, 628–630

WILHELMUS, K.R., ROBINSON, N.M., FONT, R.A., HAMILL, M.B. and JONES, D.B. (1988) Fungal keratitis in contact lens wearers. *American Journal of Ophthalmology*, **106**, 6, 708–714

WILLIAMS, C.E. (1986) Soft contact lens toxic occlusion phenomenon. *Contact Lens Spectrum*, Nov., 14–18

WILLIAMS, D.F. and ROAF, R. (1973) *Implants in Surgery*. Saunders, Philadelphia

WILSON, L.A. and AHEARN, D.G. (1986) Association of fungi with extended wear soft contact lenses. *American Journal of Ophthalmology*, **101**, 434–436

WILSON, L., SCHLITZEER, R. and AHEARN, D. (1981) Pseudomonas corneal ulcers associated with contact lens wear. *American Journal of Ophthalmology*, **92**, 546–554

WOLOSCHAK, M. (1983) The corneal endothelial appearance in unilateral contact lens wearers. *Master's Thesis*, the Ohio State University (J. Schoessler adviser)

WOOD, T.S., STEWART, R.H., BOWMAN, R.W., MCCULLEY, J.P.

and REAVES, T.A. (1988) Suprofen treatment of contact lens-associated giant papillary conjunctivitis. *Ophthalmology*, **95**, 6, 822–826

WRIGHT, P. and MACKIE, I.A. (1982) Preservative related problems in soft contact lens wearers. *Transactions of the Ophthalmological Society of the UK*, **102**, 3–6

WRIGHT, P., WARHURST, D. and JONES, B.R. (1985) Acanthamoeba keratitis successfully treated medically. *British Journal of Ophthalmology*, **69**, 778–782

WRIGHT, W.L. (1982) Scuba divers delayed toxic epithelial keratopathy from commercial mask defogging agents. *American Journal of Ophthalmology*, **93**, 470–472

YEOH, R.L.S., COX, N. and FALCON, M.G. (1989) Spontaneous intracorneal haemorrhage. *British Journal of Ophthalmology*, **73**, 363–364

ZANOTS, S.G. and HOLDEN, B.A. (1977) Transient endothelial changes soon after wearing soft contact lenses. *American Journal of Optometry and Physiological Optics*, **54** (12), 856–858

Appendix 13.I

Processing smears of corneal scrapings

Fix by immersion in methanol for five minutes.

1   Gram stain

- Flood the slide with 0.5% crystal violet for one minute then rinse with tap water.
- Flood the slide with Gram's iodine for one minute then rinse with tap water.
- Decolorize with a few drops of ethanol-acetone or 95% ethanol, then rinse thoroughly with tap water.
- Flood the slide with safranin for one minute then rinse with tap water.
- Blot dry and examine with oil immersion microscopy.

2   Giemsa stain

- Prepare fresh Giemsa stain by mixing 45 ml distilled water, 2 ml buffer (pH 6.5) solution and add 1 ml Giemsa stain.
- Immerse slide into staining jar for 45–60 minutes.
- Dip slide into 95% ethanol briefly.
- Blot gently and air dry.

3   Calcafluor white stain

- Prepare staining solution of 0.1% calcafluor white and 0.1% Evans blue in distilled water.
- Flood slide with stain for five minutes.
- Apply coverslip and examine with fluorescent microscopy.

Appendix 13.II

Flow plan for consecutive staining of a single microscope slide smear (D.V. Seal):

1. Gram stain (for staphylococci, streptococci, coliforms, pseudomonas and aerobic bacteria) (Destain with acetone or acid/alcohol)
2. Modified Ziehl-Nielsen stain (for Nocardia and various Actinomycetes) (Destain with acid/alcohol)
3. Full Ziehl-Nielsen stain (for Mycobacteria) NB Nocardia and Actinomycetes are decolorized by this stain. (Destain with acid/alcohol)

Then there is a choice of three stains which cannot be destained:

(a) Periodic Acid Schiff (for fungi)
(b) Methenamine silver stain (Grocott stain) (for fungi) NB This is a good stain for hyphal cell walls but needs experience.
(c) Acridene orange stain (for all types of bacteria and fungi) NB Fresh 1% solution must be used and visualization is for yellow/orange fluorescence under UV light. The stain is difficult to use on cellular material, but good for fluids, e.g. aqueous or vitreous.

Appendix 13.III

Culture of corneal scrapings and solutions

In standard media for 48 hours

Chocolate agar
Sabouraud agar
Brain-heart infusion broth

Re-incubate negatives in 5% CO_2 (for Nocardia) for 5 days.

Re-incubate negatives at 30° + 25° (for fungi) for 2 weeks.

Rescrape for special media after cessation of treatment for 24 hours.

Non-nutrient *E. coli*-seeded agar (Acanthamoebae).

Lowenstein-Jensen (Mycobacteria).

Sabouraud with vegetable matter or dung (plant fungi).

Virus transport media.

14

Therapeutic uses of contact lenses

One of the first hard scleral lenses, produced by F. Ad. Muller Sohne at Wiesbaden, in the 1880s, was for a patient of Dr Theodore Saemish whose eye was exposed because of lupus vulgaris of the lids. Since then scleral lenses have been repeatedly used for therapeutic reasons.

Over the past 20 years soft hydrophilic contact lenses have been increasingly used in the management of external eye disease. They have been termed 'bandage lenses' because of their protective role. However, the precise way in which they function is far from clear. They have largely replaced tarsorrhaphy as a mode of therapy.

Tarsorrhaphy has long been used in the treatment of corneal disease and is most effective if it is performed centrally. It is, however, a blinding procedure and if there is no vision in the other eye it is hardly acceptable as a treatment. Tarsorrhaphy also has the disadvantage that is obscures the eye and little indication is obtainable from inspection as to whether and when it can be undone. Lateral tarsorrhaphy may contribute to the wellbeing of a cornea, but it may actually interfere with the normal pattern of blinking and thus lead to more exposure of the cornea.

It might appear that closure of an eye would exacerbate a disease process by diminishing the available oxygen to the cornea, but in such conditions as neuroparalytic keratitis and persistent epithelial defect the only satisfactory treatment at present is closure. In experiments on rabbits, Ali and Insler (1986) have established that corneal epithelial wound healing is increased by tarsorrhaphy and decreased by bandage soft lenses. Zimny and Salisbury (1982) have compared two types of contact lenses (high and low water content) with regard to epithelial migration. They

were able to correlate low water content with inhibition of cell migration, and higher water content with cell migration beginning at 16 hours. Zimny and Salisbury (1982) believe that other treatment modalities should precede the use of a therapeutic bandage lens whenever a patient presents with an acute epithelial defect.

The management of such corneal disease with soft lenses is certainly not without its dangers and before this avenue of approach is contemplated it is well worth considering temporary closure of the eye with tape. Immobilization of the eyelid in this way may present less trauma to healing epithelium. The author's preference is for Blenderm (3M Company). A two and a half inch (64 mm) portion of one inch (25 mm) wide tape is used to close the eye. Before the tape is applied, the eye should be in a relaxed, closed state. The tape is usually applied horizontally, but some patients may find it more convenient to apply it vertically (Figure 14.1). The skin should be clean and dry. Cutting the lashes greatly facilitates the application and ensures better closure. Another suitable tape is Transpore (3M Company).

Tape closure has the advantage that it can be used according to the patient's needs. Thus, if a patient has a persistent epithelial breakdown as a feature of neuroparalytic keratitis it can be used to close the eye during waking hours. After the epithelial defect has healed, uncovering the eye for, perhaps, one-third of the day can be tried to see the effect this has on epithelial integrity. The time of opening can be further increased according to the clinical findings. This is a safe method of management.

A further method of closing an eye, and thus obviating tarsorrhaphy, has recently been found

164

to be effective in some cases which do not heal with taping (Adams, Kirkness and Lee, 1987). Botulinum toxin A (Dysport, supplied by Porton Products Ltd, Porton House, Vanwall Road, Maidenhead, Berkshire, SL6 4UB) is used. Dysport is supplied as a white, freeze-dried pellet containing 500 units of the toxin and this is mixed with 2.5 ml of sodium chloride injection BP (0.9%). This yields a clear solution containing 200 units/ml of Dysport. A dose of 0.05 ml (10 units) or 0.10 ml (20 units) is injected into the levator palpebrae superioris. This is reached by passing a 25 gauge, one inch (25 mm) long, orange needle through the skin of the upper lid midway and just under the superior orbital rim. The needle should be mounted on a 1.0 ml syringe. The patient should look down. The needle is directed straight back as far as it will go in line with the orbital axis and the orbital roof. This procedure produces a profound ptosis in three to four days which lasts up to six weeks. This short-term effect is a disadvantage in long-term disease.

A therapeutic soft contact lens is usually thought of as a lens designed with oxygen transmission characteristics such that it is suitable for extended wear. However, it should always be borne in mind that extended wear is not a prerequisite for therapeutic effectiveness. A number of diseases, for example, Thygeson's superficial punctate keratitis and Meesmann's dystrophy, can be managed with daily wear therapeutic lenses. The pain and photophobia in these diseases are absent when the eyes are closed, as in sleep. The daily wear therapeutic lens should still have high oxygen transmission and this can be achieved by manufacturing very thin lenses of low water content as well as by using necessarily thicker lenses of higher water content. The water content of a material roughly determines its oxygen permeability.

There are many thin (0.05 mm approximate centre thickness) low water content lenses available commercially for cosmetic use and these can be used for daily, or extended, therapeutic wear, in plano form. The author's current preference is for the CSI therapeutic lens usually of radius 8.3 or 8.6, power plano and diameter 13.8 mm (Pilkington Barnes Hind). For high water content, extended wear therapeutic use the author's preference is for the Sauflon 85 afocal lens of radius 8.4 mm and diameter 15.4 mm (the PCM, protective corneal membrane, Cantor and Silver, Brackley, Northants).

In disorders characterized by gross corneal or limbal surface irregularity, thin membrane lenses may not possess sufficient rigidity either to centre or improve the optical properties of an irregular surface. On the other hand, high water content lenses, which are thicker, and thus may centre more readily and provide a better optical surface, soil with greater rapidity, especially in an inflamed eye. Hydrogel contact lenses, it must be remembered,

1. induce variable degrees of hypoxia
2. produce low grade continuous mechanical trauma to the corneal epithelium and thus promote the entrance of organisms into the cornea
3. alter the tear film distribution and functions over the corneal surface

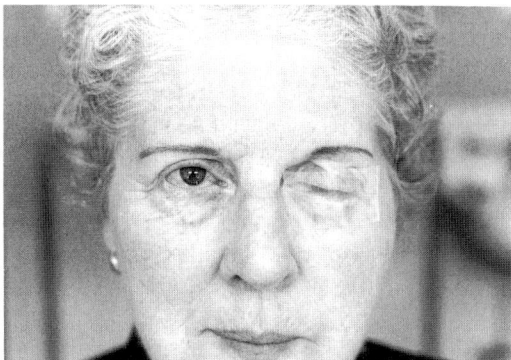

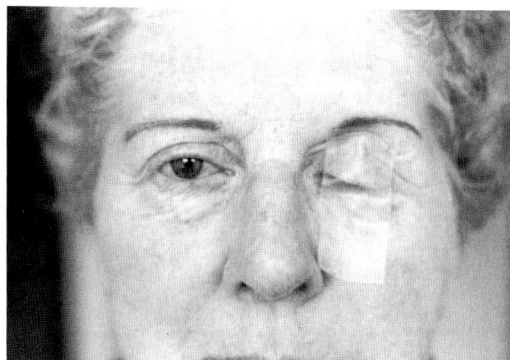

Figure 14.1 Closing the eye with tape. One inch (25 mm) tape (usually Blenderm 3M) is cut to a length of two and a half inches (64 mm) and applied either vertically or horizontally, whichever gives the best closure. Closure is facilitated by cutting the lashes

4. occlude the cornea and elevate the corneal tissue temperature and metabolic rate (Cavanagh, 1975).

Hydrogel lenses can provide a protective barrier, for example in eye lid abnormalities, with or without trichiasis, metaplasia, or cicatrization. They can insulate the corneal epithelium from the deleterious effects of blinking. They can splint or fortify weak areas such as descemetoceles, or ruptures, and they can stabilize loosely adherent epithelium. Soft lenses can greatly ameliorate symptoms which are experienced in external eye disease and can, within a very short time, abort the severe pain associated with such corneal diseases as bullous keratopathy or wet filamentary keratitis.

Although the overwhelming majority of non-optical therapeutic applications involve hydrogel lenses, other modalities of lenses can be used. For example, hard PMMA lenses can be used in Thygeson's superficial punctate keratitis. Silicon rubber lenses can be used. They have unusually high oxygen permeability with Dk values 10 to 20 times higher than hydrogel lenses. They have negligible water content and so they do not dry out in a bone dry eye. They are soft and have excellent optical properties. They have, however, serious deficiencies that limit their clinical use. They are intensely hydrophobic and for this reason have to undergo a surface treatment to induce hydrophilicity. This surface treatment wears off with time. The lenses show dimensional changes with ageing. They also absorb lipid-containing substances and this is a great disadvantage (Refojo, 1979). Rigid corneal lenses may be the only method of restoring a patient's visual acuity in quiet external eye disease, but that aspect of therapy will be dealt with in other chapters.

Therapeutic indications

Acute glaucoma

A soft contact lens soaked in pilocarpine can be used effectively in the treatment of this condition (Hillman, 1974). A suitable lens would be a high water content, therapeutic contact lens. Relief from the pain is prompt and pupil constriction is achieved rapidly without the repeated instillation of drops. This regimen can be supplemented by topical timolol 0.5% and/or oral glycerol 1 ml/kg body weight, mixed in equal proportion with lemon juice.

Amblyopia

Contact lenses have been shown to be of use in amblyopia in childhood (Catford and Mackie, 1968). One can be faced with an unapproachable child with an obvious squint of some duration where assessment of the visual acuities and conventional occlusion is not possible. The child can be swaddled with the parents holding the legs and arms and a soft contact lens of the type used for aphakia, and of about plus 16 D power, can be inserted in the good eye. The lens should be of high water content since it will, of necessity, be thick. The lens can be worn on a daily wear or an extended wear basis. Daily wear should be strived for, but this depends on the ability of the parents to insert and remove the lens. Every effort should be made to teach them. After a month or so of this occlusion the squint can be operated on and the restored acuity of the squinting eye will favour the establishment of binocular vision.

Uniocular high myopia, which often results in amblyopia, can be corrected by a contact lens and the good eye occluded with such an aphakic type lens. Personal experience of the author suggests that contact lens occlusion is more effective than conventional patch occlusion.

Aniridia keratopathy

Aniridia is usually an autosomal dominant disease. The corneal problems are superficial vascularization, stromal opacification and indolent epithelial ulceration. Seefelder (1909) drew attention to conjunctival goblet cell hyperplasia in this condition. Jay and Lee (1981) reported that this occurs in the conjunctiva in aniridia before clinical signs of corneal or conjunctival abnormality. In histological specimens they found the corneal epithelium replaced by an epithelium of conjunctival type.

It is in episodes of indolent ulceration that

therapeutic soft lenses may be of value in facilitating re-epithelialization. An extended wear, high water content contact lens should be used.

Tinted soft lenses, and soft lenses with coloured opaque pseudo-irides (e.g. Durasoft, Wesley-Jessen) which are now commercially available in various colours, may be used on a daily basis to lessen glare.

Atopic conjunctival disease with keratopathy

Atopic conjunctival disease, which is sometimes seen in association with eczema, especially when the face, or lids, are involved, usually manifests as a cellular infiltration of the palpebral conjunctiva. Occasionally the disturbing feature of keratinization of the posterior lid margins appears and this produces an erosive corneal epitheliopathy which can, in the long term, markedly reduce the visual acuity. Catastrophic destructive corneal disease can occur. Hard scleral lenses, perhaps of the slotted type, or soft contact lenses, can be used to protect the corneas from the abrasive effect of the lid margins. The scleral lenses are worn on a daily basis. The soft contact lenses can be used on a daily basis or extended wear basis, according to the indications. The author's preference is for a thin, low water content soft contact lens.

Keiselbach and Gensluckner (1987) report that all children suffering from juvenile atopic keratoconjunctivitis and seen at the Innsbruck University Eye Clinic in recent years have so far been satisfactorily treated with therapeutic contact lenses and locally applied antibiotics and steroids.

Bullous keratopathy

This is, potentially, a very painful condition and its onset may be agonizing for the patient. In such circumstances a soft therapeutic contact lens may be applied and the patient may become asymptomatic within 15 minutes. The lens is a cure for the pain, but not for the bullous keratopathy, and it seldom leads to any improvement in the visual acuity. It is interesting that the same degree of bullous keratopathy in the same eye may be completely painless when the therapeutic lens is removed after a few months. The author's preference is for a high water content extended wear soft lens.

There is a considerable risk of suppurative keratitis in patients treated for bullous keratopathy with soft lenses and patients should be warned to seek advice immediately if the eye should become red or painful. In most cases the contact lens is an interim measure and a corneal graft should be performed, if feasible, when convenient. Failing this, the lens should be removed after a period of, say, three months to ascertain whether the eye remains painless without the contact lens.

Long-term wear of the soft lens ultimately produces corneal vascularization which may become considerable. Pain is seldom a feature when the cornea is vascularized.

Aphakia

Aphakia is the commonest condition associated with corneal oedema (Ruben, 1975) and is most often due to operative trauma to the corneal endothelium. The pain can be relieved by an extended wear, high water content therapeutic lens until grafting can be performed.

Buphthalmos

Intermittent fine bullous keratopathy occurring at some part of the day, usually the morning, and giving rise to blurred vision, may be encountered in this condition and is related to endothelial decompensation. Baldone and Kaufman (1983) advocate the use of a high water soft contact lens for this phenomenon. They suggest that the use of soft contact lenses with a high water content provides a mechanism for corneal dehydration in these patients. To them it appears that, as the water evaporates from the anterior surface of the high water content lenses, a sort of 'wicking' action draws water from the cornea into the lens, thereby reducing oedema and improving vision.

Fuchs' corneal dystrophy

This is a bilateral corneal disease characterized by endothelial degeneration (cornea guttata) leading to corneal stromal oedema and the ultimate development of bullous keratopathy. There is a dominant transmission and females are affected three times as often as males. If discomfort is severe a therapeutic soft contact lens may be used to alleviate the pain before corneal grafting can take place. The object of the corneal graft is to replace corneal endothelial cells and a minimum diameter of 8 mm is indicated.

Ice syndrome

In the iridocorneal endothelial syndrome there is an alteration of the corneal endothelium which gives a fine hammered silver appearance when seen by slit lamp microscopy. Characteristic changes are seen in this endothelium by specular microscopy (Laganowski *et al.*, 1991). The endothelial disorder may present as a unilateral bullous keratopathy in the absence of iris atrophy, iris nodules, or glaucoma (Shields, 1979). The bullous keratopathy may be localized. It is frequently painful and the pain may be relieved by the application of an extended wear therapeutic soft contact lens of high water content until a penetrating graft is performed.

Posterior polymorphous dystrophy

This is an autosomal dominantly inherited bilateral corneal disease characterized by lesions which appear like snail tracks on the posterior corneal surface. These snail tracks are bounded by a grey line which borders abnormal endothelial cells. The disease is only very slowly progressive, but progression can occur so that bullous keratopathy results. A soft high water content extended wear therapeutic contact lens can be applied to relieve pain until keratoplasty can be performed.

Chemical injuries

Alkali burns

Alkalis usually penetrate the eye rapidly and cause toxic, proteolytic and collagen synthesis defects. Important prognostic features are loss of epithelium and limbal ischaemia. Eyes are usually lost because the epithelium does not regenerate or there is corneal or stromal lysis. A cornea without an epithelium may remain clear for several weeks, but ultimately the stroma will opacify and will be covered by an opaque membrane of conjunctival type.

Soft contact lenses have been advocated to promote epithelial healing in such circumstances, but there is no evidence that they do this. In fact, there is evidence to the contrary by Ali and Insler (1986) and it might be better, according to their findings, to induce a botulinum toxin ptosis, as discussed earlier in this chapter. Total epithelial loss is seldom restored by the application of a soft contact lens in such circumstances, and furthermore, as these eyes are not painful, pain is not an indication. Far more appropriate is the operation of Kenyon and Tseng (1989), referred to in Chapter 13 under the section on Thimerosal keratopathy. This operation restores corneal epithelial 'stem cells' (Schermer, Galvin and Sun, 1986) which have been destroyed.

Little can be done to reverse stromal or scleral lysis.

Acid burns

Acids coagulate and precipitate protein, causing tissue destruction and they do not tend to penetrate in the same manner as alkalis. The burns are usually limited and localized. Coagulated epithelial cells may also serve as a barrier to the penetration of acid. Again, epithelial loss and scleral ischaemia are important to the prognosis. The corneal epithelial stem cells may again be lost and the same indications for treatment apply as in alkali burns.

Cicatricial conjunctival disease

Cicatricial conjunctival disease may be progressive or non-progressive and it is important to make this distinction. There is no evidence that hard scleral lenses halt the progression of symblepharon or fornix shallowing and, although there is a dearth of literature on the subject, impressions may be gained on the effectiveness of such a procedure merely because of the slowly progressive nature of the disease or wrong diagnostic labelling.

The ocular manifestations of cicatricial pemphigoid and linear IgA disease are examples of progressive disease. They are diagnosed by *bulbar* conjunctival biopsy (Wright, 1986). Graft host disease, which causes cicatrizing conjunctival disease, is diagnosed by a history of transplantation. Graft host disease occurs in two forms – a severe form, which is usually associated with a rapid fatal outcome, and a mild form, which exhibits a cicatrizing conjunctivitis which often shows little sign of progression and is associated with dry eyes. Punctal occlusion, lubricants and the management of secondary infection is usually all that is required in such cases.

Post-membranous conjunctivitis, Stevens–Johnson syndrome, pseudopemphigoid (when identified) and old trachoma are examples of non-progressive conjunctival scarring and are diagnosed by the appropriate history. In these diseases, not characterized by progression, it is pointless to fit contact lenses unless there is corneal destructive disease and a substantial visual improvement can only be obtained by these devices.

In all these cicatricial diseases soft therapeutic lenses can be helpful in promoting re-epithelialization when there is an epithelial defect. A high water content lens may be used, but if there is some degree of dryness it may be better to use a thin, low water content lens as it will be less likely to dry. There are few other indications for soft contact lenses and their use is fraught with the dangers of vascularization or suppurative keratopathy. Ingrowing lashes, together with lid deformities, can be corrected by surgery (Jones *et al*. 1976; Wright and Collin, 1983) or cryotherapy (Collin, Coster and Sullivan, 1978).

In cases where there has been much corneal

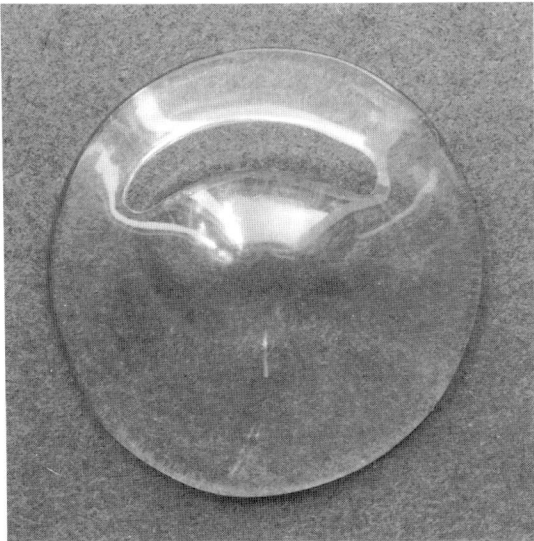

Figure 14.2 Slotted scleral lens (courtesy K.W. Pullum)

destructive disease leading to a significant decrease in visual acuity a scleral lens may be indicated. Corneal irregularity is more important than corneal opacification as a cause of diminished acuity and the use of a scleral lens in such cases will often greatly improve the vision. They are much safer than soft contact lenses, but they do lead to and exacerbate corneal vascularization. This may have to be accepted and will, in itself, not affect the visual acuity so long as the lens is worn and as long as lipid keratopathy does not develop. The lens used should be of the fenestrated type, but this is often technically very difficult to fit.

The technique of fitting a wearable scleral lens has been made easier by the development at Moorfields Eye Hospital of slotted scleral lenses (Pullum, 1984, Pullum and Trodd, 1984). These lenses have a superior limbal slot extending up to one-third of the circumference of the corneal scleral junction (Figure 14.2). This provides a far greater tear exchange underneath the lens. It also allows a much greater depth of limbal clearance and the lens does not seem to settle back, and lead to poor tear exchange, as much as a conventional scleral contact lens. The non-hyrophilic, soft silicone corneal contact lens (Wohlk) has sometimes a part to play in improving the vision in these patients where there is destructive corneal disease, especially when the eye is dry. It is more comfortable than a scleral lens and can be fitted in the presence of shallowed fornices. Having a negligible water content it does not dry out. These lenses can lead to severe complications when they become tightly adherent to the cornea – a process which Refojo and Leong (1981) attribute to water pervaporation. Dow Corning have withdrawn their silicone lenses from the American market.

Corneal dystrophies

Epithelial basement membrane dystrophy

This comprises so-called map-dot-finger print line dystrophy (Trobe and Laibson, 1972), Cogan's microcystic dystrophy (Cogan *et al*., 1964) and bleb dystrophy (Bron and Brown, 1971). Most patients with these dystrophies are asymptomatic, but about 10% develop painful recurrent epithelial erosions, usually upon awakening in the morning. These erosions usually heal within a day. A characteristic sign of a recent erosion is a collection of epithelial cysts, sometimes transparent, but often white and opaque, which are usually located in the intermediate zone of the lower half of the cornea. The epithelial cysts seldom stain. If the cornea is stained with fluorescein and viewed with cobalt light a black ring of epithelium uncovered with fluorescein film is often seen and this is, presumably, the boundary of the area of loose epithelium.

The recurrent epithelial erosions may develop once every few weeks or two or three times a week, but after a few years the symptoms usually cease.

Initial treatment should be with 5% sodium chloride ointment, or Adsorbonac 5% (Alcon, USA) drops at night. These preparations are hypertonic and may act by decreasing physiological nocturnal corneal oedema. Foulks (1981) has recommended a topical osmotic colloidal solution. If this treatment does not succeed, then a soft extended wear, therapeutic lens should be fitted. If there is a large area of opaque, apparently loose epithelium, it is safer to tape the lids for a few days until this has attached as, otherwise, there may be a marked reaction the day after the lens is fitted. The author usually uses an extended wear, high water content soft lens. However, Mobilia and Foster (1978) recommend an ultra thin, low water content lens. The lens should have very little movement on the cornea. The patient should be warned that the first few days are the most difficult and that the eye may become very uncomfortable, necessitating removal of the lens. The author often uses fluoromethalone drops 0.1% three times daily for the first few days to lessen any stromal inflammatory reaction and then reduces the dosage so that the patient is not instilling steroid after two weeks.

The patient should be seen the day after insertion of the lens. A warning sign of an unfavourable response is lid swelling, although nothing much untoward may be seen on examining the cornea through the contact lens. It is very difficult to come to any conclusion regarding corneal haze when the soft lens is in situ.

Further lid swelling over the next few days is an indication to remove the lens and, in this case, it will usually be found that a large area of corneal epithelium is loose and comes away with the lens. A broad spectrum antibiotic ointment, such as gentamicin or tobramycin, together with a topical mydriatic, should be inserted and the eye should be padded and a two inch (50 mm) crepe bandage applied.

The pad and bandage should be maintained until the cornea has re-epithelialized. At that time tape should be used on a daily basis to close the eye. It is not necessary to use it during the night. The tape closure should be continued for two months and it will usually be found that the tendency to recurrent erosion situation has resolved. If a single site for the recurrent erosion can be identified, either by a collection of epithelial cysts, or, more important, a black ring of epithelium uncovered with fluorescein stain, the techniques of needle puncture or Yag application as outlined in the section on Recurrent corneal erosions (traumatic), page 180, may be implied.

Despite a report to the contrary (Williams, 1985), the present author has found treatment with a therapeutic soft lens over a period of up to six months a successful treatment in a large number of patients. These patients are often in a highly nervous state about their eyes and need sympathetic and individual attention.

Reis-Bücklers superficial corneal dystrophy

This is an autosomal dominant corneal dystrophy characterized by whorl patterned accumulations of fibrous connective tissue in the area of Bowman's membrane which decrease the visual acuity. The disease starts in the first decade of life and features painful recurrent erosions which may continue to occur for as long as 30 years. The recurrent erosions may be treated with extended wear therapeutic soft lenses until the cornea has healed.

Lattice dystrophy

This is a bilateral, symmetrical, autosomal dominant stromal dystrophy (Biber, 1890). The lattice lines in the stroma are characteristic and vary from a few flecks to large irregular strands. Histologically, the lines are composed of amyloid and stain with Congo red.

The disease is characterized by episodes of recurrent erosions separated often by years. The erosions are quite unlike those of basement membrane dystrophies and result in a profound loss of visual acuity and much stromal swelling and inflammation. In such circumstances, it is imperative to close the eye. This is best done by taping, but botulinum toxin may also be used, as described above.

After the cornea has re-epithelialized it may take many months for the stromal inflammation to resolve and for the visual acuity to be restored. It is important that no corneal graft be done after an erosion until a year has elapsed because the vision will probably return to its original level.

The episode of erosion is usually very painful and there may be a case for inserting a therapeutic soft extended wear lens to promote re-epithelialization and relieve pain, but this should be done under close medical supervision. In this case, the author would use a high water content extended wear therapeutic lens.

Meesmann's juvenile epithelial dystrophy

This is a bilateral, symmetrical, autosomal dominant dystrophy appearing in very early life. The corneal epithelium appears to be covered with minute clear vesicles which are actually epithelial cysts containing degenerated cell debris. The application of fluorescein to the cornea shows rough, and sometimes confluent, staining. With minor disease the patient may be largely asymptomatic, but irritation and photophobia may be troublesome. The visual acuity is frequently reduced. If the patient presses for something to be done, daily wear therapeutic soft contact lenses may be tried to lessen the irritation and photophobia and improve the vision. The author's preference in this case is for a thin, daily wear, low water content, therapeutic, soft contact lens. This lens is best accepted when there is a degree of ametropia which can be corrected. Some patients find that a lens actually increases the discomfort. On no account should a penetrating, or lamellar, corneal graft be done since this graft will rapidly be epithelialized with dystrophic epithelium. Burns (1968) advocates keratectomy removing Bowman's membrane. He believes that this membrane plays some part in the production of dystrophic epithelium. In future the keratectomy may be done by excimer laser ablation which can produce an optical surface.

Saltzmann's nodular dystrophy

This is really a degeneration and is a late sequel to other corneal diseases, such as phlyctenulosis, trachoma and interstitial keratitis. The disease occurs more often in women than in men and is characterized by elevated nodules of epithelium under which Bowman's membrane is missing and replaced by a basement membrane like material (Vannas, Hogan and Wood, 1975).

There is sometimes a complaint of discomfort and photophobia. If there are central nodular lesions the visual acuity may be reduced.

Soft contact lenses may be used in an attempt to increase comfort and to improve vision. Corneal irregularity is more important than opacity as a cause of diminished acuity. The soft lens will tend to flatten the nodule and improve the acuity. A daily wear, thin, low water content therapeutic contact lens can be used, but it is often not tolerated.

Drug delivery

It has been noted that contact lenses soaked in pilocarpine can be used in the management of acute glaucoma. Contact lenses soaked in glaucoma medications have been used in the management of chronic disease but this idea was superseded by the advent of hydrophilic polymer inserts which were placed in the inferior fornix (Ocuserts, May & Baker).

Arthur *et al*. (1983) reported on the ultrastructural effects of topical timolol on the rabbit cornea – the outcome with the medication alone and in conjunction with a gas permeable contact lens. Corneas treated with either timolol or contact lens alone showed mild to moderate oedema or degeneration of epithelial and endothelial cells. However, the combined use of a contact lens and timolol produced marked alterations in both the corneal epithelium and endothelium.

In the future the delivery of drugs may be increasingly performed by the use of soft contact lenses. The section on Persistent corneal epithelial defects, page 179, notes that epithelial growth factor and fibronectin can be kept in contact with the eye by this means.

Busin and Spitznas (1988) soaked 10 bandage contact lenses (HEMA 38.6% water content) overnight in an 0.5% solution of sterile, unpreserved, commercially available gentamicin and fitted them thereafter on 10 eyes of healthy adult volunteers. Gentamicin concentrations in the tear film were determined 10, 30 and 60 minutes and 4, 8, 24, 48, 72 and 96 hours after fitting, using agar diffusion bioassay. Bactericidal concentrations were found up to three days after contact lens fitting in all subjects, and no toxic or systemic effects were seen.

Reccia *et al*. (1985) have reported on the treatment of 14 patients with primary and recurrent herpetic keratitis with human leucocyte interferon at low concentration using therapeutic contact lenses. All the patients recovered in a medium-short time of seven days, including some who had not benefitted by previous treatments. They concluded that continuous treatment with human leucocyte interferon increased its effectiveness.

Drug induced keratopathy

This condition is seen after the long-term administration of ophthalmic drops in the treatment of major or minor eye disease. It may be caused by the medicaments in the drops or by the preservatives used in them. These substances may cause a primary keratopathy or a secondary keratopathy caused by dysplastic changes in the palpebral conjunctiva. The reaction is toxic rather than allergic, and in the case of primary keratopathy, represents the destruction of limbal epithelial stem cells by the drug, or its preservatives, or a hypersensitivity reaction to them.

The primary keratopathy can be seen in the absence of any palpebral conjunctival change. It is seen, typically, after the use of tear substitutes in dry eye states, but also after the habitual use of antibiotics, decongestants and anti-inflammatory drugs. The cornea may be in an advanced state of disease before the case is correctly diagnosed, during which time the same drops may still be being used in a futile attempt to control the keratopathy. The keratopathy is mainly an epitheliopathy. The epithelium is thickened and opacified. There is coarse staining with fluorescein. Sometimes dellen develop centrally in the cornea and epithelial defects are common. The condition does not improve after withdrawal of the toxic substance. There may be periods when a therapeutic soft contact lens is indicated. The usual indication is the development of a large epithelial

defect. Re-epithelialization is usually very slow with the ever present danger of stromal ulceration or sterile hypopyon. An extended wear high water content therapeutic soft contact lens can be used as an alternative to taping in this condition.

The operative procedure advocated by Kenyon and Tseng (1989) can be performed in an attempt to restore the corneal epithelium. Their operative technique involves the transfer of limbal tissue (epithelial stem cells) from the uninjured or less injured donor eye of the patient to the severely injured recipient eye, the latter having been prepared by limited conjunctival resection and superficial dissection of fibrovascular pannus without keratectomy. The procedure is a modification of the operation of keratoepithelioplasty described by Thoft (1984) whereby healthy limbal epithelium is obtained by fresh donor eyes in which the epithelium is intact and clear.

The secondary keratopathy is caused by conjunctival dysplasia. This is seen typically after the use of guanethidine drops in glaucoma. The conjunctival dysplasia takes the form of plaques of soggy keratinization which abrade the cornea. Withdrawal of the toxic compound ultimately results in the disappearance of these soggy plaques and their replacement by conjunctival scarring, or a dry, glistening conjunctival dysplasia much like that described and illustrated here in relation to radiation keratopathy. A soft extended wear high water content contact lens can be used to protect the cornea.

Dry eyes

Soft contact lenses are sometimes used in the treatment of dry eyes. There is a dearth of recent literature on the subject. Most of the published papers relate to the late 1960s or early 1970s. The only current report is by Hasegawa *et al*. (1979). They treated one eye in each of 15 patients with keratoconjunctivitis sicca and compared the treated eye with the untreated eye. Corneal objective findings were improved in all treated cases. They used drops in conjunction with the lenses. Seven patients discontinued lens wear, while eight patients continued to wear the lenses. The authors were enthusiastic about the treatment.

Cederstaff and Tomlinson (1983) measured tear evaporation rates in five subjects wearing soft contact lenses ranging in water content from 38%

to 70%. They found that contact lenses produced a significant increase in tear evaporation not related to the initial water content of the lens. They also found that the water lost by dehydration of the lens material made a relatively minor contribution to the increase in evaporation from the eye during lens wear. This means that the fitting of a soft contact lens should stress a dry eye.

Sheridan and Walker (1983) studied the changes in the water content of hydrogel lenses during wear. They found that lenses partly dehydrate during wear and they observed that the amount of water lost during the first hour of wear was not related to the diameter of the lens. They also found that high water content lenses showed a weight loss almost double that of low water content lenses.

The present author has shown (Mackie, 1985) that the thickness of soft contact lenses does not influence their rate of dehydration and that a lower water content lens will, in the absence of a fluid surround, remain hydrated to a reasonable extent for a longer period than one of higher content.

The soft lens of choice would appear to be a thin, low water content one which can be worn on a daily basis. The author has used the CSI T (Pilkington Barnes Hind) which, because of its low water content and small pore size, is particularly resistant to dehydration.

Baldone and Kaufman (1983) believe that patients with dry eyes benefit from wearing soft contact lenses with lower water content. They state that these lenses provide a barrier to evaporation to the corneal surface and do not seem to have the same water requirements as high water content lenses. They have gone so far as to fit an extended wear therapeutic soft lens with a very low water content (the Revlens, available from Bio Contacts Inc., San Francisco, made of soft acrylic rubber with a water content of zero to 1%).

Although it has recently been shown that dry eyes are no more prone to infection than normal eyes (Seal *et al.*, 1986), the danger of suppurative keratitis is probably increased, because of the lack of corneal epithelial integrity in these cases.

A painful filamentary keratitis, resistant to all treatment, is probably the most logical reason for the use of soft lenses. Relief from pain is almost instantaneous and the filaments seem to melt away under the lens (Lamberts, 1983).

The lenses can be kept moist by instillation of sterile normal unpreserved saline or by tear substitutes, but a careful watch should be kept for signs of preservative toxicity if the latter are used.

No case of keratoconjunctivitis sicca should be treated with soft contact lenses until the effect of occlusion of all four punctae has been observed. This often brings about a marked improvement in the condition and is much more cost effective. It is done by passing a cautery wire far into the canaliculus after dilatation with a Nettleship dilator. The current should have been adjusted so that the wire is at black heat at the point just before redness is observed. The current should be applied for three seconds while the cautery wire is in the canaliculus and this is repeated once or twice. The cautery wire should be left in the canaliculus until it can be felt adherent to its lining. This procedure is frequently unsuccessful in occluding the punctum, even in experienced hands, and often needs to be repeated. Lacrymal syringing is the only way to confirm if the procedure has been successful. Punctal occlusion should not be performed in young people with associated diseases of the autoimmune type because it is not easily reversible and sometimes there is a return of tear production when the systemic disease has improved. Care should be taken that the diagnosis of dry eyes is correct because other diseases can mimic dry eyes in the absence of a marked reflex tear flow (Mackie and Seal, 1981).

In the author's opinion there is very little indication for the use of soft lenses in keratoconjunctivitis sicca. Most cases do not progress in severity and are easily managed with punctal occlusion and tear substitutes. An increase in the keratopathy associated with the dry eyes should alert the ophthalmologist to the possibility of a toxic reaction produced by the preservatives in the tear substitute solutions.

Epidermolysis bullosa

Epidermolysis bullosa is not one, but a family of disorders that share the common feature of reduced resistance of the skin to shear and frictional injury. The basic lesions of the different forms occur at various anatomical sites in epidermal and subepidermal tissues. Some forms of epidermolysis bullosa are associated with ocular diseases –

blepharitis, bullous lesions of the eyelids and corneal erosions.

Gans (1988) reported on the eye lesions observed in a series of 78 patients of varying ages. Three consistent types of ocular involvement were identified – recurrent corneal erosions, punctate staining in the lower third of the corneas and blepharitis. Recurrent corneal erosions occurred with and without corneal scarring. These erosions were heralded by the sudden onset of pain and photophobia in one or both eyes, associated with tearing and a red eye. Tape could not be used in these patients to close the eyes because the skin would blister under the tape. Contact lenses were used in older patients to minimize frequent recurrences of the erosions.

Cicatricial conjunctivitis has been reported in patients with epidermolysis bullosa (Cohen and Sulzberger, 1935; Sorsby, Roberts and Brain, 1951; Wright, 1986) but none of the patients in the study by Gans had this complication.

Adamis, Schein and Kenyon described the ultrastructure of the conjunctiva and anterior cornea in epidermolysis bullosa in Scientific Poster No. 14 at the 1990 Annual Meeting of the American Academy of Ophthalmology. The transmission electron microscopy findings were similar to those seen in recurrent corneal erosions and the conjunctiva appeared normal. Their case was successfully treated with soft contact lenses.

Eyelid defects

In the past, eyelid defects such as colobomata, trichiasis, dystichiasis and entropion were often managed by the insertion of scleral lenses. In the opinion of the author there is now very little indication for such treatment, with the advent of oculoplastic surgery as a sub-speciality. These defects can be managed satisfactorily by surgery or cryosurgery, which is much more cost effective.

Facial nerve palsy

This commonly results in exposure problems for the eye and soft therapeutic lenses have little part to play in the management of this condition, although patients are often referred for their fitting. Just as the cornea is exposed, so will be the

contact lenses, and they will dry, shrink and be ejected.

If the palsy is temporary, exposure can be treated by taping, as described above. The tape should be worn during the night as well as the day and it is important that it is properly applied so that it does not damage the cornea. If taping is impracticable, the eye can be closed by creating a profound ptosis with botulinum toxin (see above). A moist chamber is a possible means of treatment with a Guibor transparent plastic shield (Guibor shield, Concept Inc., Clearwater, Florida) during the day and this may be particularly applicable if it is the only seeing eye. A cheaper alternative is the use of kitchen cling film and Micropore tape (3M Company).

If the palsy is going to be permanent, other means of managing it must be considered. Intracranial transplant of a segment of the sural nerve from the lower leg at the time of any destructive operative procedure on the facial nerve, as performed by King, T.T. and Morrison, A.W. at the London Hospital, London, England (unpublished), is a possibility. Hypoglossal nerve transplantation (Bucheit and Delgardo, 1985) is another possible approach and is done a month after the operation which has destroyed the nerve. The latter procedure results in the restoration of some facial tone and movement.

Finally, there is the operation described by Harrison (1985, 1990) in which a segment from the sural nerve from the leg is anastomosed to a branch of the facial nerve on the contralateral side and fed under the upper lip to the maxillary region on the other side. About six months later a pectoralis minor muscle transplant is inserted in the cheek on the affected side. The operation usually results in good facial movement on the affected side after about a year. It is more effective in younger patients.

In permanent facial palsy where the eye is exposed it is always worth considering the insertion of a small, sausage-shaped gold weight into the upper lid of the affected eye. Gold weights can be obtained from the dental department of a hospital. Varying weights are taped on to the margin of the upper lid until the precise weight is found which just allows the patient voluntarily to close his eye. This weight is then inserted in the middle of the lid, under the skin and muscle next to the tarsal plate, as close to the lid margin as possible. The skin incision is made at the lid crease. Extrusion may be a problem and it has been pointed out that the gold weight does not assist closure while the patient is recumbent. One disadvantage of this procedure is that the upper lid cannot be everted for examination should an external eye disease problem present.

An alternative to this procedure to assist closure of the eye is the recession of the upper lid retractor muscles (Collin, 1983). This, of course, results in ptosis.

Familial dysautonomia

This is an inborn error of metabolism inherited almost exclusively in Ashkenazi Jews in an autosomal recessive fashion. The disease has many systemic features, including an indifference to pain. The ocular disease is a neuroparalytic keratitis often exacerbated by poor reflex tear production. The neuroparalytic keratitis is best managed by lid closure as described at the beginning of this chapter as frequently both eyes are not affected at the same time. Soft contact lenses may have a place in the treatment of the neuroparalytic keratitis when otherwise bilateral eye closure would be indicated, but their use is associated with the greatest danger.

Glaucoma surgery

Zalta and Wieder (1991) reported the management of five leaking filtering blebs, occurring between 10 months and 25 years after trabeculectomy. Filtering bleb integrity was preserved in four cases so that additional microsurgery was avoided. The conjunctival bleb leaks were identified using Seidel's test. The eyes were anaesthetized. A lid speculum was inserted to prevent lid closure during and after the application of tissue adhesive (see section on Perforation of the cornea, page 178). The leak was positioned perpendicular to the vertical direction of application of the glue. The conjunctival fistula site was dried with a cotton tip applicator just prior to the application of one to three drops of Histoacryl Blue. Antibiotic and/or antibiotic-steroid ointments were instilled. The eye was pressure patched for 24 hours, with or without a bandage soft contact lens, according to the needs of the patient.

Blok *et al*. (1990) have evaluated the use of a newly developed, large diameter (20.5 mm), therapeutic soft contact lens (the Megasoft Bandage Lens – a lathe cut lens especially developed for their research product by Procornea, The Netherlands) in five patients with shallow anterior chambers and 10 patients with leaking filtering blebs after trabeculectomy. All patients with shallow anterior chambers developed deep chambers after a mean treatment period of five days. Of the 10 patients with leaking filtering blebs, in eight the leak closed after a mean treatment period of 2.2 months. They see the use of this new therapeutic device as an improvement in the treatment of complications after trabeculectomy.

Keratoplasty management

Contact lenses have a part to play in the management of keratoplasties, not only in improving the patient's acuity, but in dealing with the complications which can follow the operative procedure.

Cheesewiring of sutures

In this condition the sutures erode through the host cornea, which may be friable, and there is imminent danger of wound dehiscence. A soft extended wear, high water content contact lens can be applied to protect the graft.

Elevation of the graft

This can be treated with a flush scleral lens (see Chapter 3) or a soft hydrophilic therapeutic lens. Ideally, Sauflex 55, which is probably the firmest soft contact lens material available, should be used. These lenses are worn on a daily basis. There is sometimes an associated dellen formation at three o'clock or nine o'clock on the recipient cornea and the fitting of a soft contact lens will control this.

Failure of graft epithelialization

Where there is a high chance of rejection the surgeon often decides to remove the epithelium from the donor button. If there is a failure to epithelialize within the first few days postoperatively, a soft extended wear lens can be applied to encourage this.

Where there is considerable chronic conjunctival disease the decision is often made to preserve the epithelium on the donor button. Within the first few days this epithelium may be seen to become lustreless and then desquamate, at first from the centre of the graft, and then moving peripherally, so that only a fringe of it is visible at the edge of the graft. This is an indication of imminent graft failure and for the application of an extended wear, high water content, therapeutic soft contact lens. This lens must be kept on the eye for a considerable length of time. It may not be possible to manage without a soft lens in highly compromised eyes.

Tilting of the graft

This usually produces considerable astigmatism. It may be due to cheesewiring of sutures, badly placed sutures, or to the fact that the donor button chosen had dimensional parameters quite different to that of the recipient cornea. At an early stage a scleral lens can be fitted to regularize the graft. This scleral lens can be of the flush, fenestrated or slotted type. A soft, extended wear, high water content contact lens may also be effective in this situation. Alternatively, a daily wear lens of Sauflex 55 material may be fitted.

Wound dehiscence

This can occur following trauma at any time after graft surgery has been performed, or it may occur in some corneas which do not heal well because of too early removal of sutures. It may result from the premature removal of sutures which are causing discomfort or vascularization. Then the anterior chamber is rapidly lost. It can usually be reformed by the application of a high water content extended wear soft lens which is left in position for some months.

Mooren's ulceration

This is a chronic painful ulceration of the cornea which starts at the periphery and progresses centrally and circumferentially to involve the entire cornea. It is bilateral in about 25% of cases and may be responsive or resistant to steroid therapy. The bilateral cases usually do not respond to topical steroid therapy.

There is usually a marked limbitis which precedes the ulceration. The advancing ulcer undermines the corneal stroma, producing the typical overhanging edge. Blood vessels rapidly grow into the ulcer site. The central cornea remains clear until it is involved in the ulcerative process. Therapeutic soft hydrophilic contact lenses can be used to relieve the pain during treatment and may potentiate the effect of local steroid. They bridge the diseased tissue and prevent trauma caused by a blinking lid.

Neuroparalytic keratitis

Neuroparalytic keratitis is a potential sequel to trigeminal anaesthesia. The three most common causes are surgery for the trigeminal neuralgias, surgery for acoustic neuromata and herpes zoster ophthalmicus. In the latter disease about 8% of patients develop neuroparalytic keratitis. There are other causes for trigeminal nerve damage – trauma, tumours, multiple sclerosis, toxic chemical reactions, leprosy and brainstem haemorrhages. There is a congenital form (Hewson, 1963). It occurs in familial dysautonomia (Riley–Day syndrome).

About 15% of patients with anaesthetic eyes develop serious complications which may develop at any time after the initiation of trigeminal insensitivity. The potential of developing neuroparalytic keratitis can wax and wane and this must always be borne in mind in the long-term management of these patients.

The author believes that, to develop a true neuroparalytic keratitis, one must have an insensitive cornea, together with an insensitive conjunctiva. Palpebral conjunctival sensation can be tested by the prick of a hypodermic needle.

All patients with trigeminal anaesthesia produce excess mucus. This mucus is produced by subvillous vesicles in the surface epithelial cells (Dilly and Mackie, 1981). Its presence must not be taken as evidence of infection.

Neuroparalytic keratitis is a disease of abnormal epithelial cell turnover. Epithelial thinning (Alper, 1975) has been shown, together with decreased mitotic rates (Mishima, 1957; Schimmelpfennig and Beuerman, 1981).

Cavanagh and Colley (1989) believe that the endogenous proliferation of corneal epithelial cells is regulated by a bidirectional control process, characterized by an adrenergic cAMP-dependent 'off' and a cholinergic, muscarinic cGMP dependent 'on' response. Mishima (1957) found that the decreased mitotic rate was accompanied by a fall in intracellular levels of acetycholine.

About 50% of patients with trigeminal anaesthesia can be seen to have some corneal abnormality.

Stage one of the disease is a punctate epitheliopathy of greater or lesser extent which can wax and wane. Its long time presence can lead to epithelial opacification and thickening of Bowman's membrane so that the corneal surface becomes irregular. This reduces visual acuity.

Stage two of the disease develops as an acute episode and is characterized by corneal epithelial detachment. This detachment is often in an area covered by the top lid. The patient is usually first aware of a marked reduction in his visual acuity and the eye becomes slightly red. The gap seen in the corneal epithelium is surrounded by an area of undermined epithelium extending some distance beyond (Figure 14.3). Folds in Descemet's membrane develop rapidly and are accompanied by aqueous flare and cells.

Stage three of the disease develops when stromal lysis takes place which frequently leads to perforation.

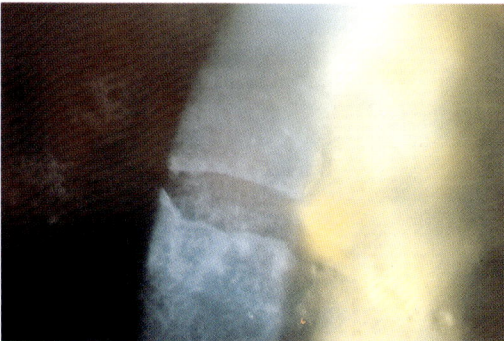

Figure 14.3 Stage two neuroparalytic keratitis showing characteristic corneal epithelial detachment, in this case, in the upper half of the cornea. Visual acuity is reduced and the eye becomes slighty red. A gap is seen in the corneal epithelium surrounded by an area of undermined epithelium extending some distance beyond. Descemet's folds develop rapidly and are accompanied by aqueous flare and cells. A soft therapeutic contact lens is contraindicated. It will result in a hypopyon within 12 hours. Closure of the eye is indicated

Treatment with soft lenses presents considerable difficulties and dangers, and taping or botulinum toxin (Adams, Kirkness and Lee, 1987) should always be employed as an alternative unless there are overriding reasons why they cannot be used. The patient cannot feel the contact lens and reflex tearing is not present because of the lack of an afferent pathway. The lens tends to dry. It is frequently lost without the patient being aware of the fact and this often happens during sleep. Since the eye is insensitive the patient is unaware of corneal inflammation and must rely on the appearance of the eye to let him know that a complication has developed. These patients are often old and viewing the eye is difficult through reading spectacles.

Such are the dangers of the use of soft lenses in this condition that a relative or friend should be trained in the examination of the eye on a twice daily basis to detect abnormality at an early stage. The relative or friend should be taught focal illumination with a strong light in a darkened room and instructed that the early signs of a potential problem are a red eye and a white spot on the cornea. Regular assessment of the vision at home is also helpful.

In stage one a thin, low water content, daily wear, therapeutic lens may be used to control the punctate epitheliopathy and prevent the possible development of stage two with epithelial detachment. Where a daily wear schedule is not practicable, or effective, an extended wear, low water content, therapeutic lens can be fitted. The author prefers the low water content, drying and soil resistant CSI T lens (Pilkington Barnes Hind) for both daily and extended wear in this disease.

In stage two, with epithelial detachment and anterior chamber involvement, there is no place for the use of soft contact lenses. Their use will lead to the development of intense flare and marked sterile hypopyon within 12 hours. The essential treatment is the instillation of atropine 1% drops and the closure of the eye with tape, having first cut the lashes. The classical treatment for this stage of the disease was tarsorrhaphy. Neurosurgeons were always quick to perform it because they knew the great dangers of leaving the eye open. With the advent of taping and botulinum toxin availability, tarsorrhaphy is rarely necessary.

Stage three is treated, bearing in mind that it may be secondarily infected, by measures which are appropriate for a suppurative keratopathy (see Chapter 13). The eye is closed with tape or botulinum toxin, as previously described. It is opened only for the application of medicaments. There was a vogue for the use of anti-collagenases, such as L-cysteine in such cases, but this practice appears to have passed. There may be an indication for the use of systemic tetracycline as an anti-collagenase agent, following the report by Seedor *et al.* (1987). However, exceedingly high dosage of tetracycline was used by those investigators and this may not be appropriate in humans.

Steroids should not be used since they potentiate collagenase activity (Berman, Cavanagh and Gage, 1976). Soft contact lenses should not be used at this stage, except as outlined below.

In stage three the patient may present with a perforation of the cornea. This is likely to be ragged and may require the application of glue and a contact lens. This procedure is described in a following paragraph dealing with perforation of the cornea.

Nystagmus

Allen and Davies (1983) have reported the use of contact lenses in the management of congenital idiopathic nystagmus, a condition usually associated with poor vision which has generally proved resistant to treatment. Their study involved the use of contact lenses in eight patients, five of whom achieved an improvement in their visual acuity of three lines on the Snellen's chart.

From 1973 to 1978, 210 contact lenses were fitted in 112 patients (Golubovic *et al.*, 1989). These patients were suffering from nystagmus and a refraction anomaly. In 79% it was possible to correct myopia, or a myopic, or mixed form of astigmatism. In these cases the visual acuity improved significantly. The hard contact lenses were well tolerated in all patients and these authors stated that the intensity of the nystagmus can be reduced through this treatment.

Pellucid marginal degeneration of the cornea

This degeneration (Schaeppi, 1975) begins in the inferior portion of the cornea, near the limbus.

There is an uninvolved area between the thinned area and the limbus. There is no vascularization and no associated arcus. The corneal sensation remains normal. It is probably a connective tissue anomaly and often gives rise to pseudokeratoconus. The visual acuity can be restored with the use of hard corneal lenses or, in advanced cases, with scleral lenses.

Varley, Macsai and Krachmer (1990), on the basis of observing 12 eyes of 11 patients over a 14 year period, reported that penetrating keratoplasty offers an excellent surgical result for patients with this disease.

Perforation of the cornea

This occurs with trauma, stromal lysis in neuroparalytic keratitis, autoimmune disease and suppurative keratopathy.

When the perforation is not suitable for suturing because of the friability of the surrounding tissues and corneal grafting is not a practicable alternative, a soft contact lens is often effective with, or without, the use of glue.

The contact lens used is a high water content therapeutic soft lens. The application of this will often result in a reformation of the anterior chamber within a few hours.

If the perforation is ragged, glue will have to be used. The glue used is 2-butylcyanoacrylate (Histoacryl Blau, manufactured by B. Braun, Melsungen AG, D-3508, Melsungen, Germany), the so-called 'blue glue'. The glue is conveniently applied in the following manner. Retract the lids with a speculum and dry the cornea with a small sponge. De-epithelialize the margins of the perforation with a knife. Take an orange stick approximately 8 mm in length and with a small amount of KY jelly attach, to one end of it, a small piece of plastic film (Steridrape, 3M is ideal). There should be enough film to cover the perforation and a little beyond. With the orange stick held upright, so that the plastic film is on top, apply the glue sparingly to the plastic film. The glue will not set on it. Invert the orange stick and apply the glue and the film to the area of the perforation. The glue sets rapidly. A therapeutic soft contact lens of high water content should then be applied over the glue and the film. The large diameter (15.5 mm) PCM (protective corneal membrane), manufactured by A.S. Optics, Cheam, Surrey, or, Cantor and Silver, Brackley, Northants., is ideal.

Reformation of the anterior chamber is usually rapid. Prior to the application, the cornea should be scraped for microscopy and bacterial culture and sensitivity so that appropriate antibiotics can be used.

Persistent corneal epithelial defects

These occur notably in stromal herpes simplex disease, but also in association with other stromal disease such as herpes zoster and chemical burns. A high water content, extended wear therapeutic lens can be applied to the cornea to protect and, perhaps (despite the results of the rabbit experiments of Zimny and Salisbury (1982), quoted at the beginning of this chapter), promote epithelialization.

Epidermal growth factor has been found to promote rapid healing of epithelial wounds in alkali burned rabbit corneas (Singh and Foster, 1987). These authors found that the healing was only maintained as long as the substance was used.

Nishida *et al.* (1988) studied the influence of epithelial growth factor on the healing of epithelial defects. They found that it is only effective for the first few days in which it is used. It would appear that fibronectin is also necessary for the healing to continue. Fibronectin is a basement membrane glycoprotein and a sort of natural tissue glue which can easily be isolated from blood drawn from the patient. It has been found that some method has to be used to keep these substances in contact with the eye and that a soaked soft contact lens is at present the best way to do this.

Post-radiation keratopathy

This may develop after X-ray treatment to the whole head, the orbit or the lids. It is characterized by a gross confluent punctate keratopathy which usually diminishes the visual acuity considerably. It is accompanied by focal dysplasia of the conjunctival epithelium so that white plaques of soggy keratinization replace the normal palpebral conjunctiva (Figure 14.4). Some months

after the radiation the white plaques resolve to reveal smaller areas of squamous metaplastic, dry conjunctiva (Figure 14.5). Whether the corneal disease is secondary to the conjunctival disease or caused by the radiation is not certain. However, in cases where the cornea alone is given high doses of irradiation with a Beta ray applicator (strontium 90) which is shielded on its external surface corneal problems are seldom encountered (J. Hungerford, personal communication). The discomfort of the condition can be greatly alleviated by the fitting of a therapeutic soft lens, preferably of the high water content, extended

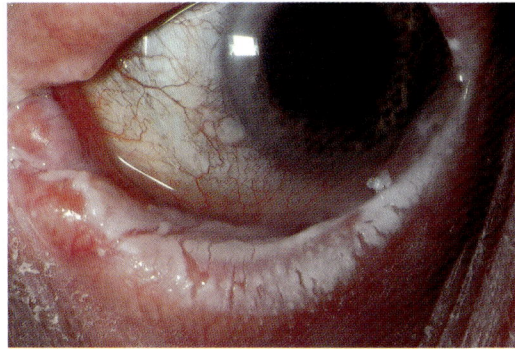

Figure 14.4 Soggy keratinization of the conjunctiva after whole head radiation for secondary breast cancer. There was a gross erosive keratopathy. A soft therapeutic lens was inserted and was responsible for a rapid improvement in the visual acuity and comfort

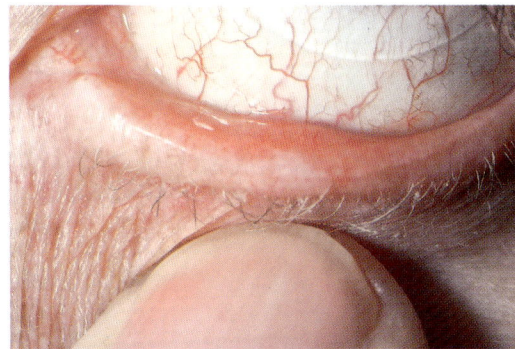

Figure 14.5 The same case as Figure 14.4 three months later. A small area of squamous metaplastic, dry conjunctiva is seen below

wear type. This usually brings about a considerable improvement in the visual acuity. Before the advent of soft contact lenses scleral lenses were used for this condition, but this is now unnecessary. In such a compromised eye there is a great danger of suppurative keratitis and measures should be taken so that it can be diagnosed and treated early, should it occur.

Ptosis

Scleral contact lenses have been used for a long time to correct ptosis where surgery is contraindicated. Originally a shelf was constructed on the upper portion of the scleral part of the lens, to hold the lid in the open position. This technique has been superseded at Moorfields Eye Hospital by the use of slotted lenses (Pullum and Trodd, 1984). These lenses, which adequately support the ptotic lid, are easier to fit and facilitate greater tear exchange than conventional scleral lenses (see Figure 14.2).

Recurrent corneal erosions

Traumatic

These, classically, occur after a baby's finger has scratched a mother's cornea, but any mild trauma can cause this condition. Its treatment with therapeutic contact lenses does not differ from that described earlier under Epithelial Basement Membrane dystrophy.

Further modalities of treatment have recently been advocated for traumatic recurrent erosion, which may be applicable to some erosions in basement membrane dystrophies. Recurrent erosions usually occur at one site only, which is usually in the intermediate zone of the lower half of the cornea, where the Hudson–Stahli line may be seen. The area may be distinguished by a black ring in the fluorescein film for a short time after an attack and there are usually epithelial cysts in the vicinity.

McLean, MacRae and Rich (1986) were the first to advocate multiple anterior stromal punctures with a 20 gauge hypodermic needle, to the area of recurrent erosion. Approximately 15 to 25 punc-

tures, through Bowman's membrane and spaced 0.5 mm to 1.0 mm apart, were made. The direction of the needle was perpendicular to the plane of the cornea and enough pressure was exerted to indent the cornea one-quarter to one-third of the depth of the anterior chamber. The procedure was performed at the slit lamp with topical anaesthesia. Following treatment, a pressure patch was used for two to four days.

Rubinfeld *et al.* (1990) have modified the procedure and introduced a new commercially available instrument (Look Inc., Norwell, Mass., USA) designed to standardize the technique, minimize scarring and prevent corneal perforation. They pointed out that E.N. McLean, in a personal communication, had related that he had had two cases in which the cornea was perforated. These authors stained the cornea with fluorescein to enhance visualization of the puncture sites, which stained brightly during the procedure.

An instrument similar to the one described and illustrated by Rubinfeld *et al.* can be constructed from a 27 gauge × half inch (1.25 cm) needle. Using a needle holder, the needle can be bent some 4 mm along its shaft, in the direction of the obliquity of its point, to approximately 45°. The 27 gauge needle tip can then be inserted into the lumen of a 21 gauge × 1.5 inch (3.8 cm) needle so that the obliquities of the tips face each other. The extreme tip of the 27 gauge needle can then be bent to an angle of approximately 90° away from the obliquity of its tip. The modified 27 gauge needle can then be fixed on a 1.0 ml syringe from which the plunger has been removed. Such an instrument, used so that the bent cutting tip is perpendicular to the cornea, avoids the hazard of corneal penetration and contributes to a standard depth penetration. The barb on the commercially available instrument, which can be obtained from Look Inc., is stated to be from 0.1 to 0.3 mm in length.

Geggel (1990) has reported the successful treatment of three patients by Nd:YAG. Multiple applications to the erosion area were used with energy levels between 1.8 and 2.2 mJ. The erosions of all patients healed without complications and the patients remained symptom free for four to six months. One of these patients had a previous stromal puncture with a bent 25 gauge needle. Compared with needle puncture, the laser punctures were more reproducible, shallow and translucent.

Diabetic recurrent corneal erosions

These typically occur after vitreous surgery in the diabetic eye. A soft extended wear therapeutic lens of high water content can be used to control this condition.

Recurrent erosions after chemical burns

In this case the stroma is always involved and topical steroids are often used to control the corneal inflammation. A soft lens can be applied to control the recurrent erosions but, at this time, the steroid medication must not be stopped or reduced as, otherwise, a marked stromal inflammatory response will ensue. The lens used should be a high water content extended wear therapeutic soft contact lens.

Retinitis pigmentosa

Damage to photoreceptors by hereditary degeneration has been reported to be accelerated by light exposure in the rat (La Vail and Battelle, 1975). On the basis of this finding, light deprivation with an opaque contact lens to one eye has been advocated in this disease so that one eye may be preserved, as it were, for future use (Berson, 1971). Berson (1980) disproved this theory on examining two patients who had worn one opaque scleral lens for approximately six to eight hours a day for a period of five years. Miyake *et al.* (1990) examined a 37-year-old man who had had trauma to one eye 30 years earlier and whose pupil was largely occluded by iris. There was a pinhole pupil through which could be seen a thick white membrane. The left eye showed early features of retinitis pigmentosa. Twelve years later, when the man was 49, the right pupil was opened, using a vitrectomy instrument. The fundus appearances were the same in both eyes. Cone, rod, flicker and single bright flash electroretinograms were no longer recordable in either eye.

Rosacea keratitis

This disease is seldom seen in the absence of rosacea conjunctivitis. Perilimbal vessels advance into the cornea, superficially, and subepithelial infiltrates develop, often in a triangular fashion with the base at the limbus. The cornea becomes irregular in thickness and then the visual acuity is grossly impaired. The keratitis of rosacea is seldom seen now that the effectiveness of systemic tetracycline given over long periods is known. In cases of old keratitis the visual acuity can often be greatly improved by fitting scleral or soft silicone lenses.

Terrien's ectatic marginal dystrophy

This is a marginal degeneration of the cornea which occurs at any age and usually in men. It is usually bilateral and very slowly progressive. There is usually a peripheral corneal opacification resembling an arcus senilis which leaves a clear zone between itself and the sclera. Within this clear zone there is a progressive thinning of the peripheral cornea and, unlike Mooren's ulceration, the gutter so formed remains epithelialized and becomes lightly vascularized (Figure 14.6). In contrast to Mooren's ulceration, the condition is painless. Pseudo pterygia can develop. Perforation, with prolapse of the iris, can occur. The condition gives rise to ectasia of the cornea so that a secondary type of keratoconus results. This can be treated with hard corneal lenses which usually need to be of small diameter, fitting in much the same way as for true keratoconus. Advanced disease requires scleral lenses.

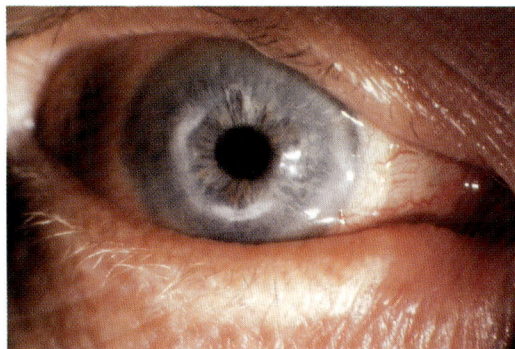

Figure 14.6 Terrien's marginal degeneration. There is mid-zone corneal opacification resembling an arcus senilis and a clear zone between this and the sclera. Within this peripheral clear zone there is progressive thinning of the peripheral cornea and the gutter so formed remains epithelialized and becomes lightly vascularized

Theodore's superior limbic keratoconjunctivitis

This condition is characterized by inflammation and keratinization of the superior bulbar conjunctiva and the superior limbus so that they freely stain with Rose Bengal. The superior limbus is sometimes so swollen that it hangs like an apron over the superior cornea. The superior cornea can show a punctate epithelial keratitis and frequently filaments appear in this area. These intensify the pain associated with this condition. The upper palpebral conjunctiva is infiltrated, papillary and keratinized.

Superior limbic keratoconjunctivitis is associated with thyroid disease in about one-third of cases.

The classical treatment advocated by Theodore (1963) is the local application of 0.5 to 1.0% silver nitrate to the superior palpebral conjunctiva. In the author's experience, this results in a much more uncomfortable patient for some two days, followed by a period of relief of about one week before the symptoms return. Nelson (1989) believes that this treatment usually results in the relief of symptoms for four to six weeks.

Although it is a painful disease it does not interfere with the patient's sleep. The pain disappears when the eyes are closed. Alternate taping of one eye and then the other is a method of dealing with a severely painful episode (Mondino, Zaidman and Salamon, 1982).

Acetyl cysteine 5%, 10% or 20% is often prescribed because of its mucolytic property (Wright, 1972), but the author has not found it to be of much use in cases of even moderate severity.

Cryotherapy to the superior palpebral conjunctiva has been advocated by Osler (1987a).

Undell *et al*. (1986) have used thermocauterization of the superior bulbar conjunctiva as a treatment for 13 eyes in 11 patients. Under local anaesthesia a disposable microsurgery cautery was used to apply 30 to 50 brief focal applications to the superior bulbar conjunctiva between the 10 o'clock and 2 o'clock positions from the limbus to 8 mm posteriorly. Each burn was of sufficient intensity to involve the entire epithelial layer and produce stromal shrinkage without injuring the underlying sclera. Their overall response rate to thermocautery was 73% (eight patients). Of the positive responders, 63% (five patients) had been considered silver nitrate treatment failures.

Superior limbic bulbar conjunctival resection has been advocated as a treatment by Donshik *et al*. (1978) and Passons and Wood (1984). The former authors treated four patients by this method with relief of symptoms. They stated that after the resection the corneoscleral limbus was smooth and flat. This has not been the present author's experience; a few months after the procedure, the thickening and Rose Bengal staining of the bulbar conjunctiva can be seen to return.

The latter authors reviewed 10 patients who underwent superior limbic conjunctival resection. With a follow-up of greater than one year (one to three years), five of 10 patients remained asymptomatic after conjunctival resection. Three patients were much improved, but had some persistence of complaints and two patients had little or no improvement of symptoms, despite healing of the conjunctiva. Interestingly, the two eyes showing no improvement had a marked decrease in Schirmer's test as did two of three patients showing much improvement, but some persistence of symptoms.

The surgical procedure for conjunctival resection involves anaesthetizing the conjunctiva with topical anaesthetic and then giving an injection of local anaesthetic beneath the superior bulbar conjunctiva so that a wheal is created above the limbus. The affected area of conjunctiva is then excised, conveniently with a sharp pointed de Wecker's scissors. The cut is at first along the limbus from two to ten o'clock and then backward to the extent of 5 mm so that a crescent of conjunctiva is resected. Tenon's capsule should be included. This is the only treatment which has been effective in the author's hands.

The author has found that soft contact lenses are poorly tolerated in these patients, although there would appear to be an indication for them, especially when filaments are present.

Mondino, Zaidman and Salamon (1982) found that wearing soft contact lenses prevented the recurrence of signs and symptoms of superior limbic keratoconjunctivitis in six patients whom they treated with pressure patching.

Thygeson's superficial punctate keratopathy

This is a condition affecting the epithelium of the cornea. Usually both corneas are involved, but the disease may be unilateral. The lesions are characteristically small, granular, elevated and transient. They do not usually stain with fluorescein, but rather break the fluorescein film and appear as black spots within it. There is no stromal component and the conjunctiva is not involved. The eye is painful and yet it is white. The pain is relieved by topical steroid administration which should always be the minimum necessary. It is debatable whether steroid administration has any effect on the resolution of the lesions since they disappear in any case in a few days. Contrary to the original description of Thygeson (1950), the disease may last for over 30 years. There are exacerbations and remissions of pain even while the lesions continue. Osler (1987b) suggests that the use of topical steroids prolongs the course of the disease.

Painful and incapacitating as the white eyes can be in this disease, they do not interfere with sleep. That is, when the eyes are closed there is no pain. If steroids are contraindicated because they elevate the ocular pressure, taping of the lids can serve as a stop-gap procedure. Forstot and Binder (1979) reported the use of soft contact lenses in three cases of the disease. Two of their cases used daily wear soft lenses. One of their cases was intolerant of continuous wear Bausch and Lomb plano T lenses, but tolerant of continuous wear Softcon lenses. All three cases became asymptomatic.

Goldberg, Schanzlin and Brown (1980) described four patients who were fitted with extended wear soft lenses and obtained symptomatic relief. In all four cases the lesions disappeared and topical steroids could be discontinued. One of their cases turned himself into a daily wear patient and another became intolerant of continuous wear lenses.

Williams and Mackie (1981) described the use of daily wear soft therapeutic lenses in seven cases with success in five cases. One patient who failed was thought to be psychologically unsuited to wearing contact lenses and the other had disease of 27 years' duration.

The author's subsequent experience of daily wear therapeutic soft contact lenses in this condition has forced him to the conclusion that the lenses are most acceptable where they are employed early in the disease and where there is a refractive error. Concurrent topical steroid administration may have to be used during marked exacerbations. The lenses are highly effective in relieving pain.

The author has seen three patients who developed Thygeson's superficial punctate keratopathy while they were already established wearers of hard corneal lenses. Referral for an ophthalmological opinion led to the cessation of contact lens wear and this in its turn led, in the course of a few weeks, to pain and photophobia developing, which had not been experienced before the lens had been discontinued. One of these patients developed steroid glaucoma as a consequence of the medication which had to be introduced. All three patients became asymptomatic when hard corneal lens wear was resumed. Although the author has had no personal experience of the therapeutic fitting of hard corneal lenses in patients with this disease, this possibility should be considered, especially when significant astigmatism is also present which would necessitate the use of toric soft lenses, the fitting of which is time consuming and expensive.

Trachoma

This disease leads to conjunctival and corneal scarring. In stage 4 of the disease (MacCallan, 1931) there may be trichiasis, entropion, corneal opacities, vascularization and corneal irregularity, together with dry eyes. This may be treated with scleral or silicone soft lenses. The corneal irregularity is often more important than the opacities in producing visual impairment and a substantial improvement may be obtained in the visual acuity with the use of contact lenses. The soft silicone lens has the advantages that being soft it is better tolerated and since it has virtually zero water content does not have to be kept hydrated. The dangers associated with the use of such lenses have been dealt with above.

Wet filamentary keratitis

This condition occurs, for example, in association with herpes simplex keratitis, recurrent erosions, cataract surgery, albinism, midbrain strokes producing nystagmus, essential orbicularis spasm and Theodore's superior limbic keratoconjunctivitis. There is also an idiopathic variety.

Wet filamentary keratitis is distinguished from the more common filamentary keratitis which occurs in dry eyes. This keratitis is much more painful than that occurring in the latter and the pain is often accompanied by profuse watering. Long, and often globular shaped, filaments, attached to the corneal surface, move like tassels in the precorneal film. The eye becomes very red and the palpebral conjunctiva shows a marked papillary response with gross hyperaemia. There is often a mucopurulent discharge. The picture resembles a bacterial conjunctivitis, but treatment with appropriate antibiotics is of little use. It is important not to waste time in this direction.

Therapeutic soft contact lenses are very effective in controlling the condition. The filaments disappear and the eye whitens within a very short time. A therapeutic soft lens need only be worn on a daily wear basis, provided its insertion and removal are practicable, and the author prefers a thin, low water content lens.

After two or three months of use the soft lens wear can be discontinued and often the filaments do not reappear. If they do, it is an indication to re-insert the lens. There is often a latent period of a few days before the filaments reappear and it may only be necessary for the soft therapeutic lens to be worn on every second or third day. The only exception in wet filamentary keratitis is that seen in association with Theodore's superior limbic keratoconjunctivitis. In this condition there is often gross superior palpebral conjunctival infiltration and the lenses are seldom tolerated.

Sinha and Sinha (1986) have described the treatment of filamentous keratitis with supersaturated saline. The supersaturated saline used was from a plastic container (the proprietary name is Miniflex – commonly used for the termination of pregnancy). In a double blind trial with normal saline it was found that the cases which recovered had been treated with supersaturated saline. The cases which showed no change had received normal saline.

Complications of therapeutic contact lenses

Corneal wrinkling

Thinner therapeutic soft lenses have been shown to cause little or no corneal thickening when worn continuously (Mobilia, Dohlman and Holly, 1977), and have increased the potential for safe and effective therapeutic use of these lenses. A

'rippling phenomenon' which may involve these extremely thin lenses and the underlying corneal surface has been reported (Mobilia, Yamamoto and Dohlman, 1980). Slit lamp microscopy reveals a variety of patterns, star burst, regular diagonal folds and irregular creases. When the lenses are removed the corneal surfaces are found to have a corresponding rippled figuration, and visual acuity with and without the lenses is unsatisfactory. The wrinkling of the cornea is temporary and appears to be related to lens thickness factors.

Vascularization

Sooner or later, with the use of a soft or a hard scleral contact lens, the cornea will vascularize and the rate at which it develops depends on the state of the cornea. Thus, if there is oedema, as in bullous keratopathy, it will develop fairly rapidly and if there is already an area of cellular activity in the stroma it will soon encourage the growth of vessels towards it. The vessels may be in a superficial layer, in which case the vascularization seems to be largely reversible, or they may occur as a brush of vessels at the level of the deep stroma, in which case they usually result in marked stromal oedema. Apart from the latter type, vascularization does not normally have much influence on the visual acuity unless a lipid keratopathy forms. It has been pointed out that vascularization of a cornea prevents its ulceration (Conn *et al.*, 1980).

Sterile corneal infiltrates

These infiltrates can occur without much in the way of symptoms and tend to be located peripherally or in the mid zone. There is always the question of whether they really are sterile. Scraping of the cornea and bacteriology reveals no pathogens. They resolve with the use of local steroid. They tend to recur and they may give rise to local vascularization.

Sterile hypopyon

This begins as an apparent uveitis with flare and is typically seen when a soft lens is applied to an eye with stage two neuroparalytic keratitis, or the neuroparalytic keratitis of herpes zoster. It is not necessarily associated with infiltration of the cornea, but when this is present there is always the possibility that one is dealing with a suppurative keratopathy. The eye becomes very red. It is imperative that the lens be removed and the case should be treated as if it were infected. It may be appropriate to perform a tap of the anterior chamber for bacteriological examination. The cause of this intense uveitis is not known.

It is possible that the basis of this reaction and the sterile infiltrates is an initial allergic response which releases inflammatory mediators and sets off the activation of complement by the alternative pathway (Mondino, Brown and Rabin, 1978). Perhaps the soft lens prevents the dispersal of inflammatory substances and products of metabolism.

Suppurative keratitis

This not infrequently occurs as a complication of therapy with soft contact lenses. The eye becomes painful and red. It may occur at the site of a previous epithelial defect or nebula. The tell-tale sign that there is new active pathology is the presence of stromal cellular activity in the area surrounding the previous defect or nebula and this is seen with the fine beam of the slit lamp. Measures should be taken as outlined in the section on Suppurative keratitis in Chapter 13.

Collagen corneal shields

A section on collagen shields is added here as a postcript, not because they are contact lenses, but because they rival therapeutic soft contact lenses as a therapeutic modality.

These shields are fashioned to fit over the eye and are made from porcine sclera (Bausch and Lomb Pharmaceuticals Inc., Clearwater, Florida) or bovine skin (Chiron Ophthalmics, Irvine, California). Baush and Lomb market their collagen shields under the trade name BioCor and they are available in 12, 24 or 72 hour maximum approximate dissolution rates. The Chiron Collagen Shield is of one type and is completely biodegradable over approximately 24 hours. Both porcine and bovine shields are clear and permit clinical

observation of the eye, provided pus or organic matter does not accumulate under them. The BioCor shields have a diameter of 14.5 mm and a posterior curve radius of 9.0 mm. The Chiron Collagen Shields have a diameter of 14 mm and a posterior curve of 9.1 mm.

Weissman and Lee (1988) studied the oxygen transmissibility, thickness and water content of the three types of BioCor collagen shields. They found that the water content was about 63% and that, so far as oxygen permeability was concerned, they behaved like 63% water content hydrogel contact lenses. They found that the central thickness of the 12 hour shields was significantly greater than the central thickness of the other two types.

The Chiron Collagen Shield is stated to have a water content of 80% when fully hydrated.

These devices are well accepted by the majority of patients and may be used in the following situations after they have been hydrated with sterile fluid:

1. Acute epithelial defects.
2. Persistent epithelial defects.
3. Postoperatively.
4. Drug delivery systems.

Bausch and Lomb claim, and have data on file to support this claim, that their shield speeds corneal epithelial healing as much as 50% or more. Chiron claim that their shield provides patient comfort during epithelial resurfacing of the cornea following surgery, accidental trauma or other insults.

Frantz et al. (1989) evaluated the effect of a collagen shield on epithelial wound healing in keratectomy wounds on rabbit eyes. They found that epithelial healing was significantly faster in corneas treated with corneal shields compared to untreated corneas. Scanning electron microscopy of the collagen shields after eight hours of wear showed a large number or polymorphonuclear leucocytes entrapped in the collagen matrix.

Shaker et al. (1989) studied epithelial wound healing in cats and found a significantly greater healing response in the group treated with collagen shields than in the control group. However, they found that the shield did not increase the speed of epithelial cell migration. Rather, the effect of the shield was most pronounced during the first eight hours after wounding, there being earlier wound closure in the treated group. They suggested that this may be due to protection and lubrication of the epithelial cells at the margins of the fresh wound.

Ruffini, Aquavella and LoCascio (1989) evaluated the effects of collagen shields on corneal epithelialization following keratoplasty. Donor corneas treated with collagen demonstrated significantly less epithelial staining and smaller epithelial defects on the first day following surgery compared with controls.

Fourman and Wiley (1989) have reported the use of a collagen shield to treat a spontaneous glaucoma filter bleb leak. A previous leak had been resistant to patching and bandage contact lens use and the patient had gone on to develop a *Staphylococcus epidermidis* endophthalmitis. A 24-hour collagen shield which had been soaked in gentamicin was used for the new leak. Two days later the leak was sealed and remained sealed. Collagen shields can be rehydrated in a solution containing antibiotics to deliver these to the eye.

Unterman *et al*. (1988) demonstrated that collagen shields that had been immersed in tobramycin produced higher concentrations of antibiotic in the cornea and aqueous humour of rabbit eyes than did subconjunctival injections.

Sawusch *et al*. (1988) found that the use of tobramycin-containing collagen shields, to treat *Pseudomonas aeruginosa* keratitis in the rabbit eye, was more effective than treatment with topically applied tobramycin drops.

Hobden *et al*. (1988) showed that corneas infected by intrastromal injection of *Pseudomonas aeruginosa* and receiving shields rehydrated with 4% tobramycin which were applied for four hours, demonstrated significantly reduced numbers of bacteria compared with those infected corneas without shields which were treated with half hourly 4% tobramycin drops. They further observed that the addition of 4% tobramycin to shields in situ was as effective as exchange with a new shield containing 4% tobramycin.

Phinney *et al*. (1988) studied the corneal shield delivery of gentamicin and vancomycin. In vitro studies showed that presoaked shields released the majority of gentamicin within the first 30 minutes of elution while vancomycin was released gradually over six hours of elution. Their experiments in rabbits compared the gentamicin and vancomycin levels produced at five time points in tears, cornea and aqueous humour by shields soaked in antibiotics versus frequent drop

therapy. The corneal shields soaked in gentamicin, vancomycin, or a combination of the two, produced tear, cornea and aqueous humour levels that were generally higher or, at least, comparable with those achieved with frequent drop therapy.

Schwartz *et al*. (1990) have studied the corneal shield delivery of amphotericin B. In vitro studies showed that presoaked collagen shields released most of the amphotericin B within the first hour of elution. Collagen shields soaked in amphotericin B produced corneal levels that were higher than those produced by frequent drop therapy at one hour, equivalent to drop therapy at two and three hours and lower than drop therapy at six hours. There were no differences in amphotericin B levels in aqueous humour at any time point between rabbits treated with collagen shield delivery and rabbits treated with frequent drop therapy.

O'Brien *et al*. (1988) compared the use of collagen shields versus soft contact lenses to enhance penetration of topical tobramycin in rabbits. The contact lenses used were of 38.6% water content. Topical tobramycin was applied to 16 eyes in all – six with collagen shields, six with soft lenses, and four with neither shield nor contact lens. Samples of aqueous humour were removed at 15 and 60 minutes following the last dose. Collagen corneal shields allowed a significant increase in tobramycin penetration into the anterior chamber at 60 minutes compared with hydrophilic soft contact lenses or controls.

Collagen shields may be soaked in other drugs apart from antibiotics with advantage.

Murray *et al*. (1990) studied collagen shield heparin delivery to the rabbit eye utilizing radiolabelled heparin as well as fibrin inhibition assay. A single collagen shield soaked in heparin achieved anterior chamber anticoagulant levels that paralleled the time course of the radiolabelled heparin delivery and resulted in fibrin inhibition during the six hour study period. Subconjunctival heparin injection did not alter baseline aqueous anticoagulant activity. Their studies suggested that a heparin-hydrated collagen shield may prevent postoperative fibrin formation in eyes at risk from this complication, including eyes undergoing surgery for the complications of proliferative diabetic retinopathy, proliferative vitreoretinopathy and glaucoma filtration surgery.

Hwang *et al*. (1989) showed that collagen

shields enhanced the ocular penetration of topical dexamethasone. Treatment with presoaked collagen shield, plus hourly drops, resulted in peak and cumulative drug delivery to the cornea, aqueous, iris and vitreous that was twofold to fourfold higher than that achieved with hourly drops alone.

Chen *et al*. (1990) in rabbit experiments studied rejection of 37 keratoplasties placed in vascularized beds. Cyclosporine was delivered in presoaked collagen shields or in olive oil. Treatment was begun immediately after grafting or at the first sign of immune reaction. The mean survival time of the grafts in the collagen shield treated eyes was significantly longer than in the eyes treated with drops. In the eyes treated at the first sign of graft reaction, cyclosporine in collagen shields halted the rejection process: seven of these eyes survived the 120-day observation period compared to one of the eyes treated with drops.

The use of cyclosporine as an ophthalmic preparation has been hampered by its low solubility and poor ocular penetration. Both topical preparations formulated in various vegetable oils and systemically administered cyclosporine have produced relatively low drug levels in the eye. Reidy *et al*. (1988) mixed cyclosporine powder into a 1% collagen gel (40 μg/ml collagen) and then fashioned 12 corneal shields containing 4 mg of cyclosporine each, in the initial experiments on the penetration of the drug into cornea and aqueous.

Chen *et al*. (1990) used collagen shields that were prepared by Bausch and Lomb Pharmaceuticals, Clearwater, Florida, and contained 4 mg cyclosporine.

References

ADAMS, G.G.W., KIRKNESS, C.M. and LEE, J.P. (1987) Botulinum toxine A induced protective ptosis. *Eye*, **1**, 5, 603–608

ALLEN, E.D. and DAVIES, P.D. (1983) Role of contact lenses in the management of congenital nystagmus. *British Journal of Ophthalmology*, **67**, 12, 834–836

ALI, Z. and INSLER, M.S. (1986) A comparison of therapeutic bandage lenses, tarsorrhaphy, and antibiotic and hypertonic saline on corneal epithelial wound healing. *Annals of Ophthalmology*, **18**, 22–24

ALPER, M.G. (1975) The anaesthetic eye; an investigation of the changes in the anterior ocular segment of the monkey caused by interrupting the trigeminal nerve at various levels along its course. *Transactions of the American Ophthalmological Society*, **73**, 323–365

ARTHUR, B.W., HAY, B.J., WASAN, S.M. and WILLIS, W.E. (1983) Ultrastructural effects of topical timolol on the rabbit cornea. Outcome alone and in conjunction with a gas permeable contact lens. *Archives of Ophthalmology*, **101**, 10, 1607–1610

BALDONE, J.A. and KAUFMAN, H.E. (1983) Soft contact lenses and clinical disease. *American Journal of Ophthalmology*, **95**, 6, 851–852

BERMAN, M., CAVANAGH, H.D. and GAGE, J. (1976) Regulation of collagenase activity in the ulcerating cornea by cyclic AMP. *Experimental Eye Research*, **22**, 209–218

BERSON, E.L. (1971) Light deprivation for early retinitis pigmentosa. A hypothesis. *Archives of Ophthalmology*, **85**, 521

BERSON, E.L. (1980) Light deprivation and retinitis pigmentosa. *Vision Research*, **20**, 1179

BIBER, M. (1890) Uber einige seltene Hornhautkrankugen. *Thesis*, Zurich

BLOK, M.D.W., KOK, J.H.C., VAN MIL, C,. GREVE, E.L. and KIJLSTRA, A. (1990) Use of Megasoft bandage lens for treatment of complications after trabeculectomy. *American Journal of Ophthalmology*, **110**, 264–268

BRON, A.J. and BROWN, N.A. (1971) Some superficial corneal disorders. *Transactions of the Ophthalmological Society of the UK*, **91**, 13–29

BUCHEIT, W.A. and DELGARDO, T.E. (1985) Tumors of the cerebellopontine angle: clinical features and surgical management. In *Neurosurgery*, pp. 720–729 (Wilkins, R.H. and Rengachary, S.S., eds). McGraw-Hill, New York

BURNS, R.P. (1968) Meesman's corneal dystrophy. *Transactions of the American Ophthalmological Society*, **66**, 530–635

BUSIN, M. and SPITZNAS, M. (1988) Sustained gentamicin release by presoaked medicated bandage contact lenses. *Ophthalmology*, **95**, 6, 796–798

CATFORD, G.V. and MACKIE, I.A. (1968) Occlusion with high plus corneal lenses. *British Journal of Ophthalmology*, **52**, 342–345

CAVANAGH, H.D. (1975) Herpetic ocular disease: therapy of persistent epithelial defects. *International Ophthalmology Clinics*, **93**, 1047–1048

CAVANAGH, D. and COLLEY, A.M. (1989) The molecular basis of neurotrophic keratitis. *Acta Ophthalmologica*, **67** (Suppl 192), 115–134

CEDERSTAFF, T.H. and TOMLINSON, A. (1983) A comparative study of tear evaporation rates and water content of soft contact lenses. *American Journal of Optometry and Physiological Optics*, **60**, 167–174

CHEN, Y.F., GEBHARDT, B.M., REIDY, J.J. and KAUFMAN, H.E. (1990) Cyclosporine-containing collagen shields suppress couneal allograft rejection. *American Journal of Ophthalmology*, **109**, 132–137

COGAN, D.G., DONALDSON, D.D., KUWABARA, T. and MARSH-

ALL, D. (1964) Microcystic dystrophy of the corneal epithelium. *Transactions of the American Ophthalmological Society*, **62**, 213–225

COHEN, M. and SULZBERGER, M.B. (1935) Essential shrinkage of conjunctiva in a case of probable epidermolysis bullosa dystrophica. *Archives of Opthalmology*, **13**, 374–390

COLLIN, J.R.O. (1983) *A Manual of Systemic Eyelid Surgery*. Churchill Livingstone, Edinburgh, p.70

COLLIN, J.R.O., COSTER, D.J. and SULLIVAN, J.M. (1978) Cryosurgery for trichiasis. *Transactions of the Ophthalmological Society of the UK*, **98**, 81–83

CONN, H., BERMAN, M., KENYON, K., LANGER, R. and GAGE, J. (1980) Stromal vascularization prevents corneal ulceration. *Investigative Ophthalmology and Visual Science*, **19**, 362–370

DILLY, P.N. and MACKIE, I.A. (1981) Surface changes in the anaesthetic conjunctiva in man, with special reference to the production of mucus from a non-goblet cell source. *British Journal of Ophthalmology*, **65** (12), 833–842

DONSHIK, P.C., COLLIN, H.B., FOSTER, C.S., CAVANAGH, H.D. and BORUCHOFF, S.A. (1978) Conjunctival resection treatment and ultrastrucural histopathology of superior limbic keratoconjunctivitis. *American Journal of Ophthalmology*, **85**, 101–110

FORSTOT, S.L. and BINDER, P.S. (1979) Treatment of Thygeson's superficial punctate keratopathy with soft contact lenses. *American Journal of Ophthalmology*, **88** (2), 186–189

FOULKS, G.N. (1981) Treatment of recurrent erosion and corneal edema with topical osmotic colloidal solution. *Ophthalmology (Rochester)*, **88**, (8), 801–803

FOURMAN, S. and WILEY, L. (1989) Use of a collagen shield to treat a glaucoma filter bleb leak. *American Journal of Ophthalmology*, **107**, 673–674

FRANTZ, J.M., DUPUY, B.M., KAUFMAN, H.E. and BEUERMAN, R.W. (1989) The effect of collagen shields on epithelial wound healing in rabbits. *American Journal of Ophthalmology*, **108**, 524–528

GANS, L.A. (1988) Eye lesions of epidermolysis bullosa. *Archives of Dermatology*, **124**, 762–764

GEGGEL, H.S. (1990) Successful treatment of recurrent corneal erosion with Nd:YAG anterior stromal puncture. *American Journal of Ophthalmology*, **110**, 404–407

GOLDBERG, D.B., SCHANZLIN, D.J. and BROWN, S.I. (1980) Management of Thygeson's superficial punctate keratitis. *American Journal of Ophthalmology*, **89**, 22–24

GOLUBOVIC, S., MARJANOVIC, S., CVETKOVIC, D. and MANIC, S. (1989) The application of hard contact lenses in patients with congenital nystagmus. *Fortschritte der Ophthalmologie*, **86**, 5, 535–539

HARRISON, D.H. (1985) Pectoralis minor vascularized muscle graft for the treatment of unilateral facial palsy. *Plastic and Reconstructive Surgery*, **75**, 2, 206–213

HARRISON, D.H. (1990) Current trends in the treatment of facial palsy. *Annals of the Royal College of Surgeons of England*, **72**, 94–98

HASEGAWA, E., MATSUO, N., SARADA, K. and MIYAGAWA, K. (1979) Studies on the treatment of keratoconjunctivitis sicca. *Acta Medical Okayama*, **33**, 21–28

HEWSON, E.G. (1963) Congenital trigeminal anaesthesia. *British Journal of Ophthalmology*, **47**, 308–311

HILLMAN, J.S. (1974) Management of acute glaucoma with pilocarpine-soaked hydrophilic lens. *British Journal of Ophthalmology*, **7**, 674–679

HOBDEN, J.A., REIDY, J.J., O'CALLAGHAN, R.J., HILL, J.M., INSLER, M.S. and ROOTMAN, D.S. (1988) Treatment of experimental pseudomonas keratitis using collagen shields containing tobramycin. *Archives of Ophthalmology*, **106**, 1605–1607

HWANG, D.G., STERN, W.H., HWANG, P.J. and MACGOWAN-SMITH, L.A. (1989) Collagen shield enhancement of topical dexamethasone penetration. *Archives of Ophthalmology*, **107**, 1375–1380

JAY, J.L. and LEE, W.R. (1981) Aniridia keratopathy. *Proceedings of 6th Congress of European Society of Ophthalmology*, Brighton, 1980 (Trevor-Roper, P.D., ed.). The Royal Society of Medicine, London

JONES, B.R., BARRAS, T.C., HUNTER, P.A., DAROUGER, S. and MOHSENINE, M. (1976) Neglected lid deformities causing progressive corneal disease. *Transactions of the Ophthalmological Society of the UK*, **96**, 1, 45–51

KENYON, K.R. and TSENG, S.C.G. (1989) Limbal autograft transplantation for ocular surface disorders. *Ophthalmology*, **96**, 5, 709–723

KIESELBACH, G.F. and GENSLUCKNER, W. (1987) Die Behandlung der atopischen Keratokonjunktivitis im Kindesalter. *Klinische Monatsblatter fur Augenheilkunde*, **191**, 380–381

LAGANOWSKI, H.C., SHERRARD, E.S., KERR MUIR, M.G. and BUCKLEY, R.J. (1991) Distinguishing features of the iridocorneal endothelial syndrome and posterior polymorphous dystrophy. Value of endothelial specular microscopy. *British Journal of Ophthalmology*, **75**, 212–216

LAMBERTS, D.W. (1983) Dry eyes. In *The Cornea* (Smolin, G. and Thoft, R., eds). Little, Brown & Co., Boston, pp 293–309

LA VAIL, M.M. and BATTELLE, B.A. (1975) Influence of eye pigmentation and light deprivation on inherited retinal dystrophy in the rat. *Experimental Eye Research*, **21**, 167

MACCALLAN, A. (1931) The epidemiology of trachoma. *British Journal of Ophthalmology*, **15**, 369–441

MACKIE, I.A. (1985) Contact lenses in dry eyes. *Transactions of the Ophthalmological Society of the UK*, **104**, 477–483

MACKIE, I.A. and SEAL, D.V. (1981) The questionably dry eye. *British Journal of Ophthalmology*, **65**, 2–9

MCLEAN, E.N., MACRAE, S.M. and RICH, L.F. (1986) Recurrent erosion. Treatment by anterior stromal puncture. *Ophthalmology*, **93**, 6, 784–788

MISHIMA, S. (1957) The effects of the denervation and the

stimulation of the sympathetic and trigeminal nerve on the mitotic rate of the corneal epithelium in the rabbit. *Japanese Journal of Ophthalmology*, **1**, 65–73

MIYAKE, Y., SUGITA, S., HORIGUCHI, M. and YAGASAKI, K. (1990) Light deprivation and retinitis pigmentosa. *American Journal of Ophthalmology*, **110**, 305–306

MOBILIA, E.F., DOHLMAN, C.H. and HOLLY, F.J. (1977) A comparison of various soft contact lenses for therapeutic puposes. *Contact and Intraocular Lens Medical Journal*, **3**, 1, 9–15

MOBILIA, E.F. and FOSTER, C.S. (1978) Management of recurrent corneal erosions with ultrathin lenses. *Contact and Intraocular Lens Medical Journal*, **4**, 1, 25–29

MOBILIA, E.F., YAMAMOTO, G.K. and DOHLMAN, C.H. (1980) Corneal wrinkling induced by ultra-thin soft contact lenses. *Annals of Ophthalmology*, **12**, 4, 371–375

MONDINO, B.J., BROWN, S.I. and RABIN, B.S. (1978) Role of complement in corneal inflammation. *Transactions of the Ophthalmological Society of the UK*, **98** (3), 363–366

MONDINO, B.J., ZAIDMAN, G.W. and SALAMON, S.W. (1982) Use of pressure patching and soft contact lenses in superior limbic keratoconjunctivitis. *Archives of Ophthalmology*, **100**, 1932–1934

MURRAY, T.G., STERN, W.H., CHIN, D.H. and MACGOWAN-SMITH, E.A. (1990) Collagen shield heparin delivery for prevention of postoperative fibrin. *Archives of Ophthalmology*, **108**, 104–106

NELSON, J.D. (1989) Superior limbic keratoconjunctivitis (SLK). *Eye*, **3**, 180–189

NISHIDA, T., NAKAGAWA, S., WATANABE, K. *et al.* (1986). Pathobiology of epithelial defects. Peptide (GRGDS) of fibronectin cell binding domain, inhibits corneal epithelial attachment and spreading on fibronectin. *Investigative Ophthalmology and Visual Science*, **27** (Suppl. 3) abst. 7, p.53

O'BRIEN, T.P., SAWUSCH, M.R., DICK, J.D., HAMBURGH, T.R. and GOTTSCH, J.D. (1988) Use of collagen corneal shields versus soft contact lenses to enhance penetration of topical tobramycin. *Journal of Cataract and Refractive Surgery*, **14**, 505–507

OSLER, H.B. (1987a) Superior limbic keratoconjunctivitis. In *The Cornea* (Smolin, G. and Thoft, R.A., eds). Little Brown, Boston, pp 269–298

OSLER, H.B. (1987b) Superficial punctate keratitis. In *The Cornea* (Smolin, G. and Thoft, R.A., eds). Little Brown, Boston, pp. 221–224

PASSONS, G.A. and WOOD, T.O. (1984) Conjunctival resection for superior limbic keratoconjunctivitis. *Ophthalmology*, **91**, 8, 966–968

PHINNEY, R.B., SCHWARTZ, S.D., LEE, D.A. and MONDINO, B.J. (1988) Collagen-shield delivery of gentamicin and vancomycin. *Archives of Ophthalmology*, **106**, 1599–1604

PULLUM, K.W. (1984) Development of slotted scleral lenses. *Journal of the British Contact Lens Association*, **7**, 92–95

PULLUM, K.W. and TRODD, T.C. (1984) Development of slotted scleral lenses. *Journal of the British Contact Lens Association*, **7**, 28–38

RECCIA, R., DEL PRETE, A., BENUSIGLIO, E. and ORFEO, V. (1985) Continuous usage of low doses of human leukocyte interferon with contact lenses in herpetic keratoconjunctivitis. *Ophthalmic Research*, **17**, 4, 251–256

REFOJO, M.F. (1979) Contact lenses. In *Encyclopedia of Chemical Technology*, 3rd edn (Kirk, R.E., Othmer, D.F., eds). Wiley Press, New York, vol. 6, p. 720

REFOJO, M.F. and LEONG, F.L. (1981) Water pervaporation through silicone rubber contact lenses: a possible cause of complications. *Contact and Intraocular Lens Medical Journal*, **7**, 226–233

REIDY, J.J., GEBHARDT, B.M., PADUMANE, K. and KAUFMAN, H.E. (1988) Ocular pharmacokinetics of cyclosporine and delivered by collagen corneal shields. *Presentation No. 8 at the 22nd Annual Meeting of the Ocular Microbiology and Immunology Group* in October, 1988

RUBEN, M. (1975) Soft contact lens treatment of bullous keratopathy. *Transactions of the Ophthalmological Society of the UK*, **95**, 75–78

RUBINFELD, R.S., LAIBSON, P.R., COHEN, E.J., ARENTSEN, J.J. and EAGLE, R.C. (1990) Anterior stromal puncture for recurrent erosion: further experience and new instrumentation. *Ophthalmic Surgery*, **21**, 5, 318–326

RUFFINI, J.J., AQUAVELLA, J.V. and LOCASCIO, J.A. (1989) Effect of collagen shields on corneal epithelialisation following penetrating keratoplasty. *Ophthalmic Surgery*, **20**, 1, 21–25

SAWUSCH, M.R., O'BRIEN, T.P., DICK, J.D. and GOTTSCH, J.D. (1988) Use of collagen shields in the treatment of bacterial keratitis. *American Journal of Ophthalmology*, **106**, 279–281

SCHAEPPI, V. (1975) La dystrophe marginale inferieure pellucide de la cornée. *Problemes Actuels d'Ophthalmologie*, **1**, 672

SCHERMER, A., GALVIN, S. and SUN, T.T. (1986) Differentiation related expression of a major 64K corneal keratin in vivo and in culture suggests limbal location of corneal epithelial stem cells. *Journal of Cell Biology*, **103**, 49–62

SCHIMMELPFENNING, B. and BEUERMAN, R.W. (1981) Trophic changes in corneal epithelium after controlled thermocoagulation of the trigeminal ganglion. *Proceedings of the European Society of Ophthalmology*, Brighton, 1980 (Trevor-Roper, P., ed.). The Royal Society of Medicine, London, pp. 287–289

SCHWARTZ, S.D., HARRISON, S.A., ENGSTROM, R.E., BAWDON, R.E., LEE, D.A. and MONDINO, B.J. (1990) Collagen shield delivery of amphotericin B. *American Journal of Ophthalmology*, **109**, 701–704

SEEDOR, J.A., PERRY, H.D., MCNAMARA, T.F., GULUB, L.M., BUXTON, D.P. and GUTHRIE, D.S. (1987) Systemic tetracycline treatment of alkali-induced corneal ulceration in rabbits. *Archives of Ophthalmology*, **105**, 268–271

SEEFELDER, R. (1909) Die Aniridie als eine Entwicklungshemmung der Retina, *Von Graefe's Archive for Clinical and Experimental Ophthalmology*, **70**, 65–87

SEAL, D.V., MCGILL, J.I., MACKIE, I.A., LIAKOS, G.M., JACOBS, P. and GOULDING, N.J. (1986) Bacteriology and tear protein profiles of the dry eye. *British Journal of Ophthalmology*, **70**, 122–125

SHAKER, G.J., UEDA, S., LOCASCIO, J.A. and AQUAVELLA, J.V. (1989) Effect of a collagen shield on cat corneal epithelial wound healing. *Investigative Ophthalmology and Visual Science*, **30**, 7, 1565–1568

SHERIDAN, M. and WALKER, P.R. (1983) Changes in the water content of hydrogel lenses during wear. *Journal of the British Contact Lens Association*, **6**, 8–12

SHIELDS, B. (1979) Progressive essential iris atrophy, Chandler's syndrome and the iris naevus (Cogan Reese syndrome): a spectrum of disease. *Survey of Ophthalmology*, **24**, 1, 3–20

SINGH, G. and FOSTER, C.S. (1987) Epidermal growth factor in alkali-burned corneal epithelial wound healing. *American Journal of Ophthalmology*, **103**, 6, 802–807

SINHA, A. and SINHA, A.K. (1986) Treatment of filamentous keratitis with supersaturated saline. *Proceedings of the XXVth International Congress of Ophthalmology*, Rome, 1986. Kugler Publications, Berkeley, and Ghedini Editore, Milan, pp 1368–1369

SORSBY, A., ROBERTS, J.A.F. and BRIAN, R.T. (1951) Essential shrinkage of the conjunctiva in a hereditary affliction allied to epidermolysis bullosa. *Documenta Ophalmologica*, **5**, 118–150

THEODORE, F.H. (1963) Superior limbic keratoconjunctivitis. *Eye, Ear, Nose and Throat Monthly*, **42**, 25–28

THOFT, R.A. (1984) Keratoepithelioplasty. *American Journal of Ophthalmology*, **97**, 1–6

THYGESON, P. (1950) Superficial punctate keratitis. *Journal of the American Medical Association*, **144**, 1544–1549

TROBE, J.D. and LAIBSON, P.R. (1972) Dystrophic changes in the anterior cornea. *Archives of Ophthalmology*, **87**, 378–382

UDELL, I.J., KENYON, K.R., SAWA, M. and DOHLMAN, C.H. (1986) Treatment of superior limbic keratonconjunctivitis by thermocauterisation of the superior bulbar

conjunctiva. *Ophthalmology*, **93**, 2, 162–166

UNTERMAN, S.R., ROOTMAN, D.S., HILL, J.M. and KAUFMAN, H.E. (1988) Enhanced corneal tobramycin delivery using cross-linked collagen shields. ARVO abstracts, *Investigative Ophthalmology and Visual Science*, **29** (Suppl.), 52

VANNAS, A., HOGAN, M.J. and WOOD, I. (1975) Saltzmann's nodular degeneration of the cornea. *American Journal of Ophthalmology*, **79**, 211–219

VARLEY, G.A., MACSAI, M.S. and KRACHMER, J.H. (1990) The results of penetrating keratoplasty for pellucid marginal degeneration. *American Journal of Ophthalmology*, **110**, 149–152

WEISSMAN, B.A. and LEE, D.A. (1988) Oxygen transmissibility, thickness and water content of three types of collagen shields. *Archives of Ophthalmology*, **106**, 1706–1708

WILLIAMS, H.P. and MACKIE, I.A. (1981) Current management of Thygeson's superficial punctate keratopathy. *Proceedings of the 6th Congress of the European Society of Ophthalmology*, Brighton, 1980 (Trevor-Roper, P., ed.). Royal Society of Medicine, London

WILLIAMS, R. (1985) Pathogenesis and treatment of recurrent erosion. *British Journal of Ophthalmology*, **69**, 6, 435–437

WRIGHT, P. (1972) Superior limbic keratoconjunctivitis. *Transactions of the Ophthalmological Society of the UK*, **92**, 555–560

WRIGHT, P. (1986) Cicatrizing conjunctivitis. *Transactions of the Ophthalmological Society of the UK*, **105**, 1, 1–17

WRIGHT, P. and COLLIN, J.R. (1983) The ocular complications of erythema multiforme (Stevens Johnson syndrome) and their mangement. *Transactions of the Ophthalmological Society of the UK*, **103** (3), 338–341

ZALTA, A.H. and WIEDER, R.H. (1991) Closure of leaking filtering blebs with cyanoacrylate tissue adhesive. *British Journal of Ophthalmology*, **75**, 170–173

ZIMNY, M.L. and SALISBURY, C. (1982) Effects of soft contacts on corneal wound healing in rabbits. *Cornea*, **1**, 301–307

15

Keratoconus

The earliest sign of keratoconus is seen on oph-thalmoscopy with the instrument held 12 inches (30 cm) from the patient's eye. A 'black blob' is observed in the red reflex and this moves against the movement of the ophthalmoscope. At this time there is usually a typical 'skew' distortion of the mires of the Javal Schiotz keratometer, but this may be absent in early disease or where the cone is not central.

Maguire and Bourne (1989) suggest that corneal topography analysis systems are useful in the detection and description of corneal irregularity in the early stages of keratoconus and they warn the radial keratotomy surgeon that normal results on slit lamp examination and normal keratometry and refractive data do not rule out the presence of early keratoconus.

Thinning of the cornea is not a reliable early sign. Later signs are Vogt lines (Vogt, 1919) and Fleischer rings (Fleischer, 1906). Vogt lines are vertical striae seen centrally on the posterior sur-face of the cornea. They disappear on gently pressing the eye with the finger against the sclera. Fleischer rings are often seen as an incom-plete ring, usually below, at the base of the cone. They are formed by the deposition of haemo-siderin superficial to Bowman's membrane. They are yellow or olive green in colour and are best detected while using the cobalt filter of the slit lamp.

Visible thinning of the cornea is a later sign and it has been pointed out by Buxton (1973) that the cones that result may be of two types. First, there is the round or nipple type cone (Figure 15.1a) whose apical centre is close to the visual axis. Secondly, there is the oval or sagging type cone (Figure 15.1b) whose apical centre is in the lower part of the cornea remote from the visual axis. This distinction has important implications so far as corneal contact lens fitting is concerned. The round or nipple type cone can usually be fitted with a small diameter lens, whereas the oval or

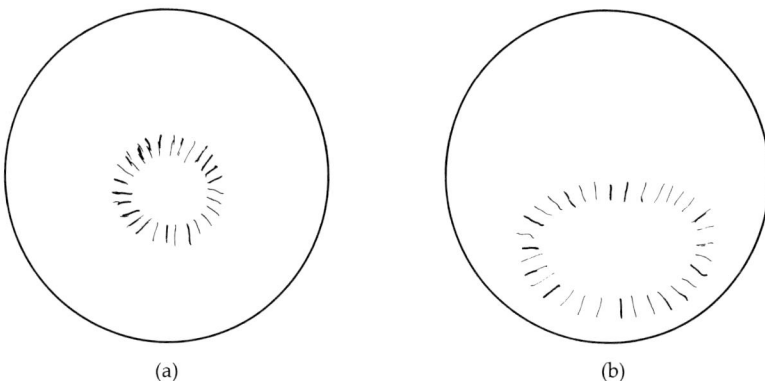

(a)   (b)

Figure 15.1 (a) Round or nipple cone in keratoconus (After Buxton). (b) Oval or sagging type cone in keratoconus (After Buxton)

sagging type cone requires a much larger lens. Fortunately, the oval or sagging type cone is a much rarer entity than the round or nipple type one. A round nipple type cone tends to stay in the same site however much the protrusion may increase.

Munsen's sign, where an angular curve is assumed by the lower lid margin when the patient looks down, is a feature of late disease.

There is a high prevalence of atopy among patients with keratoconus (Davies *et al.*, 1976; Rahi *et al.*, 1977; Harrison *et al.*, 1989) and problems arise with the tolerance of contact lenses when there is, in addition, atopic conjunctival disease. Papillary conjunctivitis is sometimes a problem. Korb *et al.* (1983) in a study of 15 keratoconus patients, with papillary conjunctivitis, found that the use of an enzymatic cleaner (papain) on their rigid PMMA lenses increased the wearing time in nine and diminished the symptoms of mucus and itching in 12. In 13 control keratoconus patients, three had a decrease, four had an increase and six had no change in lens wearing time. Only one of the controls had a diminution of symptoms. They concluded that the use of an enzyme cleaner was of value, but it did not, however, influence the biomicroscopic appearance of the papillary conjunctivitis.

Treatment

The first consideration in treatment with contact lenses is whether to treat at all. Unilateral keratoconus occurs from time to time. Sometimes it is found in a patient who was previously thought to have an amblyopic eye. If such a patient has been happy with his previous vision then there may be no point in treating him. If a corneal contact lens is prescribed for the eye it will presumably be worn on a daily basis for a long time. This may bring about, perhaps, a ptosis on the affected side or contact-lens-related chronic conjunctival disease. There is also the problem of the development of corneal opacification related to the contact lens wear. This will be dealt with later. There is no evidence that corneal lenses halt the progression of the disease. Sometimes it is possible to correct the patient with spectacles which give reasonable acuity. It is inadvisable to rely on retinoscopy. A subjective refraction should be done. If the visual acuity is less than 6/60 start with a minus 6.0 D cylinder and rotate it in the trial frame until the best acuity is obtained. Use the Jackson cross cylinder to determine the precise axis, then try to improve the acuity by using plus and minus spheres. Then adjust the cylindrical power in steps of one dioptre, always adjusting the spherical component afterwards. A final adjustment is made, again using the Jackson cross cylinder, to correct both the axis and the powers of the sphero-cylindrical combination. It must be realized that many keratoconus patients who have been fitted with hard corneal lenses do not achieve 6/5, or even 6/6, with the better eye and the more affected eye may only have an acuity of 6/12. A cylindrical spectacle over-correction may improve this and should always be tried.

The success rate of contact lens fitting and rate of progression to keratoplasty has been evaluated for 115 consecutive patients with keratoconus (Smiddy *et al.*, 1988). Of 190 non-operated eyes that needed to be fitted, 25 (13%) could not be fitted, whereas 165 eyes (87%) could be fitted. Most of these eyes had been referred for keratoplasty after previous contact lens fittings had no longer been successful. Of the 165 eyes that could be fitted, 51 (31%) ultimately needed keratoplasty after an average of 38.4 months of lens wear, and 114 eyes (69%) did not require keratoplasty over an average follow-up interval of 63 months of wearing contact lenses. Of 88 postoperative eyes, 53 (60%) wore contact lenses for best vision. They considered that keratoplasty can be delayed, or avoided, in many keratoconus patients by using specially designed lenses and that keratoconus eyes often needed contact lenses after keratoplasty.

A similar experience was reported by Fowler, Belin and Chambers (1988). They conducted a two and a half year retrospective review of all newly referred keratoconus patients to determine the treatment regimen of previously diagnosed 'contact lens failures'. Forty-eight patients were reviewed. Thirty-nine patients had been diagnosed as contact lens failures. Seven of these eyes were excluded from evaluation (because of prior grafts, unilaterality and dense central scar). Of the remaining 71 eyes of these patients, 57 (80%) were successfully refitted with contact lenses, all obtaining daily wearing time of 12 hours or more and a visual acuity of 20/40 or better. Their data suggested that the vast majority of keratoconus patients previously thought to be contact lens intolerant can be successfully refitted and achieve excellent visual acuity and prolonged wearing times.

Belin, Fowler and Chambers (1988) retrospectively reviewed, over a period of two years, 33 'contact lens failures' who were referred for surgical intervention. Twenty-nine of these patients were successfuly refitted with contact lenses. All achieved wearing times of 12 hours and a visual acuity of 20/40, or better. Sophisticated methods must be used for fitting keratoconus.

Scleral lenses

Since their development in the 1880s scleral lenses have played an important part in the management of keratoconus. It is true that many patients cannot tolerate them, but those who do go on to wear them can do so for a lifetime. Cross (1949) reviewed patients fitted with scleral lenses by five prominent contact lens practitioners prior to 1945 and found that 74% were wearing the lenses for more than eight hours daily, 15% were not wearing, 5% wore sometimes and 6% wore one lens only.

The lens is fitted after a corneal mould has been taken in the same way as has been already outlined (see Chaper 3), but steeper back central optic radii are required. The object is to achieve clearance of the cone, but often a light central touch developing after the lens has 'settled back' has to be accepted. The lens is channelled, or preferably, fenestrated in the conventional way.

Recently, slotted scleral lenses have been used in the management of the disease (Pullum, 1984; Pullum and Trodd, 1984).

Scleral lenses are rarely fitted nowadays. One of the problems is the scarcity of fitters and the long time they take to fit. It has been estimated that a chair time of 15 hours is necessary before a patient can wear these lenses. Corneal lenses are equally well accepted and it is probably true that the patients who do not accept a corneal lens will not accept a scleral lens.

Scleral lenses are indicated in variations of keratoconus pathology such as keratotorus and keratoglobus. They have also a place in the management of the secondary keratoconus which occurs in Terrien's dystrophy.

Corneal lenses

Corneal lenses are easy to fit in keratoconus. Different practitioners have their own methods, but little critical assessment has been made at follow up.

History of corneal lens fitting methods for keratoconus

Large alignment lens

Bier (1957) described an alignment method using what is now considered a large total diameter (10–10.5 mm) lens which had a relatively small back optic zone diameter (BOZD) of 5–6 mm. His object was to get an alignment fitting with as even a fluorescein pattern behind the lens as possible.

Such an alignment is only possible in relatively early keratoconus. Furthermore, as the back optic zone radius of the contact lens is reduced to achieve this alignment the plus power effect of this highly concave surface must be neutralized by a minus power on the front surface. Thus, typically, a lens of

BOZR 6.80 needs a power of −6.50
        6.20   −10.40
        5.60   −14.50
        5.0   −22.00

Figure 15.2 is a scale drawing which shows what happens when a −14.50 D lens is 10.0 mm in total diameter. The edge thickness is enormous, being more than twice that of a lens of 7.0 mm total diameter. This can, perhaps, be diminished by a wide back peripheral curve, a large edge lift and front peripheral reduction. Bier did not specify his edge lift.

Other methods were used for achieving an alignment lens. Salvatori personally described to the present author in 1963 a 'tailored fit'. This was a technique of starting with a steep lens and then adding peripheral back curves until the lens fitted the cornea. The problem here is that the lens has to be thick to start with in order to accommodate potentially added back peripheral curves.

Ruben (1966) described a technique of projecting a silhouette of the cornea, or a cast of it, and using this as a basis for determining central and peripheral curves.

Te = 5.5 mm at 10.0 mm TD

Te = 2.5 mm at 7.0 mm TD

C2 7.60/8.0/8.40/10.0
Power −14.50 D

Tc 0.05

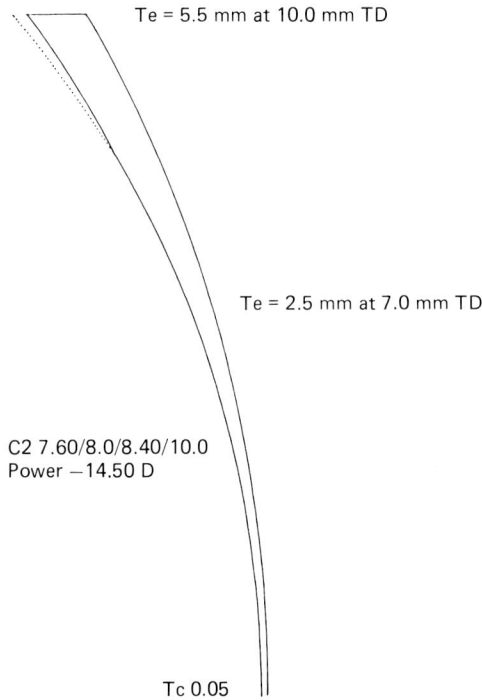

Figure 15.2 Scale drawing of a minus 14.50 D corneal lens at 10.00 mm overall diameter which shows the excessive edge thickness. It is more than twice the thickness of a 7.0 mm overall diameter lens

In a series of papers Chiquiar Arias (1963) described his techniques of topographical analysis using the fluorescein technique. Small lenses of 5 or 6 mm diameter, called Minicon lenses, were used to assess the fitting of the cone and he aimed at a three point touch, that is, a fluorescein pattern which demonstrated corneal touch in at least three areas (Figure 15.3a). The white areas represent corneal touch. A pressure rod was used on the lens as an elaboration of this test.

CA rings (that is, Chiquiar Arias rings) were used to assess the fitting at the periphery (Figure 15.3b). These rings were 2 mm wide. The central apertures varied from 4 to 7 mm in width and the outer diameters from 8 to 11 mm. The radii of curvature varied from 6.5 to 9.0 mm. The lids were kept apart while fitting these lenses, so no account was taken of the action of the lids.

Large flat lenses

Kemmetmuller (1962) described the technique of fitting a large flat fitting lens and this was again described by Clifford Hall (1963). They believed that they were forcing back the cone with a large flat lens. Clifford Hall used lenses of 9.5 to 11.5 mm in diameter. The back peripheral curve was 0.5 to 1 mm wide. He told the present author that he usually started with a lens of 8 mm back optic zone radius. He stated that the lens would occupy a 'north of the equator' position and that

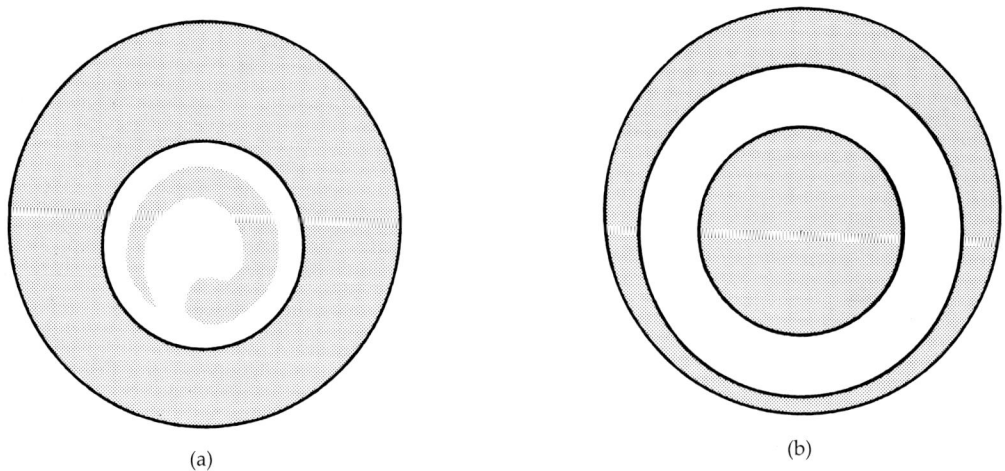

(a)   (b)

Figure 15.3 (a) Fitting of the Chiquiar Arias minilent with the three point touch. The white areas represent corneal touch and the shaded areas fluorescein pooling. (b) Chiquiar Arias ring

he depended on the upper lid to keep the lens in place. He described how the lower segment of the lens would stand away from the cornea. Large flat fitting corneal lenses did not have excessive edge thickness.

These large, flat lenses were fitted mostly in Austria (Kemmetmuller) and Scandinavia (Clifford Hall) and the author has not seen any patients wearing them. Keratoconus apices which are continually abraded by lenses which are too flat ultimately develop nebulae and this will be dealt with later.

Fitting the apex

Voss and Liberatore (1962) described a technique of fitting a small thin corneal lens of about 8 mm in total diameter – the Minilent. This lens was fitted about 0.25 mm flatter that the flattest radius of the cornea. They judged the flatness by seeing a central touch of about 4 to 5 mm in diameter on inspection after fluorescein instillation. The actual total diameters of the lenses ranged between 7.5 and 8.3 mm. This is the basis of the technique which is generally used today.

Contemporary corneal lens fitting methods

The small thin lens is usually chosen today, except where the cone is of the oval or sagging type which demands a larger lens with lens lid attachment. The lens is usually fitted flat, but this is probably undesirable. Zadnik and Mutti (1987),

using an automated visual acuity device while studying 10 eyes with keratoconus, fitted with rigid contact lenses of varying base curves and diameters, found that a small improvement in visual acuity was obtained with flat lenses equalling approximately one half line. Although this was statistically significant, they did not consider it clinically significant.

There is a useful recent review of contact lens fitting in keratoconus by Mannis and Zadnik (1989).

The small thin lens

This lens usually varies in total diameter from 6 to 8.5 mm. Appendix 15.I gives a set of such trial lenses as was manufactured by Global Contact Lenses, London. Smaller diameter lenses are used where the back optic zone is highly curved and the minus dioptric power to compensate for this is thus great.

Rosenthal (1973) pointed out that an occlusive fit with a bull's eye fluorescein pattern should not be adopted. He asserted that a ring of corneal touch beyond the apical touch (Figure 15.4a) led to stagnation of tears and corneal hypoxia. He wanted an opening in this peripheral ring of contact as an access route for tear exchange and stated that this could be achieved by progressive steepening of the back optic zone radius (BOZR), together with reduction of the lens total diameter (Figure 15.4b). He considered that the fluorescein pattern of the ideal lens–cornea relationship to be that as illustrated in Figure 15.4c with the area of contact between the lens and the cornea dis-

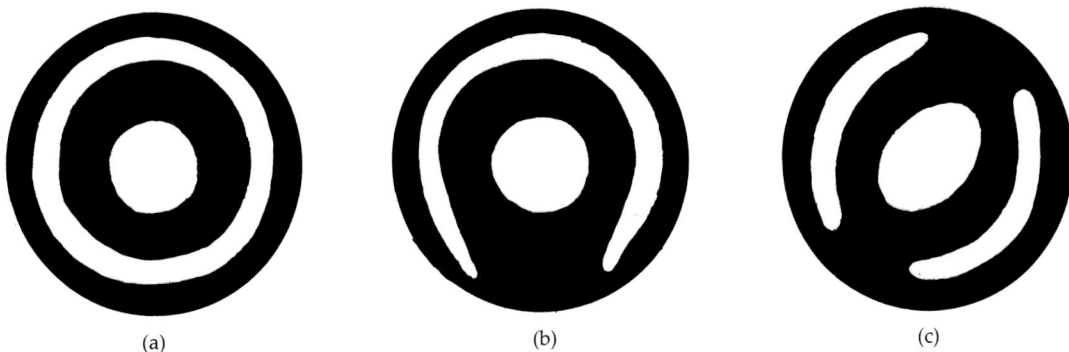

(a)   (b)   (c)

Figure 15.4 (a) Typical bull's eye fluorescein pattern (After Rosenthal). The white areas represent corneal touch and the shaded areas fluorescein pooling. (b) Opening in the peripheral ring of contact as an access route for tear exchange (After Rosenthal). (c) Fluorescein pattern of the ideal lens–corneal relationship (After Rosenthal)

tributed over much of the concave surface of the lens.

Keratoconus of the round or nipple type may be thought of as a condition in which the cornea has an exaggerated difference between the central radii and the peripheral radii. There are, thus, powerful centration forces associated with an 'overhang' meniscus below (Figure 15.5). Observation of the extent of this meniscus at the slit lamp is a means of assessing the 'flatness' of the lens and thus the pressure of the lens on the cone. If the lens is too tight then corneal epithelial problems associated with anoxia may develop and, furthermore, a steeper back central optic diameter dictates a thicker periphery in the lens since it will be more minus in power.

One of the problems associated with the fitting of keratoconus lenses is ejection when the patient blinks or moves his eye. Lens lid attachment methods may be employed to circumvent this, if the lens does not have enough bulk increase at its periphery for the upper lid to grasp. In most cases this is best achieved when using a lens of 8.6 mm total diameter.

Korb (1984) advocates that these small thin lenses should vault the apex of the cone (that is,

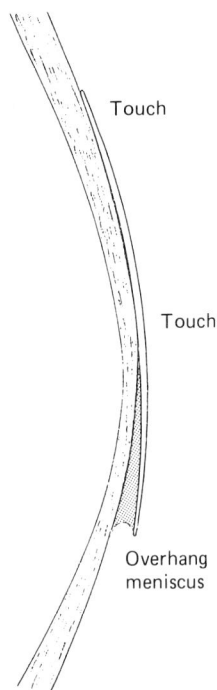

Figure 15.5 Overhang meniscus

have apical clearance) and since this method of fitting is associated with poor tear interchange, that these same lenses should be made of gas permeable material.

Korb, Finnimore and Herman (1982) studied patients with relatively symmetrical bilateral keratoconus. One eye was fitted with a large, flat-fitting, 9.4 mm total diameter design lens with an 8.0 mm back optic zone diameter and a back peripheral radius 1.5 mm flatter than the back optic zone radius (BOZR). The other eye was fitted with an apical clearance design of 8.0 mm diameter with a 5.8 mm optical zone and a secondary radius 2.5 mm flatter than the BOZR. These small lenses had an axial edge lift of approximately 0.28 mm. All lenses were of gas permeable material.

After four years, seven of the 11 eyes fitted by the flat technique developed superficial opacification. Two of these patients developed nodular scarring (proud nebulae, see below) over 1.0 mm in diameter which stained with fluorescein. There were no significant complications with the 8.0 mm diameter apical clearance design in the 11 eyes fitted.

Korb has since modified his fitting sets for keratoconus and these are given in Appendix 15.II. He believes that the steeper the keratoconus is the more the back peripheral radius needs to be flattened so that apex clearance can be maintained. As keratoconus becomes steeper the difference in radius between peripheral areas of cornea (paracentral areas) and the centre usually becomes larger.

Large thin lens

In oval or sagging cones a lens of 9.5 mm or even 10 mm total diameter has to be used. Such a lens may assume a low position (drop) on the cornea unless it has been constructed to have lens lid attachment or has sufficient bulk increase at its periphery to provide this.

The technique of lens lid attachment is discussed in Chapter 4 and the method of constructing these lenses is given.

Soper lens

In the Soper keratoconus diagnostic lens set of 10 lenses (Soper and Jarrett, 1972) (Appendix 15.III) the overall diameters vary from 7.5 mm to 9.5 mm so they are both small and large lenses. The lens has two curves on the back surface, the peripheral curve being a standard 45 dioptres (American nomenclature and equivalent to 7.50 mm radius of curvature) and the central curve varies from 48 dioptres to 60 dioptres (equivalent to 7.05 mm to 5.65 mm radius of curvature).

Gas permeable lenses

Gas permeable lenses have the disadvantage in keratoconus that they tend to warp to conform to the cone if they are too thin, and thus provide inferior vision to that provided by polymethylmethacrylate lenses. However, Korb (1984) considers that they are essential if the apex clearance method of fitting is used.

With regard to the gas permeable material to be used, the RXD material (Polymer Technology Ltd, Wilmington, Mass. 01887, USA), with its hardness (which rivals PMMA), its exceptional flexural resistance, thin design capability and Dk of 45, would seem to be the present ideal.

Toric soft lenses

These lenses may be of use in early keratoconus when the patient, whether due to atopic conjunctival disease or not, is intolerant of hard corneal lenses.

An inventory of toric lenses is desirable. Cylindrical powers are stocked in steps of 10° axis and the corresponding spherical powers in two dioptre steps so that the lens ordered will not be more than one dioptre spherical difference from the trial lens. Fitting by conventional methods is time consuming and unreliable.

Saturn lenses and SoftPerm lenses

Saturn lenses were distributed by Pilkington Barnes Hind in England. They consisted of a central portion of hard gas permeable material (pentasilcon P) 6.5 mm in diameter surrounded by a soft hydrophilic portion (hydroxyethylmethacrylate), so that the overall diameter was 13 mm.

They were useful in early keratoconus, especially where there was intolerance of hard corneal lenses and where there is atopic or other conjunctival disease.

No guidelines were given for their use in keratoconus where a reliable keratometry reading could not usually be obtained. Frequently many of the lenses in the trial set appeared to fit. High molecular weight fluorescein (Fluoresoft, 0.35% fluorexon in isotonic saline, Holles Laboratories Inc., Cohasset, Mass. 02025, USA) was useful in this respect. The author's method was to fit the flattest lens which centred and returned to the central position after slight movement caused by blinking or eye movements. The patient then wore the trial lens for eight hours and the corneal surface was examined with fluorescein and the slit lamp. The flattest lens which did not produce central corneal fluorescein staining after eight hours' wear was selected. Saturn lenses were upgraded to Saturn II lenses. Both these lenses have now been discontinued and SoftPerm lenses (see Figure 5.6) have taken their place. They are made and distributed by Sola/Barnes Hind, Sunnyvale, California, 94086, USA (a Pilkington Vision Care Company). These lenses are now available in the UK. The lenses are made from an innovative copolymer which results from polymerizing the rigid phase and the hydrophilic phase into one material. The water content of the hydrophilic skirt is 25%. The lens is made at a total diameter of 14.3 mm. The rigid centre zone is 8 mm and the optic zone is 7 mm in diameter. The available radii are 7.10 to 8.10 mm in 0.10 mm steps and powers of +6.0 D to − 13.0 D are available. Although Sola/Barnes Hind advise against its use in any eye disease that affects the cornea and conjunctiva, this lens can be of use in keratoconus.

Contact lenses after keratoconic epikeratoplasty

Lembach *et al*. (1989) have discussed the outcome of 33 epikeratoplasties performed on 31 contact lens intolerant, keratoconus patients. Thirty-two of these procedures were anatomically successful with clear lenticules and flattening of the postoperative keratometric measurements in all but one eye. Of the 32 eyes that were anatomically successful, 20 eyes in 19 patients were able to achieve satisfactory visual improvement requiring either no correction or spectacle lenses. Twelve eyes in 11 patients were successfully refitted with contact lenses for anisometropic refractive errors

(11 eyes) and residual irregular astigmatism (one eye). They recommend epikeratoplasty for contact lens intolerant keratoconus patients who can obtain at least 20/40 (6/12) visual acuity with a contact lens and have minimal or absent apical scarring.

Trial contact lenses were used for the refitting of the contact lenses. In 11 cases there were gas permeable lenses. The method of fitting was not discussed, but an illustrated fluorescein pattern, in their paper, of one of the contact lenses fitted shows a central pool of fluorescein (apex clear) and a lens centring over the epikeratoplasty lenticule. In one case a soft contact lens was used.

Specific corneal problems in keratoconus

Corneal vascularization

This is seldom seen with hard corneal lenses, but is frequently encountered with scleral lenses. It may be of the all-over pattern or related to a static bubble such as is seen in wearers for cosmetic reasons.

Corneal epithelial erosions

Corneal lens patients should routinely be examined at follow up for evidence of central corneal erosions as demonstrated by fluorescein staining. A small degree of this may have to be accepted, but if more than this it will ultimately lead to

corneal opacification with stromal involvement. A so-called 'hurricane' or 'vortex' keratopathy is evidence of too much apical pressure (Figure 15.6), but there is no doubt in the mind of the author that some keratoconic corneas are more prone to this complication than others.

Corneal lenses should always be inspected for deposit on their under-surface. This deposit produces corneal erosions and is common in lenses of keratoconus patients and in gas permeable lenses.

Corneal nebulae

Reticular nebulae

These nebulae (Figure 15.7) are characterized by reticular scarring in the stroma and occurring at the apices of cones are found in the absence of contact lenses and are a feature of the disease.

Diffuse nebulae

These nebulae (Figure 15.8) can occur with repeated trauma to the corneal epithelium and are in the superficial area of the stroma. They may be seen in patients who have never worn corneal contact lenses. They are asymptomatic and seldom add to the visual disability.

Proud nebulae

These nebulae (sometimes called nodules) are a characteristic feature of long-term corneal lens wear in keratoconus (Figure 15.9). They stain with fluorescein. They are proud of the cornea at

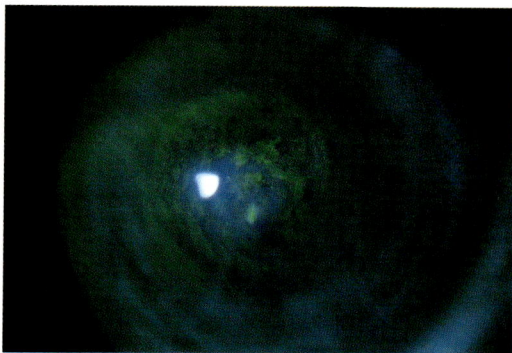

Figure 15.6 'Hurricane' or 'vortex' keratopathy

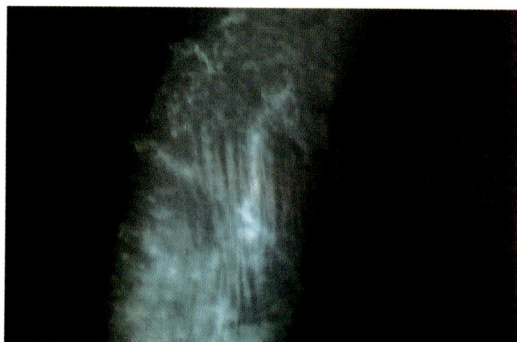

Figure 15.7 Reticular nebula. This occurs at the apex of keratoconus in the absence of corneal contact lens wear

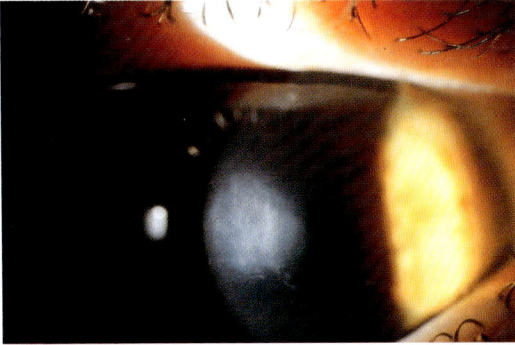

Figure 15.8 Diffuse nebula. This can occur with repeated trauma to the corneal epithelium with contact lens wear, but is also seen when contact lenses are not worn

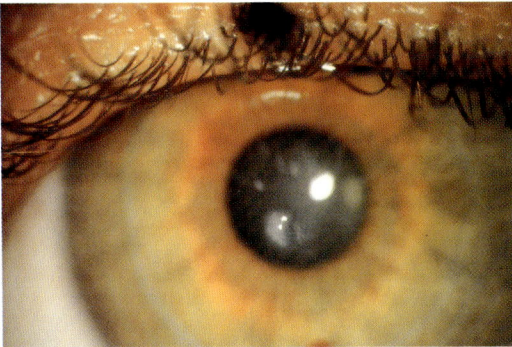

Figure 15.9 Proud nebula (corneal nodule). This is a characteristic feature of long-term corneal lens wear. It is seen at 7 o'clock within the pupil

its apex and it has been shown that over them the normal corneal epithelial microvilli are replaced by microplicae (Dilly and Mackie, unpublished). They usually appear quite suddenly and result in a marked loss of corneal lens tolerance. They may flatten after a number of months of discontinuance of corneal lens wear.

Proud nebulae are often an indication for corneal grafting. Moodaley *et al.* (1991) have described a simple technique of superficial keratectomy to remove proud nebulae. The author has found that the resulting defect healed quickly under a therapeutic hydrogel lens. Six cases were described. All patients were able to resume contact lens wear within one month of the procedure.

References

BELIN, M.W., FOWLER, W.C. and CHAMBERS, W.A. (1988) Evaluation of recent trends in the surgical and non-surgical correction of keratoconus. *Ophthalmology*, **95**, 3, 335–339

BIER, N. (1957) *Contact Lens Routine and Practice*. Butterworths, London, pp. 189–190

BUXTON, J.N. (1973) Keratoconus. In *Symposium on Contact Lenses. Transactions of the New Orleans Academy of Ophthalmology* (Dabezies, O., ed). C.V. Mosby, St Louis, pp 88–100

CHIQUIAR ARIAS, V. (1963) *Optician*. **146**, 474–451, 447–478, 501–505, 527–530, 553–559

CLIFFORD HALL, K.G. (1963) A comprehensive study of keratoconus. *British Journal of Physiological Optics*, **20**, 215–256

CROSS, A.J. (1949) Contact lenses: an analysis of the results of use. *British Journal of Ophthalmology*, **33**, 421–425

DAVIES, P.D., LOBASCHER, D., MENON, J.A., RAHI, A.H.S. and RUBEN, M. (1976) Immunological studies in keratoconus. *Transactions of the Ophthalmological Society of the UK*, **9**, 173–178

FLEISCHER (1906) Über Keratoconus und eigenartige Pigmentbildung in der Kornea. *Munchener Medizinische Wochenschrift*, **53**, 625

FOWLER, W.C., BELIN, M.W. and CHAMBERS, W.A. (1988) Contact lenses in the visual correction of keratoconus. *CLAO Journal* **14**, 4, 203–206

HARRISON, R.J., KLOUDA, P.T., EASTY, D.L., MANKU, M. and STEWART J.C.C.M. (1989) Association between keratoconus and atopy. *British Journal of Ophthalmology*, **73**, 816–822

KEMMETMULLER, H. (1962) Corneal lenses and keratoconus. *Contacto*, **6**, 7, 188–193

KORB, D.R. (1984) Recent developments in fitting contact lenses for keratoconus. *Journal of the American Optometric Association*, **55**, 172–175

KORB, D.R., FINNIMORE, V.M. and HERMAN, J.P. (1982) Apical changes and scarring in keratoconus as related to contact lens fitting techniques. *Journal of the American Optometric Association*, **53**, 3, 199–205

KORB, D.R., GREINER, J.V., FINNEMORE, V.M. and ALLAN-SMITH, M.R. (1983) Treatment of contact lenses with papain. Increase in wearing time in keratoconic patients with papillary conjunctivitis. *Archives of Ophthalmology*, **101**, 1, 48–50

LEMBACH, R.G., LASS, J.H., STOCKER, E.G. and KEATES, R.H. (1989) The use of contact lenses after keratoconic epikeratoplasty. *Archives of Ophthalmology*, **107**, 364–368

MAGUIRE, L.J. and BOURNE, W.M,. (1989) Corneal topography of early keratoconus. *American Journal of Ophthalmology*, **108**, 107–112

MANNIS, M.J. and ZADNIK, K. (1986) Contact lens fitting in keratoconus. *CLAO Journal*, **15**, 4, 282–289

MOODALEY, L., BUCKLEY, R.J., WOODWARD, E.G. and RUBEN, M. (1991) Surgery to improve contact lens wear in keratoconus. *CLAO Journal*, **17**, 2, 129–131

PULLUM, K.W. (1984) Development of slotted scleral lenses. *Journal of the British Contact Lens Association*, **7**, 92–95

PULLUM, K.W. and TRODD, T.C. (1984) Development of slotted scleral lenses. *Journal of the British Contact Lens Association*, **7**, 28–38

RAHI, A.H.S., DAVIES, P.D., RUBEN, M., LOBASCHER, D. and MENON, J.A. (1977) Keratoconus and co-existing atopic disease. *British Journal of Ophthalmology*, **61**, 761–764

ROSENTHAL, P. (1973) Use of corneal contact lenses in the management of keratoconus. In *Symposium on Contact Lenses. Transactions of New Orleans Academy of Ophthalmology* (Dabezies, O., ed). C.V. Mosby, St Louis, pp. 101–108

RUBEN, M. (1966) Unpublished paper read at a meeting of the Medical Contact Lens Association

SMIDDY, W.E., HAMBURG, T.R., KRACHER, G.P. and STARK, W.J. (1988) Keratoconus. Contact lens or keratoplasty? *Ophthalmology*, **95**, 4, 487–492

SOPER, J.W. and JARRETT, A. (1972) Results of a systematic approach to fitting keratoconus. *Contact Lens Medical Bulletin*, **5**, 50–59

VOGT, A. (1919) Reflexlinien durch Faltung spiegelnder Grenzflachen im Bereiche von Cornea, Linsenkapsel und Netzhaut. *Von Graefe's Archive for Clinical and Experimental Ophthalmology*, **99**, 296–338

VOSS E.H. and LIBERATORE, J.C. (1962) Fitting the apex of keratoconus. *Contacto*, **6**, 7, 212–214

ZADNIK, K. and MUTTI, D.O. (1987) Contact lens fitting relation and visual acuity in keratoconus. *American Journal of Optometry and Physiological Optics*, **64**, 9, 698–702.

Appendix 15.I

Fitting set for keratoconus as manufactured by Global Contact Lenses, London, at various diameters. The axial edge lift varies from 0.43 mm at 5.0 mm back optic zone radius to 0.10 mm at 7.0 mm back optic zone radius.

	Power	Tc
C3 5.00/5.00/6.25/6.00/8.00/7.50	−6.00	0.10
5.25/5.50/6.25/6.50/7.75/7.50	−7.00	0.10
5.50/6.00/6.50/7.00/8.00/8.00	−8.00	0.10
5.75/6.00/6.75/7.00/8.00/8.00	−9.00	0.10
6.00/6.00/7.00/7.00/8.10/8.00	−9.00	0.10
6.20/6.00/7.00/7.00/8.00/8.00	−10.00	0.10
6.20/6.50/6.90/7.50/7.60/8.50	−10.00	0.10
6.40/6.00/7.00/7.25/7.60/8.50	−11.00	0.10
6.40/6.50/6.90/7.75/7.40/9.00	−12.00	0.10
6.60/6.50/7.10/7.75/7.60/9.00	−14.00	0.10
6.80/6.50/7.20/7.75/7.60/9.00	−15.00	0.10
7.00/6.55/7.40/7.75/7.80/9.00	−17.00	0.10

Appendix 15.II

Korb design lenses in Polycon II at 8.2 mm total diameter with first back peripheral radius 2.2 to 2.5 mm flatter than the BOZR. The axial edge lift varies from 0.52 mm at 5.20 mm back optic zone radius to 0.20 mm at 7.0 mm back optic zone radius.

	Power	Tc
C4 5.20/6.20/7.70/7.40/10.00/7.80/11.00/8.20	−16.0	0.11
5.40/ /7.90/	−15.0	0.11
5.60/ /8.10/	−14.0	0.11
5.80/ /8.30/	−13.0	0.11
6.00/ /8.50/	−12.0	0.11
6.20/ /8.40/	−11.0	0.10
6.40/ /8.60/	−10.0	0.10
6.60/ /8.80/	−9.0	0.10
6.80/ /9.00/	−8.0	0.10
7.00/ /9.20/	−7.0	0.11

Korb design lenses in Polycon II at 8.2 mm total diameter with first back peripheral radius 1.7 mm flatter than the BOZR. The axial edge lift varies from 0.48 mm at 5.20 mm back optic zone radius to 0.19 mm at 7.00 mm back optic zone radius.

	Power	Tc
C4 5.20/6.20/6.90/7.40/10.00/7.80/11.00/8.20	−15.0	0.10
5.40/ /7.10/	−14.0	0.10
5.60/ /7.30/	−13.0	0.10
5.80/ /7.50/	−12.0	0.10
6.00/ /7.70/	−11.0	0.10
6.20/ /7.90/	−10.0	0.10
6.40/ /8.10/	−9.0	0.10
6.60/ /8.30/	−8.0	0.10
6.80/ /8.50/	−7.0	0.10
7.00/ /8.70/	−6.0	0.11

All lenses are blended to 6.0 mm BOZD with a radius 1.0 mm flatter than the BOZR.

The second BPR is applied first. The third BPR is applied last.

Korb design lenses in Polycon II at 7.6 mm total diameter with first back radius 2.4 mm to 2.6 mm flatter than the BOZR. The axial edge lift varies from 0.48 mm at 5.0 mm back optic zone radius to 0.18 mm at 7.0 mm back optic zone radius.

	Power	Tc
C4 5.00/5.60/7.60/6.80/10.00/7.20/11.00/7.60	−17.0	0.13
5.20/ /7.80/	−16.0	0.13
5.40/ /8.00/	−15.0	0.13
5.60/ /8.20/	−14.0	0.13
5.80/ /8.40/	−13.0	0.13
6.00/ /8.40/	−12.0	0.13
6.20/ /8.60/	−11.0	0.13
6.40/ /8.80/	−10.0	0.13
6.60/ /9.00/	−9.0	0.13
6.80/ /9.20/	−8.0	0.13
7.00/ /9.40/	−7.0	0.13

All lenses are blended to 5.40 mm BOZD with the radius 1.0 mm flatter than the BOZR.

The second BPR is applied first. The third BPR is applied last.

NB For these powers and back central optic radii no lenticular construction is required. If the power of the lens at the given base curve is increased in minus, then a thin edge lenticular construction will be required. These diagnostic lenses will provide an edge thickness of approximately 0.08 mm.

Appendix 15.III

Soper keratoconus diagnostic lens set

Sagittal depth (mm)	CPC (D)	Power (D)	Diameter (mm)	Thickness (mm)	CPC diameter (mm)
0.68	48/45	−4.50	7.50	0.10	6.00
0.73	52/45	−8.50	7.50	0.10	6.00
0.80	56/45	−12.50	7.50	0.10	6.00
0.87	60/45	−16.50	7.50	0.10	6.00
1.00	52/45	−8.50	8.50	0.10	7.00
1.12	56/45	−12.50	8.50	0.10	7.00
1.22	60/45	−16.50	8.50	0.10	7.00
1.37	52/45	−8.50	9.50	0.10	8.00
1.52	56/45	−12.50	9.50	0.10	8.00
1.67	60/45	−16.50	9.50	0.10	8.00

This table is given in its American nomenclature where CPC is the central posterior curve (in this case two curves) and where the concave radius of the lens is expressed in dioptral values. The Bausch and Lomb keratometer reads both corneal radius and contact lens radius in dioptral values. A conversion dial for the measurement of contact lenses is obtainable from Bausch and Lomb, UK Ltd, Crawley, West Sussex, RH10 2GB, England.

In British nomenclature the Soper keratoconus diagnostic set can be expressed as follows:

		Power	Tc
C2	7.05/6.0/7.55/7.50	−4.50	0.10
	6.50/6.00/7.55/7.50	−8.50	0.10
	6.05/6.00/7.55/7.50	−12.50	0.10
	5.65/6.00/7.55/7.50	−16.50	0.10
	6.50/6.00/7.55/7.50	−8.50	0.10
	6.05/6.00/7.55/7.50	−12.50	0.10
	5.65/6.00/7.55/7.50	−16.50	0.10
	6.50/6.00/7.55/7.50	−8.50	0.10
	6.05/6.00/7.55/7.50	−12.50	0.10
	5.65/6.00/7.55/7.50	−16.50	0.10

16

Corneal grafts and other surgical procedures

Corneal grafts

Corneal grafts often present problems to the contact lens fitter. The highly satisfactory grafts, that is the ones in which the acuity is good unaided, or easily improved by a simple spectacle refraction, are seldom referred for contact lenses unless the other eye has to wear a contact lens.

The problems are usually grafted eyes with high ametropia or high astigmatism or such distortion that spectacles cannot be used. The donor cornea may be steep or flat (Figure 16.1). The author has seen induced ametropia to the extent of −15 dioptres in the case of steep grafts and +15 in the case of (phakic) flat grafts.

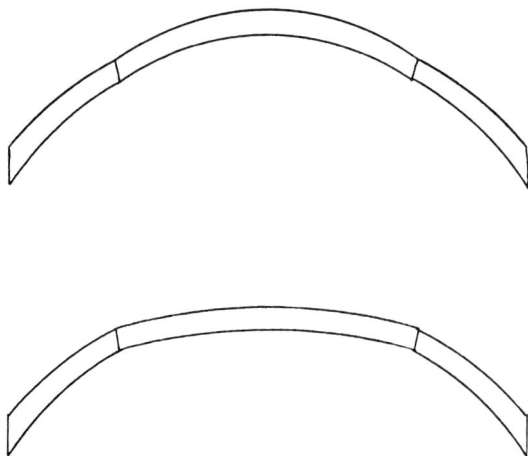

Figure 16.1 Drawings of steep and flat corneal grafts. The steep graft is more curved and the flat graft is less curved relative to the recipient cornea

Hard corneal lenses

There is no agreement as to when patients should first be fitted with corneal lenses after keratoplasty, but an intact corneal epithelium is necessary and this may be delayed postoperatively. The presence of vascularization outside the graft is unimportant. Continuous corneal sutures present no problem for fitting and prolonged tolerance of corneal contact lenses. However, a careful watch should be kept for neovascularization in the region of the sutures, which is often a trigger for a rejection episode.

Steep grafts

A steep donor cornea (see Figure 16.1) acts as a 'corneal cap' (see Chapter 4) in which case there is usually no problem with stability and centration of the corneal lens, unless the graft is eccentric. Eccentricity of the graft is a major problem in fitting. An air bubble may be seen between the lens and cornea, above the apex of the donor cornea. Progressive flatting of the back central optic radius (BCOR) of the lens will often get rid of this. Such an air bubble is usually mobile and often intermittent and therefore does not give the problems of corneal drying seen with static bubbles in the case of scleral lenses (see Chapter 11). Furthermore, since it is not in the visual axis it does not give problems with visual acuity.

A hard corneal lens, fitting very flat, seldom gives rise to a vortex keratopathy as it can do in the case of keratoconus (see Chapter 15). Gross astigmatism does not usually give problems in fitting provided the graft is small (6–7.5 mm).

The graft–host junction is usually raised after keratoplasty and fitting flat on a donor cornea, which is acting as a 'corneal cap', avoids damage to this area. Such flat lenses are usually mobile on blinking and, if they are not, the lens lid attachment technique can be used to encourage this (Chapter 4). It is important that the lens moves with blinking for if it does not tears will stagnate and the epithelium of the graft will become hypoxic with resultant oedema.

Larger convex corneal grafts (8.00 mm or more) may give rise to corneal lens instability and lack of centration because there is no 'corneal cap'. In this case a lens lid attachment technique may be successfully used. This often demands a larger corneal lens which is kept mobile by lid action.

As has already been stated, the graft–host junction is usually slightly raised and there may be problems with the corneal lens eroding suture sites and giving rise to vascularization. A corneal lens smaller than the donor cornea should be avoided as it will constantly strike the prominent graft–host junction and give rise to erosion and vascularization.

Erosion at the graft–host junction is often a prelude to an episode of rejection.

Fitting is often a trial and error procedure. Think, at first, in terms of two diameters of corneal lens, 8.6 mm and 9.5 mm, as advocated in Chapter 4.

The use of gas permeable material is advantageous, but a lot may be lost in terms of corneal lens flexure and resultant poor visual acuity. Gas permeable lenses need to be thicker to maintain their shape.

Flat grafts

Flat grafts (see Figure 16.1) produce great problems. The hard corneal lens settles over them so that an air bubble is trapped underneath. This air bubble is over the graft and thus in the visual axis. It may be possible to fit a soft contact lens in such cases and perhaps a toric soft contact lens will be needed, but often a bubble remains under the centre of the soft lens. A scleral lens gives the same problem. Happily, most of these grafts, in the fullness of time, become more convex, but fitting may have to be delayed for one or two years.

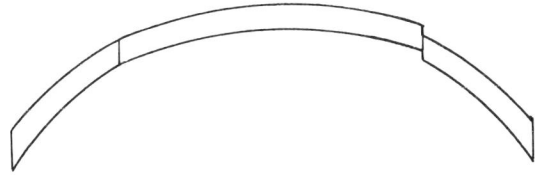

Figure 16.2 Drawing of a tilted corneal graft. There is a prominent portion of the donor cornea at its edge

Tilted grafts

A tilted graft (Figure 16.2) creates problems in hard corneal lens fitting. First, the hard lens will often position itself so that the apex is over the prominent portion of the edge of the graft. If it is fitting flat on this portion it will cause erosion of the graft with vascularization. This may well trigger off an episode of rejection. If an attempt is made to fit the lens clear of the prominent portion, an air bubble will often be introduced adjacent to the prominence.

The use of rigid contact lenses after keratoplasty is further discussed by Mannis, Zadnik and Deutch (1986) and Beekhuis *et al*. (1991).

Soft contact lenses and SoftPerm lenses

Soft lenses, or toric soft lenses, may be the preferred mode of contact lens correction after keratoplasty if they can produce a satisfactory visual outcome. Often their use is mandatory, even if the visual acuity obtained is somewhat less than that which would be obtained with a hard corneal lens.

Not infrequently a corneal graft has been performed in a patient with keratoconus, because of intolerance of a hard corneal lens. This intolerance is often related to coexisting conjunctival disease. Atopic conjunctivitis is a major problem in the case of some keratoconus patients. In this case, a soft lens, or a toric soft lens, may be tolerated. If a satisfactory standard of vision cannot be obtained with these lenses, a SoftPerm lens which has a hard gas permeable centre and a soft hydrophilic periphery (see Chapter 15) may be accepted.

If a grafted eye is aphakic, and thus requires a very thick soft lens, this lens may, in wear, gradually push back the prominent portion of a tilted graft, or a markedly steep graft. The use of a firm soft lens material such as Sauflex 55 will, at a central thickness of some 0.45 mm, eliminate some corneal astigmatism and tend to regularize what astigmatism remains. A spectacle overcorrection can be used.

Mannis and Zadnik (1988) described the use of hydrophilic contact lenses for wound stabilization in keratoplasty. They reported the use of these lenses in five cases of penetrating keratoplasty complicated by a partial wound dehiscence and anterior slippage of the donor tissue. Rather than resuturing, a soft contact lens was used as a corneal stent to realign the graft–host interface. No serious complications were encountered and all wounds were adequately reapposed.

Scleral contact lenses

Where a hard corneal lens cannot be fitted because of the topography of the cornea, or because of current problems with lid function, a scleral lens, flush, fenestrated or slotted, can be fitted (see Chapter 3). It may be used where the graft is tilted in an attempt to correct the tilt over a period of time.

Corneal lacerations

Contact lenses are useful for the visual rehabilitation of some patients after corneal laceration repair where there is often an irregular corneal surface and/or induced irregular astigmatism. Spectacles are of little use in such cases. Furthermore, aphakia is often present as a result of the accident and it gives rise to gross anisometropia if spectacles are used.

Hard corneal lenses

Hard corneal lenses can be fitted using the fluorescein pattern (see Chapter 4) as an indicator of a satisfactory back optic zone to corneal curvature relationship. A convenient start can be made by inserting a lens in which the back optic zone radius (BOZR) is that of the average keratometry found in the patient's other (good) eye. Adjustments can be made to the back optic zone radius of the lens so that there is no excessive pooling or bubble formation under it, or excessively hard touch on any prominence on the cor-

neal surface. It is a matter of trial and error. If the lens assumes a low immobile position on the cornea, the lens lid attachment technique can be used (see Chapter 4).

In aphakia the hard corneal lens, which is thick and heavy, should have a front optic reduction to facilitate lens lid attachment.

The use of gas permeable lenses will tend to prevent hypoxia in these corneas with consequent vascularization. Vascularization often occurs in suture lines and corneal nebulae would appear to attract vessels from the limbus.

Soft contact lenses

Soft contact lenses are easier to fit and are more comfortable to wear after corneal laceration. They do, however, have the tendency to induce vascularization, especially if the lacerations are near to the periphery. With central lacerations this tendency is slight.

Thin soft contact lenses will drape themselves on the corneal surface and will tend to eliminate surface irregularities there, allowing only the remaining astigmatism to manifest itself. If this is slight, the use of a non-spherical front surface lens (the SV38 Nissel lens discussed in Chapter 7) may be all that is required. This lens has the advantage of being thin overall and highly gas transmissible. Failing this, a toric soft contact lens will be required.

Lacerated eyes are often aphakic and the thickness of a soft lens for an aphakic eye is often such as to eliminate quite a measure of astigmatism.

Boghani, Cohen and Jones-Marioneaux (1991) found that contact lenses were successful in the majority of patients referred after corneal lacerations. They fitted 30 eyes of 28 patients – 13 eyes with rigid gas permeable lenses and 17 eyes with daily wear soft lenses. None of their five eyes with large peripheral lacerations could be successfully fitted with contact lenses. Now that the law in Great Britain makes seat belt wearing obligatory, corneal lacerations are much less frequently seen.

Radial keratotomy

This is a procedure in which deep, but non-penetrating radial incisions are made in the cornea, avoiding the central zone. It leads to flattening of the central zone of the cornea and, thus, decreases its refractive power. After the operation there is a marked hypermetropic shift of about 5–7 D. Over the following six to 12 months there is a return towards the original corneal shape and power as the incisions heal and the corneal rigidity increases. On settling, the average myopia reduction has been found to be 3.5 D. After the operation of radial keratotomy the corneal rigidity is decreased and the intraocular forces act on the cornea causing the mid-peripheral regions to bulge forwards.

Once the cornea has settled after the surgery there may be residual visual impairment due to diurnal variation of vision, increased sperical aberration, increased sensitivity to glare, contrast sensitivity reduction, together with ametropia. The results of radial keratotomy, then, sometimes fail to satisfy the patient. The patient may be able to get about without having to wear glasses but still has difficulty in avoiding their use. Avoiding their use is the usual *raison d'être* for the operation. On occasion there is gross undercorrection

or even overcorrection, leading to a hypermetropic shift.

Such a dissatisfied patient may present for contact lens fitting. Corneal surgery seems, in some subtle way, to increase the acceptance of contact lenses. It is not entirely a matter of sensation and may be, in part, metabolic.

Hard corneal lenses

Rigid gas permeable lenses are the preferred type for fitting after radial keratotomy. The problem is that the radial keratotomy flattens an area in the central cornea (Figure 16.3). This creates, in effect, two apices in the contour of any one plane. A small lens may centre over a superior apex and give a very high riding fit or centre over an inferior apex and give a very low riding fit. These fits often result in inadequate pupil coverage by the contact lens. Larger lenses, up to 10 or 11 mm in diameter, are often necessary.

It is probably best to start with a lens whose back optic zone radius is that of the flattest pre-

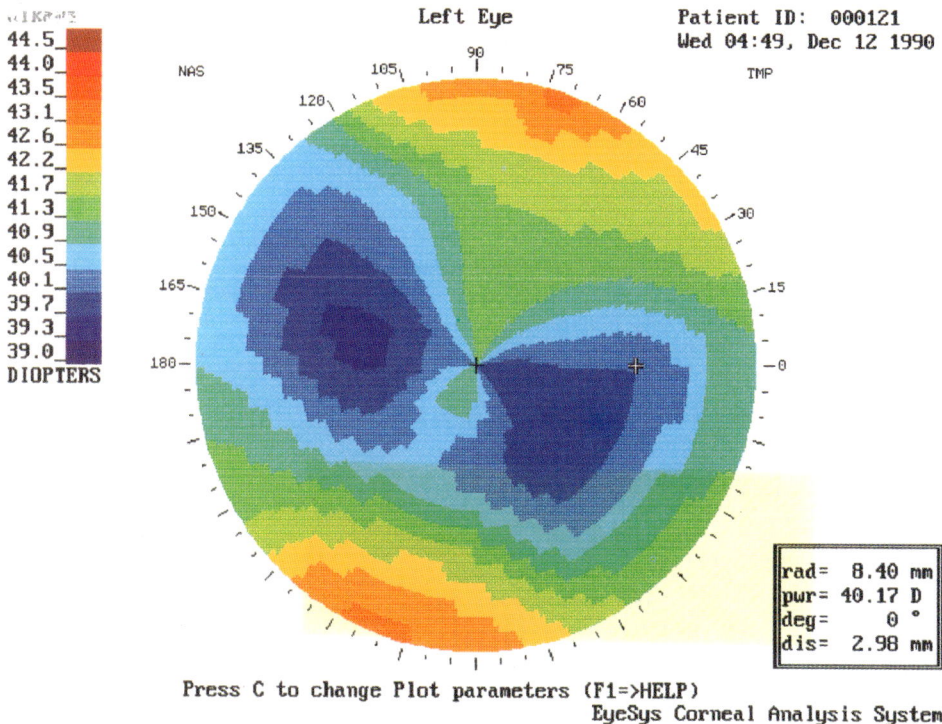

Figure 16.3 Computerized corneal imaging in a patient after radial keratotomy. The visual acuity was 6/9 uncorrected. The bowtie pattern of the astigmatism is seen in normal corneas, but the central flattening is not normal. (Courtesy of Professor Colin Kirkness)

radial keratotomy reading. Fitting flatter gives fluorescein pooling and perhaps air bubbles under the peripheral and intermediate zones of the lens. Fitting tighter will mean fluorescein pooling and perhaps air bubbles over the central flattened (and optical) zone of the cornea. The best fit is that which gives minimal pooling in the centre and this is achieved by trial and error. A small axial edge lift (see Chapter 4) helps to minimize fluorescein pooling and bubble formation at the periphery of the lens.

Rowsey and Rubin (1988) have reported problems with epithelial erosions at the junction of the central flattened and peripheral areas of corneas.

Astin (1991) discusses corneal and refractive changes that are revealed even when correctly fitting hard contact lenses are worn one to five years postoperatively. These changes indicate that lens wear may influence corneal topography and refraction, even several years after radial keratotomy.

Special methods of fitting are given by El Hage and Baker (1986), Goldberg, cited by Greco (1986), Janes and Reichle (1986), Shivitz *et al.* (1986) and Vickery (1986).

Soft lenses

Soft hydrophilic lenses are much easier to fit. They drape themselves over the cornea and give better centration and comfort. The pliability means that air bubbles are much less likely to accumulate over the central flattened zone of the cornea. However, in as much as six weeks of wear they can give rise to the ingrowth of vessels from the limbus into the radial incisions (Bores, Myers and Cowden, 1981). This is a most undesirable complication.

Shivitz, Arrowsmith and Russell (1987) found that superficial vascularization developed within the radial incisions in 33% of the eyes they fitted with daily wear soft contact lenses over a period of five months to four years. They found that the neovascularization regressed with discontinuation of the lenses. The reason for fitting these lenses was overcorrection by the radial keratotomy, resulting in a shift to hypermetropia.

Hybrid lenses (SoftPerm, Pilkington Barnes Hind) would also seem to be contraindicated since they have relatively poor oxygen transmissibility and can be seen to promote vascularization in some normal corneas.

Epikeratoplasty

Epikeratoplasty has been found equal to graft surgery in keratoconus in producing eyes with a contact lens corrected acuity of 20/40, or better, provided there was no previous central corneal scarring present (Goosey *et al.*, 1991). Both procedures increase the acceptability of contact lenses. The usual cause for these surgical procedures is intolerance of contact lenses. However, Goosey *et al.* (1991) noted that a higher percentage of eyes in their keratoplasty group had visual acuities of 20/20 than in the epikeratoplasty group, but 31% of eyes in the keratoplasty group had graft reactions whereas there were no serious complications in the epikeratoplasty group.

Lembach *et al.* (1989) found that the majority of keratoconic epikeratoplasties achieved a satisfactory visual result, either unaided or with spectacles. They performed 33 epikeratoplasties on 31 keratoconic contact lens intolerant patients. Twelve eyes in 11 of these patients were successfully refitted with contact lenses for anisometropic refractive errors (11 eyes) and residual astigmatism (one eye). All their contact lens patients were fitted using a trial lens method. The contact lenses were fitted flatter than the average keratometry reading preoperatively and steeper than the average keratometry reading postoperatively. Lembach *et al.* used commercially available gas permeable materials in 11 of the 12 fits. Only one patient required a hydrogel lens and that patient had only hypermetropic postoperative correction. Their fluorescein pattern figure for hard lenses shows a central pool of fluorescein.

Hard corneal lenses

Provided that the curvature of the lenticule is not excessive it should act as a convenient 'corneal cap' and give ideal conditions for centration, so that a hard contact lens can be fitted much in the way that one is fitted for keratoconus. It does not appear that a flat fitting technique results in a vortex keratopathy as it does in keratoconus.

Soft contact lenses

Soft contact lenses can be fitted to correct spherical ametropia and toric soft contact lenses can be used to correct astigmatism. Corneal vascularization does not appear to be a problem with these lenses.

References

ASTIN, C.L.K. (1991) Keratoreformation by contact lenses after radial keratotomy. *Ophthalmology and Physiological Optics*, **11**, 156–162

BEEKHUIS, W.H., VAN RIJ, G., EGGINK, F.A.G.J., VREUGDENHIL, W. and SCHOEVAART, C.E. (1991) Contact lenses following keratoplasty. *CLAO Journal*, **17**, 1, 27–29

BOGHANI, S., COHEN, E.J. and JONES-MARIONEAUX, S. (1991) Contact lenses after corneal lacerations. *CLAO Journal*, **17**, 3, 155–158

BORES, L.D., MYERS, W. and COWDEN, J. (1981) Radial keratotomy – an analysis of the American experience. *Annals of Ophthalmology*, **13**, 941–948

EL HAGE, S. and BAKER, R.N. (1986) Controlled keratoreformation for postoperative radial keratotomy patients. *International Eye Care*, **2**, 49–53

GOOSEY, J.D., PRAGER, T.C., GOOSEY, C.B., BIRD, E.F. and SANDERSON, J.C. (1991) *American Journal of Ophthalmology*, **111**, 145–151

GRECO, A. (1986) Fitting the postoperative keratotomy patient. *International Eye Care*, **2**, 188–190

JANES, J.A. and REICHLE, R.N. (1986) Refractive surgery and contact lenses. *Contact Lens Forum*, Oct., **11**, 10, 28–32

LEMBACH, R.G., LASS, J.H., STOCKER, E.G. and KEATES, R.H. (1989) The use of keratoconic lenses after epikeratoplasty. *Archives of Opthalmology*, **107**, 364–368

MANNIS, M.J. and ZADNIK, K. (1988) Hydrophilic lenses for wound stabilization in keratoplasty. *CLAO Journal*, **14**, 4, 199–202

MANNIS, M.J., ZADNIK, K. and DEUTCH, D. (1986) Rigid contact lens wear in the corneal transplant patient. *CLAO Journal*, **12**, 1, 39–42

ROWSEY, J.J. and RUBIN, M.L. (1987) Refraction problems after refractive surgery. *Survey of Ophthalmology*, **94**, 120–124

SHIVITZ, I.A., RUSSELL, B.M., ARROWSMITH, P.N. and MARKS, R.G. (1986) Optical correction of postoperative radial keratotomy with contact lenses. *CLAO Journal*, **12**, 59–62

SHIVITZ, I.A., ARROWSMITH, P.N. and RUSSELL, B.M. (1987) Contact lenses in the treatment of patients with overcorrected radial keratotomy. *Ophthalmology*, **94**, 8, 899–903

VICKERY, J.A. (1986) Post-RK and the soft lens. *Contact Lens Forum*, Oct., **11**, 10, 34–35

17

Aphakia

In hospital contact lens practice aphakia was by far the major indication for fitting contact lenses. The number of patients increased steadily until the late 1970s. The increase was due to the introduction of chymotrypsin which greatly facilitated the extraction of immature cataracts, together with the ready availability of contact lenses and contact lens fitters. More uniocular cataracts were thus operated upon. Prior to the emergence of these factors, there was no point in performing the operation in unilateral cataract as spectacle correction was impracticable due the anisometropia. Nowadays lens extraction with intraocular implantation is the preferred method of managing cataract.

There are still a number of patients who do not have an intraocular lens implanted. This may be due to unfamiliarity with the technique on the part of the ophthalmic surgeon, complications at the time of operation or complications experienced when the other eye was previously implanted. The age of the patient is sometimes another reason. Some surgeons are reluctant to implant young and middle-aged adults because of the fear of complications some 20 or more years afterwards.

Few would disagree that an extracapsular extraction and a daily wear contact lens is the safest procedure and one in which a visual acuity of 6/6 can more reliably be obtained. This is not to say that it is a preferable procedure to intraocular lens implantation which is cost effective and very much more convenient to the majority of patients. This was the opinion of Bernth-Petersen and Srensen (1983).

When a contact lens has to be fitted there is always the question of what type to fit. To most patients this means the choice between a hard corneal lens or a soft lens. In a survey by Astin (1984) of aphakic contact lens fitting at Moorfields Eye Hospital the lens of first choice was a rigid gas permeable lens of CAB material.

Graham et al. (1988) studied the success rate and complications for wear in 366 aphakic patients of the Contact Lens Department at Moorfields Eye Hospital, who were evaluated retrospectively over a period of 36 months. They found that 86% of unilateral aphakic patients under 70 years of age could handle a daily wear contact lens, compared with only 27% over 70 years of age. Extended wear soft lenses were fitted to patients unable to use daily wear lenses, but only 50% were successful.

They found no difference in the incidence of complications between daily wear soft and daily wear hard contact lenses or between young, middle-aged and elderly patients who wore either type of daily wear contact lens.

However, the risk of serious complications was six times greater for patients using extended wear soft contact lenses (55%) compared with those using hard or soft daily wear lenses (8.8%). They found that daily wear contact lenses of hard or soft type are a safe and successful method of aphakic correction for patients under 70 years of age and that once the ability to handle a daily wear contact lens had been learned, success was maintained when the second eye was fitted.

In private practice things may be different. The private patient tends to be more demanding, more aware of what is happening to his friends and colleagues and may return, many months after being fitted with a hard lens, asking why he was not fitted with a more comfortable soft lens.

The author's practice is to fit a soft contact lens initially in all aphakic patients except those who are near emmetropic or emmetropic in the other eye. Patients who do not wear spectacles for distance do not usually want to start doing so if it can be avoided and, after cataract extraction, a soft contact lens often needs a spectacle over-correction for astigmatism. If the other eye is not emmetropic spectacles will have to be worn for distance in any case.

If the other eye has a large degree of ametropia the soft lens power is adjusted to balance the spectacle refraction in the two eyes. In this case, when the other eye is operated upon, a soft contact lens can be fitted for maximum distance acuity to both eyes.

The author reserves extended wear soft contact lenses for those aphakes who cannot handle contact lenses and who have no help in this direction from relatives or friends in the home. Extended wear soft lenses in the aphake are associated with a considerable danger of suppurative keratopathy.

Scleral lenses

Prior to the 1950s scleral lenses were used exclusively. They are seldom used today because there are now very few practitioners who can fit them, and the fitting is very time consuming. A large number of people cannot tolerate scleral lenses. Nevertheless, a patient who has been fitted with scleral lenses in the past and has been able to tolerate them will not easily take to alternative contact lenses. Scleral lenses are easier for the aphake to see, to find if lost and to insert without a mirror. The need for an elaborate disinfection routine is avoided. They also give a constant standard of vision without the added need for spectacles.

The fitting is done in the conventional way either by the use of preformed scleral lenses, which are then adjusted for fit and power, or by moulding methods. Slight corneal apical clearance and a good limbal clearance (see Figure 3.12) is desirable. A moderate-sized air bubble which ro-

tates as the eye performs its versions and an even scleral fit are the objectives.

Hard corneal lenses

There are two ways of fitting hard corneal lenses in the aphake.

Small centring lenses

The first method is by using a small corneal lens of, say, 8.00 mm diameter designed to centre on the cornea. Because it is designed to centre, the lens does not have a reduced optic construction. That is, it does not have a front peripheral optic curve. If this were present the lens would tend to attach itself to the upper lid and thus decentre. Decentration of such a small lens would probable adversely affect its visual performance.

The mean of the two keratometric readings taken at right angles to each other is used as a starting point for the choice of back optic zone radius (BOZR) of the lens. The object is an alignment fitting (see Chapter 4). It is important to realize that this lens will centre, or not centre, according to the topography of the cornea and no amount of decreasing its back optic zone radius ('steepening') will induce it to centre. Alteration of diameter may have some effect. Decentration, which usually means a lens which drops to the lower part of the cornea, dictates abandonment of this method of fitting.

Lenses for this purpose can be constructed as follows:

C2 BOZR	/	BOZD	/	BPR	/	TD
As chosen		7.00 mm		0.8 mm flatter than BOZR		8.0 mm

Light blend on transition
BVP   as calculated from the trial lens
Tc   as in Appendix 17.I   Te 0.10

A suitable trial set for this type of lens would run in 0.05 mm steps of back optic zone radius from 7.20 mm to 8.40 mm in back vertex powers of +8.00 D, +12.00 D, +16.00 D and +20.00 D.

For reasons already stated in Chapter 4, the

author does not think that this method of fitting should be adopted unless there are special reasons for its use such as the avoidance of a filtering bleb or a cystic wound in the superior limbus above.

Larger lens lid attachment lenses

These lenses are designed to attach themselves to the upper lid. Sometimes this does not happen and the lens centres on the cornea. This may be acceptable.

The lens lid attachment is achieved by introducing a front optic reduction and a front peripheral curve which is parallel to the back peripheral curve or curves. The usual overall size is 9.50 mm and the usual front optic diameter is 7.50 mm. The reduced optic zone diameter permits a decrease in the minimum centre thickness of the lens and, thus, its weight.

Large edge lifts are not desirable in aphakic lenses as they tend to make the lenses unstable, easily ejected or displaced under the lids or into the regions of the canthi. In the absence of any indication, such as a lens which drops to the lower part of the cornea, they should be avoided.

Lenses for this purpose can be constructed in bicurve form with axial edge lifts varying from 0.11 mm for BOZR 7.20 mm to 0.07 mm for BOZR 8.20 mm as follows:

C2 BOZR / BOZD / BPR / TD
As chosen 7.50 mm 0.8 mm flatter 9.50 mm
                    than BOZR

Light blend on transition
BVP   as calculated from the trial lens
Tc   as in Appendix 17.I   Te 0.10
FOZD   7.50
FPR.   So that the peripheral optic is plano.

Suitable trial lenses would run in 0.05 mm steps of back optic zone radius from 7.20 mm to 8.40 mm and in powers +8.00 D, +12.00 D, +16.00 D and +20.00 D. It may be necessary, for example when the corneas are large or there is lateral displacement of the lens ('temporal ride'), to fit a larger diameter lens. In this case, the back optic zone diameter and the total diameter of the lens should be increased to an equal amount. Compensation should be made in the back optic

zone radius for the tighter fit produced by the increase in diameters:

e.g.   C2 7.80/8.00/8.60/10.00

The front optic zone diameter in this case would also be increased to 9.00 mm and the total diameter to 11.0 mm.

Such lens lid attachment lenses may be designed in tricurve form with larger axial edge lifts. These are useful in small eyes with narrow palpebral apertures where there will not be problems of ejection and where the lens may cause limbal staining when it comes in contact with the sclera below or above.

Such lenses may be constructed with a small BOZD or a large BOZD and back profiles for such lenses are given in Appendix 4.II.

Problems with hard corneal lenses in aphakia

1   Ejection

The lens for the aphakic eye is a thick lens and is more than usually subject to ejection due to lid action. This tendency can be avoided by making the lens:

(a) Somewhat 'steeper' in fitting, that is up to 0.15 mm steeper than the average keratometric reading.
(b) With a small edge lift.
(c) With thin edges, that is edge thicknesses of 0.08 mm or 0.10 mm.

2   Displacement

In some aphakic patients the hard lens may disappear into the upper fornix at times after a blink. Only the marginal band of the upper lid is in close contact with the globe and it can act as a very efficient sling in some patients. This is a distressing phenomenon as the patient immediately loses vision and has great difficulty in retrieving the lens.

The measures which can be taken for displacement are frequently ineffective. It may be useful to increase the weight of the lens. This is done by increasing its centre thickness, say from 0.40 mm to 0.60 mm. Centre thickness is the most important parameter governing lens mass.

3 Temporal ride

In some patients the lens moves to a temporal position on the cornea. The decentration may be so marked that the edge of the lens, or the edge of the front optic zone, is over the pupillary aperture (see Figure 4.15d). This is caused by the toricity of the cornea against the rule (the minus cylinder at or about 90°) and the bulk of the lens. Reading (1984) observed that against the rule astigmatism predominates after cataract surgery.

Attempts may be made to correct the decentration by making the back optic zone of the lens toric, but this is seldom successful. More usually the situation is accepted and the lens is made larger in diameter so that its edge, or the edge of the front optic zone, does not encroach on the pupil.

4 Endophthalmitis

This can occur when there are wound complications resulting in filtering blebs and it also occurs from time to time with soft lenses. Bellows and McCulley (1981) reported four cases occurring two weeks to 30 months after being fitted with corneal contact lenses. Three patients were wearing hard contact lenses and one wore a soft lens. Significant blepharoconjunctivitis was present and treated in two patients. All patients had bleb infection and hypopyon. Despite aggressive medical therapy, two eyes required enucleation, while two eyes survived with good vision. Bellows and McCulley recommend that eyes that have unplanned filtering blebs following cataract surgery should not have a contact lens inserted until the blebs have been closed.

Now that intraocular lens insertion is almost universally performed, contact lens fitters will tend to deal more and more with eyes in which there have been operative difficulties and often these have filtering blebs. The fitter should beware, since only a thin film of bulbar conjunctiva separates the inside of the eye from the outside.

Soft contact lenses

Soft contact lenses are fitted in the conventional way, as described in Chapter 6. Stock lenses from large manufacturers may be used. It is almost always the case that these lenses have a front optic reduced to 8.00 mm in diameter. In the experience of the author it is seldom necessary to have anything larger than a 7.00 mm front optic reduction which allows a lesser central thickness. Custom made lenses can be ordered from small laboratories with the front optic so reduced and at an overall size of 13.50 mm. The author's preference here for daily wear is for a material of 55% water content (Sauflex 55) or 61% water content (Duragel). Lenses of these materials are available from A.S. Optics, Cheam, Surrey.

Appendix 17.II gives the minimal central thicknesses of such lenses, together with the central thicknesses of lenses of 75% water content for extended wear.

The author's preference for adult extended wear is a moulded stock 78% water content lens (Incanto) distributed in England by G. Nissel and Co. Ltd, Hemel Hempstead, Herts.

Problems with soft contact lenses in aphakia

1 Ejection

This is seldom seen with the soft contact lens and if it does occur it demands a tighter fitting lens and, failing that, a lens made of a more rigid material, such as Sauflex 55.

2 Displacement

Displacement of a soft lens so that it is not sitting centrally on the cornea demands a tighter fit.

Displacement upwards into the superior fornix can be a troublesome feature with extended wear soft lenses which are usually very soft and floppy, having a high water content. In this case the only remedy is to fit the lens tighter, but this may not be effective and the fitting may have to be abandoned. In the case of a daily wear lens it should be remade in more rigid material, such as Sauflex 55.

3 Visual

Where the corneal astigmatism is high it may not be possible to fit a soft contact lens which, with a cylindrical spectacle overcorrection, achieves the same level of acuity as is obtained in spectacles alone. Aphakic spectacles, of course, give a larger image size which may benefit the patient by as much as one line on the Snellen chart compared with contact lenses, but apart from this, there is the bending, and perhaps deformation, of the soft lens as it conforms to the shape of the eye. This appears to reduce the potential visual acuity further so that a spectacle overcorrection for the astigmatism does not result in maximum acuity. This effect can be minimized by using a more rigid material such as Sauflex 55.

4   Endophthalmitis

This is dealt with above, under Problems with hard corneal lenses in aphakia.

Paediatric aphakia

Cataract in infancy is relatively rare. The major paediatric referral centre in London reported that 250 children had been fitted with contact lenses between 1976 and 1982; 105 of these were bilateral infantile aphakic patients (Taylor, 1982).

Aphakia in young children poses many problems as far as contact lenses are concerned. These contact lenses are almost always soft. There is the problem of acceptance of the contact lens by the child. Initial fitting may be very difficult to manage and the usual resort is to swaddle the child in a blanket and get both parents to hold the legs and arms while the lens is inserted. Once the soft lens is in the eye, the child does not usually object and many will allow inspection of the eye and the contact lens. It is only in this way that the fitting can be evaluated. It is useless to fit under a general anaesthetic as the lids are lax and there is little reflex tearing and therefore the fitting cannot be judged.

There may be difficulty in the objective refraction with a soft contact lens and for this a general anaesthetic is frequently required, especially in young children. Before this anaesthetic is administered it is important to ascertain that there is a sufficient gap in the capsule for retinoscopy to be performed with any degree of accuracy.

Contact lenses used for aphakia in infants usually have to be steeper in back optic zone radius than those for adults. This is because keratometric readings are steeper at birth (Asbell *et al.*, 1990). Ehlers *et al.* (1976) concluded from their investigations that corneal curvature reaches the adult range at about three years of age. The contact lenses also have to have much increased power. Powers in excess of plus 30 D are not uncommon. The reason for this is obscure. It may be that there is a different balance between the refractive powers of the crystalline lens and the cornea in the infant eye, or there may be a forward placement of the crystalline lens in the eye. It will be recalled that shallowing of the anterior chamber in adults induces myopia.

There is a further factor which adds to the power of the contact lens. The infant's world is that of near objects at a small arm's length. Consequently, allowance has to be made for this and plus 2.50 D is usually added to the predicted distance power of the contact lens. All this dictates that the lens for an infant usually has to be specially manufactured.

The aim should be to fit a daily wear soft contact lens which the parents can handle. The author's preference is to use Sauflex 55% material which is very strong, easy to handle and has a certain rigidity which overcomes the tendency to displacement. The standard total diameter used is 13.50 mm and the front optic zone is reduced to 6.00 mm in order to allow a decrease in the central thickness (see Appendix 17.III). Small infants are adept at rubbing their eyes to displace contact lenses.

It is not always possible to fit daily wear soft contact lenses. Parents with congenital cataracts and poor vision tend to produce children with congenital cataracts. Furthermore, people with blunted sight tend to marry people with blunted sight. Those parents find great difficulty in managing daily wear in a child.

Failure of the parents to cope means that extended wear soft contact lenses have to be fitted. The author's preference is to use Optima 75 material. This is available from A.S. Optics, Cheam, Surrey. It lathes well, is robust and has sufficient oxygen permeability. The standard total diameter is 13.50 mm and the front optic zone is reduced to 6.00 mm in order to minimize the central thickness (see Appendix 17.III).

Extended wear soft lenses, in infants and children, are associated with blinding corneal complications. Taylor (1982) reported five eyes of 43 patients to have residual visual defects after acute episodes of infection. The time scale is not mentioned.

In the infant, the fitting of contact lenses must

proceed with speed after the surgery to avoid the establishment of amyblyopia. Amblyopia has been reported to be the major cause of poor visual results from congenital cataract surgery (Hiles and Wallar, 1977). Visual results can be improved by prompt and vigorous optical treatment. Gelbart *et al.* (1982) reported visual acuities of 6/18, or better, in 29 eyes of 24 infants who underwent surgery for bilateral congenital cataracts. Thirteen eyes had visual acuities of 6/60 or worse. The best results occurred in patients who underwent surgery before they were eight weeks old. Only one patient of the seven operated on after the age of eight weeks achieved a visual acuity of better than 6/60. These favourable visual outcomes were the result of early surgery, short intervals between operations on fellow eyes (48 hours or less), total bilateral occlusion between operations, careful postoperative monitoring with retinoscopy and visual-evoked potentials and early correction of aphakia.

In unilateral cataract the outcome has always been thought to be much worse, but Beller *et al.* (1981) have reported obtaining 6/9 vision or better in the aphakic eye of five out of eight neonates and 6/24 vision or better in the remaining three aphakic eyes.

Cheng *et al.* (1991) have reported on the visual results after surgery for monocular congenital cataract. They found that the cases with good visual results were exclusively those whose visual rehabilitation had been achieved by 17 weeks of age.

Amblyopia can be established during the delay from surgery to contact lens fitting. The fact that the contact lens has often to be specially made compounds the difficulty. Contact lens preparation should be made before the surgery is done.

References

ASBELL, P.A., CHIANG, B., SOMERS, M.E. and MORGAN, K.S. (1990) Keratometry in children. *CLAO Journal*, **16**, 2, 99–102

ASTIN, C. (1984) Aphakic contact lens fitting in a hospital department. *Journal of the British Contact Lens Association*, **7**, 3, 164–168

BELLER, R., HOYT, C.S., MARG, E. and ODOM, J.V. (1981) Good visual function after neonatal surgery for congenital monocular cataracts. *American Journal of Ophthalmology*, **91**, 5, 559–565

BELLOWS, A.R. and MCCULLEY, J.P. (1981) Endophthalmitis in aphakic patients with unplanned filtering blebs wearing contact lenses. *Ophthalmology*, **88**, 8, 839–843

BERNTH-PETERSEN, P. and SRENSEN, T. (1983) Intraocular lenses versus extended wear contact lenses in aphakic rehabilitation. A controlled clinical study. *Acta Ophthalmologica (Copenhagen)*, **61**, 3, 382–391

CHENG, K.P., HILES, D.A., BIGLAN, A.W. and PETTAPIECE, M.C. (1991) Visual results after early surgical treatment of unilateral congenital cataracts. *Ophthalmology*, **98**, 903–910

EHLERS, N., SORENSEN, T., BRAMSEN, T. *et al.* (1976) Central corneal thickness in newborns and children. *Acta Ophthalmologica*, **54**, 285–290

GELBART, S.S., HOYT, C.S., JASTREBSKI, G. and MARG, E. (1982) Long term visual results in bilateral congenital cataracts. *American Journal of Ophthalmology*, **93**, 615–621

GRAHAM, C.M., DART, J.K.G., WILSON-HOLT, N.W. and BUCKLEY, R.J. (1988) Prospects for contact lens wear in aphakia. *Eye*, **2**, 48–55

HILES, D.A. and WALLAR, P.H. (1977) Visual results following infantile cataract surgery. In *Infantile Cataract Surgery* (Hiles, D.A., ed.). Little Brown & Co., Boston, **17**, 4, 265–282

READING, V.M. (1984) Astigmatism following cataract surgery. *British Journal of Ophthalmology*, **68**, 97–104

TAYLOR, D.S.I. (1982) Risks and difficulties of the treatment of aphakia in infancy. *Transactions of the Ophthalmological Society of the UK*, **102**, 403–406

Appendix 17.I

Minimal centre thickness of hard corneal lenses in millimetres. If there is a reduced front optic construction the *front optic zone diameter should be used as a guide* to centre thickness in this table, rather than the overall size.

Diameter (mm)

Power (D)	6.50	7.00	7.50	8.00	8.50	9.00	9.50
+20.00	0.40	0.45	0.51	0.58	0.65	0.72	0.84
+19.00	0.38	0.43	0.50	0.56	0.63	0.70	0.81
+18.00	0.37	0.42	0.48	0.54	0.60	0.68	0.78
+17.00	0.36	0.41	0.46	0.52	0.58	0.65	0.75
+16.00	0.35	0.40	0.45	0.50	0.56	0.63	0.72
+15.00	0.34	0.38	0.43	0.48	0.53	0.60	0.68
+14.00	0.32	0.36	0.41	0.46	0.51	0.57	0.64
+13.00	0.31	0.35	0.39	0.44	0.49	0.55	0.61
+12.00	0.30	0.34	0.38	0.42	0.47	0.52	0.58
+11.00	0.28	0.32	0.36	0.40	0.44	0.49	0.55
+10.00	0.27	0.31	0.35	0.38	0.42	0.47	0.52
+9.00	0.26	0.29	0.33	0.36	0.39	0.44	0.49
+8.00	0.25	0.28	0.31	0.34	0.37	0.41	0.46

Appendix 17.II

Central thicknesses of 55% water content lenses with a radius and diameter expansion factor of 1.31, wet refractive index 1.1415 and dry refractive index 1.513 and with *front optic zone diameter of 7.00 mm*, total diameter 13.50 mm, edge thickness 0.18 mm and transition thickness 1.18 mm.

Power (D)	Tc (wet state) (mm)
+8.00	0.32
+10.00	0.36
+12.00	0.39
+14.00	0.43
+16.00	0.46
+18.00	0.49

Central thickness of 61% water content lenses with a radius and diameter expansion factor of 1.385, wet refractive index 1.403 and dry refractive index 1.516 and with *front optic zone diameter of 7.0 mm*, total diameter 14.0 mm, edge thickness 0.18 mm and transition thickness 0.18.

Power (D)	Tc (wet state) (mm)
+8.00	0.33
+10.00	0.36
+12.00	0.40
+14.00	0.43
+16.00	0.47
+18.00	0.50

Note: A.S. Optics incorporate an axial edge lift in their standard 61% material lenses. This axial edge lift is 0.11 mm and the diameter of the back peripheral curve is 1.5 mm in a lens of overall diameter 14.0 mm. This edge lift dictates extra central thickness.

Central thickness of 75% water content lenses with a radius and diameter expansion factor of 1.620, wet refractive index 1.381 and dry refractive index 1.527 and with *front optic zone diameter of 7.00 mm*, total diameter 13.50 mm, edge thickness 0.23 mm and transition thickness 0.18.

Power (D)	Tc (wet state) (mm)
+8.00	0.39
+10.00	0.42
+12.00	0.46
+14.00	0.50
+16.00	0.54
+18.00	0.58

Note: Increased water content demands greater edge thickness.

Appendix 17.III

Soft contact lenses for paediatric aphakia

Daily wear

Central thicknesses of 55% water content lenses (Sauflex 55) with a radius and diameter expansion factor of 1.31, wet refractive index 1.1415 and dry refractive index 1.513, and with *front optic zone diameter of 6.00 mm*, total diameter 13.50 mm, edge thickness 0.18 mm and transition thickness 0.18 mm.

Power (D)	Tc (wet state) (mm)
+22.00	0.45
+24.00	0.48
+26.00	0.50
+28.00	0.53
+30.00	0.55
+32.00	0.58

Note: Steeper lenses (that is, smaller BOZRs) are often required in infants so that radii of 8.10 mm, 7.80 mm and 7.50 mm are common.

Extended wear

Central thicknesses of 75% water content lenses (Optima 75) with a radius and diameter expansion factor of 1.60, wet refractive index 1.381 and dry refractive index 1.525 and with *front optic zone diameter of 6.00 mm*, total diameter 13.50 mm, edge thickness 0.23 mm and transition thickness 0.23 mm.

Power (D)	Tc (wet state) (mm)
+22.00	0.53
+24.00	0.56
+26.00	0.59
+28.00	0.62
+30.00	0.64
+32.00	0.67

Note: Steeper lenses (that is, smaller BOZRs) are often required in infants so that radii of 8.10 mm, 7.80 mm and 7.50 mm are common.

18

Presbyopia

Presbyopia in the contact lens wearer is most easily dealt with by prescribing a pair of glasses to wear over the contact lenses. These are often half glasses which are conveniently small to carry and allow the wearer clear distance vision when looking over their top. These may not be cosmetically acceptable to some wearers and an alternative may be a pair of full frame progressive spectacles. In soft contact lens wearers this has the benefit that small amounts of astigmatism, not corrected by the contact lenses, can be incorporated in the distance (and reading) portion. Such lenses are often acceptable cosmetically because they have small power and look like sun glasses. They can be made photochromatic so that they indeed become sunglasses in the sun. However, a number of people do not want, or cannot wear glasses of any type, for reading. These may be inappropriate with certain items of dress, for example, a crown.

Patients may have cosmetic or other valid reasons for not wishing to wear reading glasses. They may be allergic to the plastic of spectacle frames. They may have a poor nose structure or have had a rhinoplasty which often makes spectacle wearing difficult. They may even have no pinnae as a congenital defect. In these cases reading must be done with contact lenses while allowing clear distance vision. There are two options – monovision with contact lenses and bi-focal contact lenses.

Monovision

The technique here is to plus up the contact lens in the non-dominant eye. There are various ways of assessing the dominant eye. One of the easiest is to get the patient to form a circle with the forefinger and thumb of their dominant hand (Figure 18.1). The patient should be corrected for distance, conveniently with contact lenses. Before they raise this hand in front of their eyes, explain that you want them to look at the top letter on the Snellen chart through the circle. When they do so, they will invariably choose the dominant eye

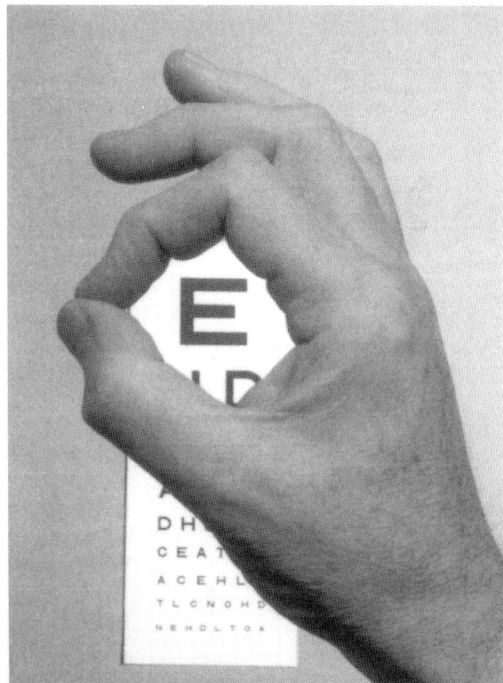

Figure 18.1 Assessment of the dominant eye. The patient looks through a circle formed by the forefinger and thumb

215

to look through the circle. Occluding one eye will establish which eye has been chosen. Dominant eyes are usually eyes with the better acuity, the lesser astigmatism and the lesser hypermetropia. Patients will often know which is their dominant eye.

High success rates have been quoted for monovision – Bayshore (1977) 85% and Scarborough and Lopanik (1976) 90%. In a study designed to compare success rates with three presbyopic contact lens systems, Back, Holden and Hine (1989) fitted 200 presbyopes with monovision, a pair of concentric centre-near bifocal lenses, or a combination of centre-near/centre-distance concentric lenses. Overall 112 subjects wore at least one system for a three-month period. Monovision was the most successful system (67% success); disrupted stereopsis was not a significant reason for failure of this system. The lower success rates with the two concentric bifocal systems (centre-near 42%, centre-near/centre-distance 37%) could be attributed to the greater visual compromise required with these lenses. Concentric bifocal systems are dealt with later on in this chapter.

Patients may have to persevere with monovision in the first few weeks, but minimal effects on spatial perception occur after adaptation. Criticism of this system has been directed at the effects of monocular blurring on binocular function. As a result, a number of studies have been undertaken comparing the stereoacuity and subjective balance responses. Bayshore (1977) commented on the ghosting of the out of focus image which is greater with higher additions. Scarborough and Lopanik (1976) found no instances where binocularity was affected after lens removal as a result of monovision.

There is an interesting study by Beddow, Martin and Pheiffer (1966). These authors showed no change in the ability of patients to walk a balance rail with monovision correction, and a greater loss of stereopsis with spectacles, than with contact lenses inducing similar amounts of anisometropia.

McGill and Erickson (1988) evaluated near point stereopsis on the Titmus stereotest for 10 presbyopic patients. Testing was done under five conditions: monovision and binocular correction with each of four marketed simultaneous bifocal contact lenses. (Simultaneous bifocal contact lenses are those in which the reading and distance portions are in front of the pupil at the same time.)

Simultaneous vision bifocals tested produced at least as much reduction in stereopsis as monovision, compared to baseline spectacle correction. Repeat testing of bifocal stereopsis with best near overrefraction suggested that a substantial portion of stereo reduction could be attributed to insufficient effective near additions with the bifocal contact lenses.

The author has physicians, surgeons, secretaries, bank officials and such who use this method of correction all their waking hours for their work and leisure with perfect ease. Often it is appropriate to supply a distance contact lens for the non-dominant eye, for occasional use for long distance driving, night driving and theatre.

Monvision is the simplest way of correcting presbyopia in a contact lens wearer and it is also the most reliable. The pupil size does not influence either the distance or near vision and near vision is possible in any direction of gaze. The ocular focusing disparity can be tolerated and even welcomed by the majority of people.

Bifocal contact lenses

When monovision is not acceptable bifocal contact lenses may have to be fitted and these may be hard or soft.

Rigid bifocal contact lenses

Rigid concentric bifocal lens

In this bifocal lens the distance correction is in the centre of the contact lens. The power of the lens for distance can be worked on the front optic zone surface, or the back optic zone surface, or a combination of the two (Figure 18.2). More commonly it is worked on the back surface only. When the addition is on the back surface allowance must be made, in calculating the appropriate curve, for the fact that it will be a tear and not an air interface and that there will be a neutralizing effect from the tears. What is required is a curve that provides approximately three times the power (when measured in air) which has to be added for near vision.

It is usually only practicable to fit this sort of lens in a hypermetropic patient where the thickness at the centre of the lens exceeds that of the periphery. Such a plus lens will usually drop (see

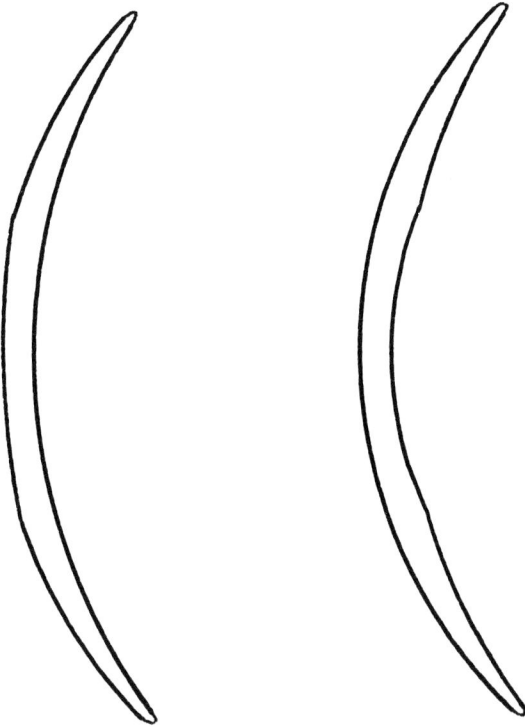

Figure 18.2 Diagrams of two hard concentric bifocal contact lenses. The central distance portion is worked on the front or the back surface of the lens or on both surfaces. Commonly the back surface only is used

Chapter 4) if it does not have a front optic reduction and this is an important fact to remember, since the distance portion of the lens will need to be over the pupil to get satisfactory vision.

The lens should be fitted from a standard single vision trial set. An idea of the size of distance portion which has to be used can be obtained by using a waterproof ink fibre pen to make an opaque circle of known diameter in the middle of the lens. Three-quarters of the pupil should be covered by the distance portion of the lens at any given time. Alternatively, a start can be made with a distance central portion of 3.5 mm and if that does not give satisfactory vision, this can be increased to 4.0 mm or even 4.5 mm. It is a matter of trial and error to get the proportions right for distance and near. It is usually enough to tell the laboratory the power required for the distance and the addition (in air) required for near, and they will do the calculations. These calculations are discussed by Stone and Francis (1980).

Rigid segment bifocal contact lenses

This type of bifocal lens is often used when the patient is myopic. A portion of plastic of higher refractive index is fused to the lens. An example is the Selecon bifocal lens (Ciba) (Figure 18.3).

This lens has a fused inset crescentic portion of higher refractive index material which is fluorescent for easy identification in fitting. It incorporates a prism ballast and the lens is truncated below. Thus, it has the possibility of being a dropping lens with all the disadvantages of such lenses (see Chapter 4). This is all the more true if the lens is a plus lens. If there is excessive vertical movement the lens will fail to provide satisfactory vision.

The lens is fitted using a Selecon prismatic lens without the bifocal segment (Figure 18.4). A tolerance test is performed with these single vision lenses over two to four weeks. These lenses have an engraved measuring line and this line should cover up to one-third of the pupil under normal room illumination.

Rigid aspheric hard bifocal contact lenses

Bifocal lenses can be made with an aspheric back surface, which has graduated steps of increasing power from the centre to the edge, and a spherical front surface. There is no segment and

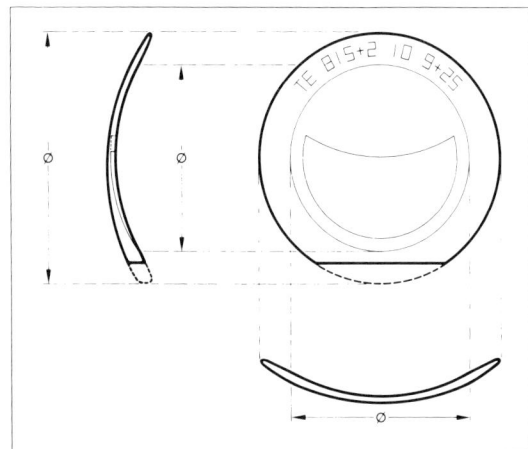

Figure 18.3 Diagram of the Selecon hard bifocal lens. The fused inset crescentic portion is of higher refractive index material and is fluorescent for easy identification in fitting. A prism ballast is incorporated and the lens is truncated below

Description:

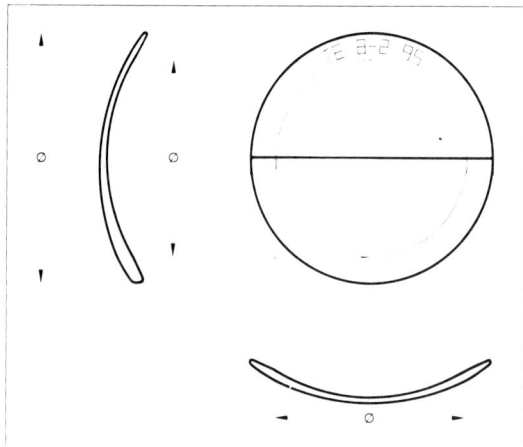

Figure 18.4 Diagram of the prismatic lens without bifocal segment used for fitting the Selecon bifocal lens

no prism. In fitting, the lenses must centre well with little movement.

Rigid diffractive bifocal contact lenses

An example of such a lens is the Diffrax bifocal contact lens (Figure 18.5) (Pilkington). It is made of Polycon II gas permeable material. It has a total diameter of 9.5 mm in various back optic zone radii. It is available in refractive powers ranging from −10.0 D to +8.0 D and near additions from +1.0 D to +3.0 D in 0.50 D steps.

Diffraction is the breaking up of light into bands. A diffractive area 5.0 mm in diameter is incorporated, centrally, on the back surface of the

lens at the time of generation. If the lens is held up to the light a series of rings can be seen in the central area. Cut in half, this area would be seen, on microscopy, to have a series of wedge-shaped formations 0.002 mm in depth on the posterior surface. These wedge shapes would be seen to lie on their sides with the sharp ends pointing to the centre of the lens. The light energy is concentrated into two focal lengths (Figure 18.6).

These lenses are designed to be fitted apex clear (that is 0.10 mm steeper than the flattest keratometer reading). If the lens is fitted flat so that the diffractive area makes contact with the cornea then the near addition function of the lens ceases to be effective.

The patient may initially report the presence of shadows or ghosting on reading, or a false stereopsis in which print appears to stand out from the page. Flare may be experienced when driving at night.

Soft bifocal contact lenses

Soft concentric bifocal contact lenses

An example of such a lens is the Weicon 38E bisoft (Ciba) (Figure 18.7). This lens is made of 38% water content hydroxyethyl methacrylate. It is obtainable in two overall diameters, 13.0 mm and 13.8 mm, with central distance zones varying from 3.2 mm to 3.8 mm. Fitting is carried out with trial lenses with clearly visible distance portion centration rings. The assessment is done under normal lighting conditions. The lens should move between 0.05 mm and 1.5 mm with a blink. The aim is to fit a lens so that three-quarters or more of the pupil area is covered by the centration ring. The refraction is done with a single vision lens.

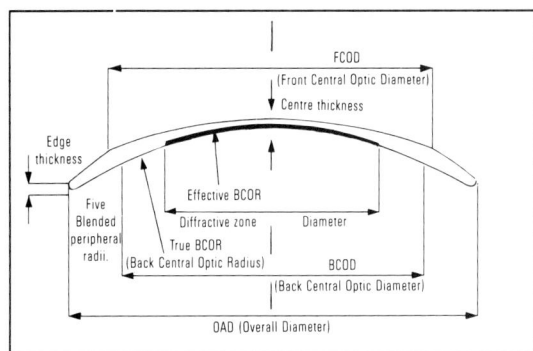

Figure 18.5 Diagram of the Diffrax bifocal contact lens. The diffractive area is in the posterior portion of the centre of the lens

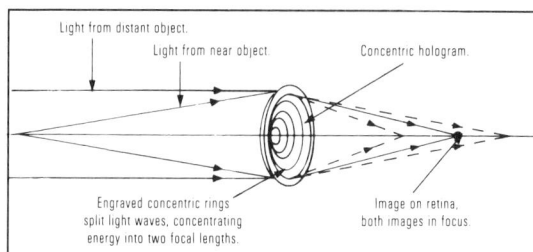

Figure 18.6 The Diffrax bifocal contact lens. The central 5.0 mm diameter diffractive portion concentrates light energy into two focal lengths

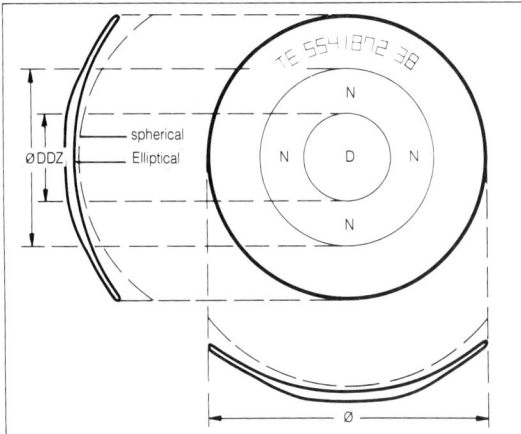

Figure 18.7 Diagram of the Weicon 38E bisoft contact lens. The lens has an elliptical, tangential back peripheral curve. There is a central distance zone surrounded by an annular near zone

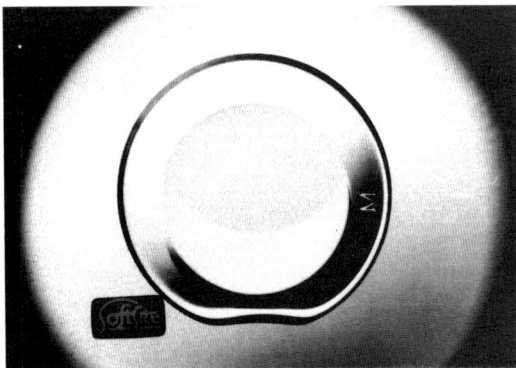

Figure 18.9 Diagram of the Softsite soft bifocal lens

Soft segment bifocal contact lenses

An example of such a lens is the Softsite bifocal contact lens (Softsite Contact Lens Laboratory, 4928 Le Jeune Road, Coral Gables, Florida, 33146, USA) (Figures 18.8 and 18.9). It is made of 45% water material, poly 2 hydroxyethyl methacrylate N-vinyl pyrrolidone.

The reading segment is crescent shaped and prism ballasted with a structural vent at the base of the prism.

The lens is made in two total diameters –

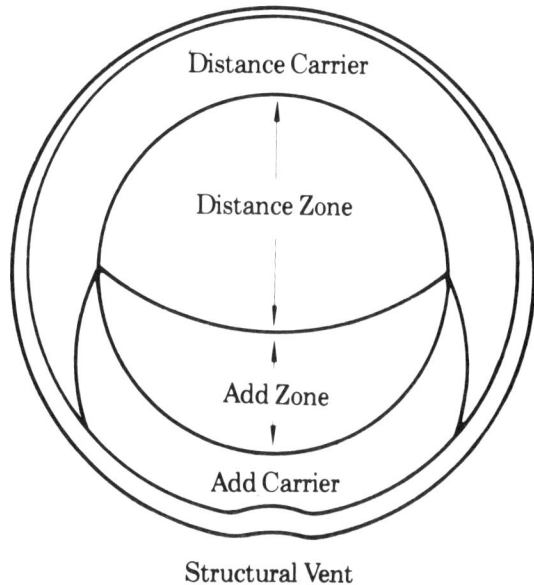

Figure 18.8 The Softsite soft bifocal lens. The segmented, crescentic near portion is prism ballasted and there is a structural vent below

13.5 mm (for plus lenses) and 14.0 mm (for minus lenses) – and three radii – F (flat), M (mid range), S (steep).

It is claimed that the success rate is best for hypermetropic and myopic contact lens wearers, slightly less for myopes between -1.50 D and -3.0 D and presbyopic emmetropes. Patients with very narrow palpebral fissures do not do as well as patients with larger palpebral fissures. Patients with the lower lid tangential to, or slightly lower than, the inferior limbus (scleral show below), adapt more easily than patients with the lower lid more than 1 mm above the inferior limbus.

The lens must fit reasonably loosely, so that it will translate into the reading mode upon down-gaze.

The flattest radius is chosen which:

1. is comfortable
2. does not fold away the cornea at the vent area
3. has the structural vent positioning at six o'clock, plus or minus 20°
4. centres on the eye.

The ophthalmoscope held at 18 inches (45 cm) from the eye can be used to evaluate the reading segment position and movement. Such lenses should not be used for persons whose acuity requirements include near objects in primary gaze, such as computer monitor operators, librarians and engineers. They are also unsuitable for patients who wish the lens primarily for working hours in which almost the full time is spent reading.

Soft non-spherical bifocal contact lenses

An example is the Nissel PS45 bifocal lens. This has a non-spherical front power curve on a spherical back curve. This 'S' form power curve, which relates directly to the spherical back curve (Figure 18.10), can, in its single vision form, maintain the same aberration-free power from lens centre to edge, unlike a normal spherical lens.

In its presbyopic form the degree of curvature undergoes constant controlled change so that, within a pre-determined power band, light rays from objects at all distances are directed to a common focal point (Figure 18.11). The brain is selective and interprets, with optimum clarity, only those impulses relevant to the object under observation. It is claimed that transfer, from one focus to another, is immediate, effortless and independent of eye position and that lateral vision is full and without distortion.

Fitting is the same as with a conventional soft lens. No more than 1.0 mm of movement should be seen with the blink. It is claimed that the lens will also reduce the effect of corneal cylinders.

The prescription powers cover an area of about 4.0 mm with the reading correction lying in the centre. This area focuses only divergent light. It is the area surrounding the central zone that deals with parallel rays. However, there is no sudden cut off of power beyond the prescription area. The maximum reading addition is plus two dioptres. The lens is made of hydroxyethyl methacryl-

Figure 18.11 The Nissel PS45 bifocal soft lens. The diagram represents the central area of the lens. The degree of curvature of the front curve undergoes constant controlled change so that, within a predetermined power band, light rays from objects at all distances are directed to a virtually common focal point

ate with ethylene glycol dimethacrylate, polymethyl methacrylate and polyvinyl pyrrolidone. Its water content is 38%.

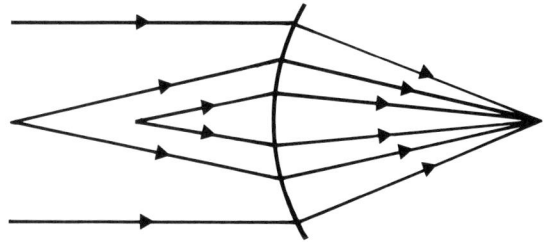

In fitting, selection of the initial trial lens should be based on power with the chosen lens being no more than 0.50 dioptres away from the final prescription (that is the distance power plus two dioptres). There is a standard back optic zone radius of 8.70 mm and a standard total diameter of 14.0 mm.

Young, Grey and Papas (1990) showed that the PS45 was, in fact, pupil dependent and Charman and Saunders (1990) showed that with the PS45 design the effective addition for near varied with the distance prescription.

Soft diffractive bifocal contact lenses

It will be remembered that the rigid diffractive lenses (Diffrax lenses) described earlier in this chapter were designed to be fitted apex clear (that is 0.10 mm steeper than the flattest keratometer reading). If these rigid lenses are fitted flat, and

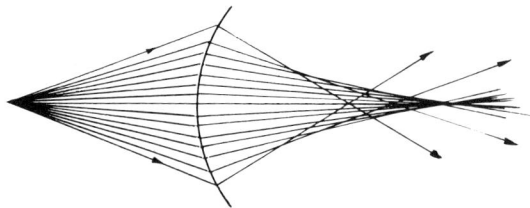

Conventional Lens   Spherical Aberration   Nissel 'S' Lens   No Spherical Aberration

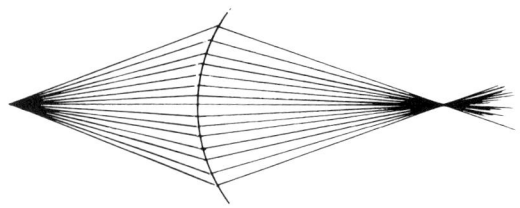

Figure 18.10 The Nissel PS45 bifocal soft lens. The 'S' form front power relates directly to the spherical back curve. In its single vision form it can maintain the same aberration free power from lens centre to edge, unlike a normal spherical lens

the diffractive area is in contact with the cornea rather than the precorneal film, then the near addition function of these lenses ceases to be effective.

Thin soft lenses drape themselves on the cornea, even if fitted moderately steeper than the corneal curvature, and emulate the corneal toricity. When they are thick or made of firm material, moderately steep lenses may bridge the cornea and thus give rise to marked fluctuation of vision when blinking takes place.

Allergan Ltd have introduced a soft contact lens (the Echelon), which in some undisclosed way, overcomes the first problem outlined above. It is a cast moulded lens which has on its back surface a series of microscopic 'echelettes' which form a diffractive phase plate across the entire optic zone (Figure 18.12). The word 'echelette' is presumably derived from the obsolete verb 'eche' which means to enlarge, augment or increase. The echelettes have a depth of less than three microns. The echelette diffractive phase plate splits light evenly between near and distant foci, maintaining both images equally bright. The lens is, of course, gaze independent, unlike segment bifocal contact lenses, and pupil size independent, unlike concentric bifocal contact lenses.

Unfortunately, there may be the problems which are encountered with hard diffractive lenses. Some patients may notice haloes around lights, especially at night. Others may notice ghost images around near objects, creating a 3D effect. The print may stand out from a printed page. There is also loss of contrast sensitivity which is most noticeable at low levels of illumination.

A diagnostic trial set is supplied with 16 lenses – eight distance powers and two addition powers – plus 1.25 D and plus 2.00 D. The lens is 13.8 mm in diameter.

Papas, Young and Hearn (1990) compared the Echelon lens with monovision. This was a crossover study involving 21 subjects and they found that the Echelon lens gave better stereopsis although monovision was subjectively preferred for reading.

References

BACK, A.P., HOLDEN, B.A. and HINE, N.A. (1989) Correction of presbyopia with contact lenses. Comparative success rates with three systems. *Optometry and Visual*

Diffractive Bifocal

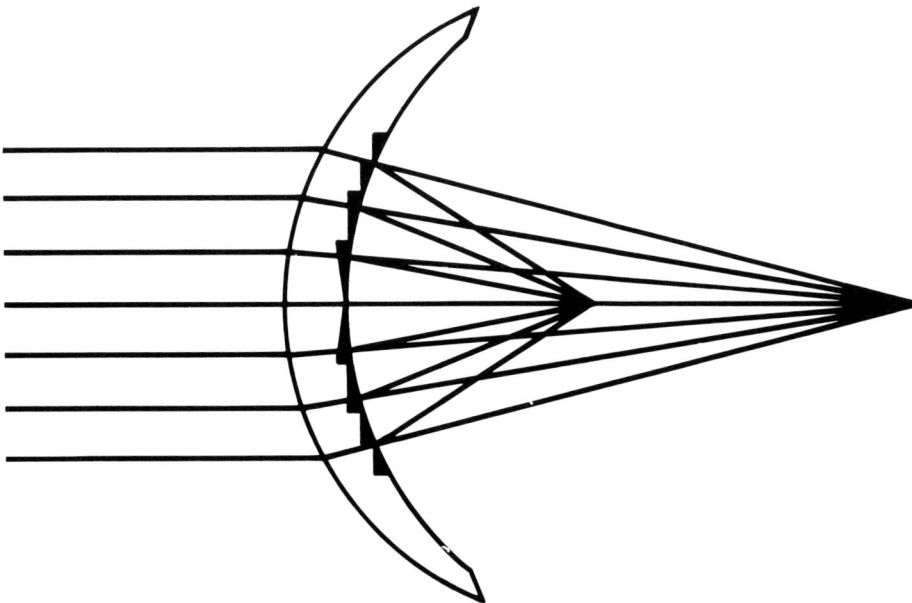

Figure 18.12 The Hydron Echelon lens. The diagram illustrates the lens which has a series of microscopic, concentric echelettes which form a diffractive phase plate across the entire optic zone of the back surface

Science, **66**, 8, 518–525

BAYSHORE, C.A. (1977) You can fit that presbyope. *Contact Lens Forum*, Dec., **2**, 12, 33–39

BEDDOW, R.D., MARTIN, J.S. and PHEIFFER, C.H. (1966) Presbyopic patients and single vision contact lenses. *Southern Journal of Optometry*, **8**, 11, 9–11

CHARMAN, W.N. and SAUNDERS, B. (1990) Theoretical and practical factors influencing the optical performance of contact lenses for the presbyope. *Journal of the British Contact Lens Association*, **13**, 67–75

MCGILL, E. and ERICKSON, P. (1988) Stereopsis in presbyopes wearing monovision and simultaneous vision bifocal contact lenses. *American Journal of Optometry and Physiological Optics*, **65**, 8, 619–626

PAPAS, E., YOUNG, G. and HEARN, K. (1990) Monovision vs soft diffractive bifocal contact lenses: a cross-over study. *International Contact Lens Clinic*, **17**, 181–186

SCARBOROUGH, S.T. and LOPANIK, R.W. (1976) A two-eyed look at the presbyopic patient. *Contact Lens Forum*, Sept., **1**, 9, 48–57

STONE, J. and FRANCIS, J.L. (1980) Practical optics of contact lenses and aspects of contact lens design. In *Contact Lenses* (Stone, J. and Phillips, A.J., eds). Butterworths, London and Boston, pp. 122–123

YOUNG, G., GREY, C.P. and PAPAS, E.B. (1990) Simultaneous vision bifocal contact lenses: a comparative assessment of the in vitro optical performance. *Optometry and Visual Science*, **67**, 339–345

Index

Acanthamoeba castellani
  chlorhexidine effect, 83
  heat disinfection, 80
  lens contamination, 75
Acanthamoeba culbertsoni, 84
Acanthamoeba keratitis, 88, 142–5
  treatment, 144–5
Acanthamoeba lens contamination, 75
Acanthamoeba polyphaga
  chlorhexidine effect, 83
  heat disinfection, 80
Acid burns, 168
Acoustic neuroma surgery, 176
Acute hypoxic keratopathy, 126
Acute toxic epitheliopathy, 126
Adrenaline, 78
Adrenochrome pigment staining, 78
Adsorbonac, 170
Aerotab, 86
Alkali burns, 168
Altered spherical power, 103
Amblyopia, 166
Amiclair, 79
Amphotericin B, collagen shield delivery, 186
Aniridia keratopathy, 166–7
Anterior stromal puncture, 180
Aphakia, 167, 208–14
  hard corneal lenses, 209–11
    displacement, 210
    ejection, 210
    endophthalmitis, 211
    minimal centre thickness, 213
    temporal ride, 211
  larger lens lid attachment lenses, 210
  paediatric, 212–13
    soft contact lenses, 214
  scleral lenses, 209
  small centring lenses, 209–10
  soft contact lenses, 211–12
    displacement, 211
    ejection, 211
    endophthalmitis, 212
    visual problem, 211–12
  water content lens, central thickness, 214
Aphakic contact lens, ulcerative keratitis associated, 90
Aquasteril, 81–2

Aseptization, 80
Aspergillus fumigatus
  heat disinfection, 80
  ultraviolet irradiation disinfection (Aquasteril), 81–2
Atopic conjunctival disease with keratopathy, 167
Autoclave, 87

Benzalkonium chloride, 78
BioCor, 185
Blenderm, 164
Blinking exercises, 115
Blue glue, 178
Botulinum toxin, 165, 177, 178
Bullous keratopathy, 167
Buphthalmos, 167

Calcium deposits, 77
Calestone, 17
Candida albicans
  Aerotab effect, 86
  Sonasept disinfection, 80
  ultraviolet irradiation disinfection, 81–2, 82
Care of contact lenses, 71–91
  gas permeable hard corneal lenses, 71–2
  hard polymethylmethacrylate corneal lenses, 71
  scleral lenses, 71
  soft hydrophilic lenses, 72
Casting materials, 17
Catarrhal ulcer, 137
Ceftazidime, 139
Cefuroxime, 139
Central corneal clouding, 102–3, 105
Central focal epithelial necrosis, 126–7
Chlorhexidine, 83
  side-effects, 83
Chronic chemical epitheliopathy, 133
Chlorine-releasing compounds, 86–7
Cicatricial conjunctival disease, 166–7
Cicatricial conjunctivitis, 174

Cicatricial pemphigoid, 168
Ciprofloxacin hydrochloride (Ciloxan), 140
Classification of contact lens materials, 50, 54
Cleaning, 79
Clen-zym, 79
Closure of eyes, 164–5
Clotrimazole, 144
Cogan's microcystic dystrophy (epithelial basement membrane dystrophy; map-dot-finger print line dystrophy), 169–70
Collagen corneal shields, 185–7
Conjunctival dysplasia, 172
Conjunctivitis, 130–1
  acute bacterial, 150
  allergic, 150
Cornea,
  acidosis, 46
  acute distortion, 133–4
  anaesthesia, 117
  cap, 24, 27
  crescentic erosions, 118
  diffuse lesions, 118
  endothelial polymegethism, 119, 149–50
  epithelial defects, 179
  epithelial dysplasia, 130
  epithelial erosion, 198
  epithelial microcysts, 135
  grafts, 89–91, 202–4
    hard corneal lenses, 202–4
      flat, 303
      steep, 202–3
      tilted, 203
    scleral contact lenses, 204
    soft contact lenses, 203–4
    SoftPerm lens, 203–4
  lacerations, 204
  lens long-term wear, 105
  mapping device, 24–7
  nebulae, 198–9
    diffuse, 198
    proud (nodules), 198–9
    reticular, 198
  oedema, 102–3, 105, 109–10, 124–5
  pellucid marginal degeneration, 178
  perforation, 178, 178–9

Cornea (cont.)
  recurrent erosions, 180–1
    diabetic, 181
    post-chemical burn, 181
    traumatic, 180
  scrappings, 162–3
  shape changes, 102
  sterile hypopyon, 138, 184–5
  sterile infiltrates, 184
  swelling response to anoxia, 47
  thickness increase, 103
  thinning, 45–6
  ulcer, 89
  vascularization, 116, 129, 143, 184
    keratoconus-induced, 189
  wrinkling, 184

Dellen formation, 114
Delayed response keratopathy,
  134–5
Deproteinization, 78–9
Desiccation staining, 128
Diffrax bifocal contact lens, 218
Disinfection, 79–87
  autoclave, 87
  chemical, 82–8
    chlorhexidines, 83
    chlorine-releasing compounds,
      86–7
    disodium edetate, 83
    polyquad, 84
    sorbic acid, 83–4
    thimerosal *see* Thimerosal
  dry heat sterilizer, 87
  heat, 79–80
  microwave, 80–1
  oxidizing systems, 85–7
    hydrogen peroxide, 85–6
  preservative-free saline, 87
  ultraviolet irradiation, 81–2
Disodium cromoglycate, 156
Disodium edetate, 83
Disposable contact lenses, 88
Doxycycline, 156
Drawing contact lenses, 40
Drug delivery, 171–2
Drug-induced keratopathy, 172
Dry eyes, 172–3
Dry heat sterilizer, 87
Durasoft, 167
D-value, 79
Dysport, 165

Elite lens, 57
Epidermal growth factor, 179
Epidermolysis bullosa, 173
Epikeratoplasty, 206–7
  hard corneal lenses, 206
  soft corneal lenses, 206–7

Epithelial basement membrane
  dystrophy (Cogan's microcystic
  dystrophy; map-dot-finger print
  dystrophy), 169–70
Erosive corneal epitheliopathy, 129
Escherichia coli disinfection, 81, 81–2
Eyelid defects, 174

Facial nerve palsy, 174–5
Familial dysautonomia (Riley-Day
  syndrome), 175, 176
Fenestration, 7
Fibronectin, 179
Filamentary keratitis, 173
Filtering blebs, 175
FLOM lens, 4–15
Fluorescein, 78
Fluroexan, 78
Fluoroquinolone antibiotics, 140
Foreign bodies, 118
Fort Dix Report, 102
Fuchs' corneal dystrophy, 167–8
Fungal keratitis, 141–12
Fusarium solarni, Aerotab effect, 86

Gas permeable lenses, 45–53, 105
  back central optic curve
    relationship, 52
  cellulose acetate butyrate lens,
    47–8
  corneal swelling responses, 48
  disadvantages of hard gas
    permeable lenses, 47–51
  fenestrations, 47
  high Dk values, 49
  lens lid attachment, 47
  lens thickness, 52
  lid attachment, 51–2
  overnight lens binding, 50
  scleral, 52
  SoftPerm, 52–3
  spontaneous movement of lens,
    50
  steepened lenses, 48
  three and nine o'clock staining, 51
  venting, 47
  wear by myopes, 50
  wettability, 51
Gas permeability (Dk value), 45
Gas transmissibility (Dk/L value), 45
Gentamicin, 140, 172
  collagen-shield delivery, 186
Giant papillary conjunctivitis, 108,
  120–1, 150–7
  atopic status of patient, 152
  clinical features, 153
  mast cells, 152
  mechanical factors, 154
  plastic as cause, 155
  protein on lens, 154–5

Glaucoma, 166, 175
Glued on syndrome, 50
Goldmann applanation tonometry,
  78
Graft-host disease, 168–9
Granular epithelial keratopathy, 133

Handling by ophthalmologist, 3–6
  inserting hard corneal lens, 3–4
  inserting scleral lens, 5–6
  inserting soft contact lens, 4–5
  removing hard corneal lens, 4
  removing scleral lens, 6
  removing soft contact lens, 5
  swan hold, 3
Hard corneal lens, 18 (fig.), 19–24
  adverse reactions, 109–21
    corneal anaesthesia, 117
    corneal deformation, 110
    corneal endothelial
      polymegathism, 119
    corneal lens intolerance, 110–11
    corneal oedema, 109–10, 111
      (fig.)
    crescentic erosions, 118
    dellen formation, 114
    diffuse corneal erosions, 118–19
    foreign bodies, 118
    giant papillary conjunctivitis *see*
      Giant papillary conjunctivitis
    nodular episcleritis, 120
    pingeculae formation, 114
    preservative keratopathy, 117
    pseudochalazion, 121
    ptosis, 121
    suppurative keratopathy, 119
    three and nine o'clock
      infiltrates, 114–15
    three and nine o'clock
      keratopathy, 112–13
    three and nine o'clock staining,
      113, 114 (fig.)
    vascularization, 116–17
  back optic zone diameter (BOZD)
    choice, 35
  back optic zone radius (BOZR), 31
  back peripheral curve/curves
    choice, 35–7
  calculation of power of fluid lens,
    32
  centring on cornea, 22, 23 (fig.),
    24–8
  collar-stud meniscus, 28
  dropping lens, 23
  edge thickness (Tea) choice, 39
  fitting, 24–44
  fluorescein patterns, 32, 33 (fig.)
  front optic zone diameter (FOZD)
    choice, 37
  front optic zone diameter/front

Hard corneal lens (cont.)
  peripheral radii for lens lid
    attachment, 43–4
  front peripheral curve/curves
    choice, 39
  froth, 21
  geometrical centre thickness (Tc),
    37–9
    advantages of minimum, 38–9
    axial edge lift, 38
    disadvantages of minimum, 39
    power of lens, 37–8
    reduced front optic zone
      construction, 38
    total diameter of lens, 38
  intolerance, 23–4
  keratometry readings *vs* back
    central radius, 32
  Korb technique, 30–1
  large back optic zone diameters,
    42
  large lens, 34–5
  lens lid attachment, 23, 29–31
  meniscus deformation, 22
  minimal geometric centre
    thickness of minus lenses, 43
  modifying, 44
  ordering, 44
  overhang meniscus, 28
  parameters calculation, 39–40
  photokeratometer calculation for
    corneal radii *vs* back optic
    zone radius of lens, 32
  preparations for use, 96
  small back optic diameters, 42
  small lens, 34
  temporal ride, 232
Hazing, 85–6
Heparin, collagen-shield delivery,
  186
Herpes zoster ophthalmicus, 176
Hibiclens, 83
Human immunodeficiency virus
  (HIV), lens contamination, 75–6
Human leucocyte interferon, 172
Hydrocare, 79
Hydrocurve II toric lens, 61–2
Hydroflex/m-T lens, 62, 63 (fig.)
Hydroflex-TS lens, 62, 63 (fig.)
Hydrogel contact lens, 165–6, 173
Hydrogen peroxide, 85–6
Hydron Echelon lens, 221
Hydron Z6T lens, 61, 64
Hypercapnia, 46
Hypermetropic patient, 105

Inferior closure staining, 128
Intracorneal haemorrhage, 148
Ionicity or ionic, 77
Iridocorneal endothelial syndrome
  (ice syndrome), 168
Iron particles, 78
Itraconazole, 144–5

Jelly bumps, 77
Juvenile atopic keratoconjunctivitis,
  167

KD plaster (Kaffir D plaster), 17
Keratan sulphate, 103
Keratoconjunctivitis sicca, 173
Keratoconus, 103, 104–5, 191–9
  associations:
    atopy, 192
    papillary conjunctivitis, 92
  corneal epithelial erosions, 198
  corneal lenses, 193–8
    fitting the apex, 194–5
    gas permeable, 197
    large alignment lens, 193
    large flat lens, 194–5
    large thin lens, 196
    post-keratoconic
      epikeratoplasty, 197–8
    small thin lens, 195–6
    Saturn lens, 197
    SoftPerm lens, 197
    Soper lens,
    toric soft lens, 197
  corneal nebulae, 198
    diffuse, 198
    proud (nodules), 198–9
    reticular, 198
  corneal vascularization, 198–9
  fitting set, 200
  Korb design lenses, 201–2
  scleral lenses
  Soper diagnostic lens set, 201
  thinning, 191
  treatment, 192–3
Keratoepithelioplasty, 172
Keratoplasty, 175–6
  cheesewiring of sutures, 175
  elevation of graft, 175
  failure of graft epithelialization,
    175–6
  Mooren's ulceration, 176
  tilting of graft, 176
  wood dehiscence, 176
Kromopan, 16

Lansche and Lee syndrome
  (overwear syndrome; two
  o'clock in the morning
  syndrome), 111–12
Lens cases, care of, 88–9
Lens contamination
  acanthamoeba, 74–5
  bacteria, 72–4
    Pseudomonas aeruginosa, 72, 73,
      74
    Serratia marcescens, 74
    Staphylococcus aureus, 74
    Staphylococcus epidermidis, 72–3
  fungi, 74

Lens contamination (cont.)
  human immunodeficiency virus
    (HIV), 75–6
Lens intolerance, 78
Lens lift, 4–5, 78
Lens spoliation, 76–8
  drug-induced, 78
Limbal follicles, 136–7
Limbitis, 129, 136–7
Linear IgA disease, 168
Linen measuring device, 36
Low water content lens, 165
Lunelle Rx lens, 65
Lysozyme, 76, 77

Map-dot-finger print line dystrophy
  (epithelial basement membrane
  dystrophy; Cogan's microcystic
  dystrophy), 169–70
Mast cells, 152
Meesmann's juvenile epithelial
  dystrophy, 165, 171
Megasoft Bandage Lens, 175
Methicillin, 139–40
Miniflex, 184
Miraflow, 79
Mirror image symmetry, 24
Mooren's ulceration, 176
Moulding materials, 16
  spatulation, 17
Mucin, 76, 77
Munsen's sign, 192
Mycobacterial (non-tuberculous)
  keratitis, 141
Myopia, 105

Neosporin, 140
Neuroparalytic keratitis, 164, 176–8
Nissel PS45 lens, 220
Nissel SV38 lens, 60–1
Nodular episcleritis, 120
Non-ionic polymers, 77
Norfloxacin, 140–1
Nummular keratitis, 137
Nystagmus, 178

Ophthalmic preparations, 96–100
Ophthalmic Zelex, 16
Optima Toric lens, 63
Overwear syndrome (Lansche and
  Lee syndrome; two o'clock in
  the morning syndrome), 111–12
Oxysept-1, 79
Oxytetracycline, 156

Papain, 79
  sensitization, 79
Papillary conjunctivitis, 192
Patient handling of contact lenses,
  67–70

Patient handling of contact lenses (cont.)
  hard corneal lenses, 67–8
  scleral lenses, 69–70
  soft lenses, 68–9
Peripheral focal arcuate epithelial necrosis, 127–8
pingeculae formation, 114
PMMA lens, 166
Polyhexamethylene biguanide (PHMB), 145
Polymegethism, 119, 149–50
Polyquad, 84
Polytrim, 140
Posterior annular keratopathy, 146–7
Posterior polymorphous dystrophy, 168
Posterior stromal opacification, 147–9
Post-membranous conjunctivitis, 169
Post-radiation keratopathy, 179–80
Presbyopia, 215–21
  monovision, 215–16
  rigid diffractive bifocal contact lens, 218
  soft concentric bifocal contact lens, 218–19
  soft diffractive bifocal contact lens, 220–1
  soft non-spherical bifocal contact lens, 220
  soft segment bifocal contact lens, 219–20
Primecare, 79
Progenitor (stem) cells, 128
Prolonged bullous keratopathy, 49
Protein deposits, 76–7
Pseudochalazion, 121
Pseudomonas aeruginosa
  keratitis, 88
  lens contamination, 72, 73
  microwave, disinfection, 81
  preservative-free saline effect, 87
  Sonasept disinfection, 80
  ultraviolet irradiation disinfection, 81–2, 82
Pseudopemphigoid, 169
Ptosis, 122, 180

Radial keratotomy, 204–6
  hard lenses, 205–56
  soft lenses, 206
Refraction problems, 101–6
  hard lenses, 101–5
  scleral lenses, 105
  soft lenses, 105–6
Reis-Bücklers superficial corneal dystrophy, 170–1
Retinitis pigmentosa, 181

Saltzmann's nodular dystrophy, 171
Sattler's veil, 105, 106
Saturn lens, 106
Sauflex 55 lens, 57
Scleral lenses, 7
  adverse reactions, 107–8
    corneal opacification, 107, 108 (fig.)
    corneal vascularization, 107
    giant papillary conjunctivitis, 108, *see also* Giant capillary conjunctivitis
    Sattler's veil, 105, 106
  fitting, 7–16
  fitting problems, 15–16
    clicking, 16
    frothing, 16
    mucus under lens, 16
    overall lens size disparity, 15–16
    rotation, 15
  flush fitting, 13
  moulded, 8–11
    moulding, 8
    preparation of cast, 8–9
    preparation of shell, 9–11
  preformed hard, 13–15
    separate lenses, 14–15
      FLOM lenses, 14–15
      offset fitting set, 14
      transcurve fitting, 14
    single lens, 13–14
  preparation, 11–13
  slotted, 169, 193
Septicon, 85
Serratia marcescens, 74
  lens case contamination, 88
  lens contamination, 74
  microwave disinfection, 81
  ultraviolet irradiation disinfection, 81–2
Sodium chloride ointment, 170
Softab, 86
Soft contact lenses, 55–6
  adverse reactions, 124–57
    acute bacterial conjunctivitis, 150
    acute corneal distortion, 133–4
    acute hypoxic keratopathy, 126
    acute toxic epitheliopathy, 126
    cararrhal ulcer, 137–8
    central focal epithelial necrosis, 126–7
    chronic chemical epitheliopathy
    corneal endothelial polymegethism, 149–50
    corneal epithelial microcysts, 135
    corneal oedema, 124–5
    corneal thinning, 145–6
    corneal vascularization, 145
    delayed response keratopathy, 134–5

Soft contact lenses (cont.)
  desiccation staining, 128
  giant papillary conjunctivitis *see* Giant papillary conjunctivitis
  granular epithelial keratopathy, 133
  inferior closure staining, 128
  intracorneal haemorrhage, 146
  limbic follicles, 136–7
  limbitis, 136–7
  nummular keratitis, 137
  peripheral focal arcuate epithelial necrosis, 127–8
  posterior annular keratopathy, 146–7
  posterior corneal complications, 146
  posterior stromal opacification, 147–9
  prolonged bullous keratopathy, 149
  sterile corneal infiltrates, 138
  subepithelial haemorrhages, 135–6
  suppurative keratitis *see* Suppurative keratitis
  thimerosal keratopathy *see* Thimerosal keratopathy
  total endothelial bedewing, 146
  visual complications, 157
  preparations for use with, 100
  therapeutic, 165
Soft contact lens fitting, 55–8
  choice of lens, 57–8
    plastic material, 57
    water content, 57–8
  technique, 56–7
Soft Lens Care Tablets, 79
Softsite lens, 219
Sonasept, 80
Sorbic acid, 83–4
Stabilizers, 85
Staphyloccocus aureus
  lens contamination, 74
  microwave disinfection, 81
  ultraviolet irradiation disinfection, 81–2, 82
Staphylococcus epidermidis, lens contamination, 72–3, 74
Stem (progenitor) cells, 128
Sterile hypopyon, 138, 184–5
Steroids, topical, 141, 156, 178
Stevens-Johnson syndrome, 169
Streptococcus mutans, 91
Stromal puncture, 180
Subepithelial hemorrhage, 116, 135–6
Subtilisin A, 79
Sulindac, 145
Sulphasalazine, 78
Suppurative keratitis, 87, 88, 120, 138–45, 185
  acanthamoebic, 142–5

Suppurative keratitis (cont.)
  bacterial, 138–41
  fungal, 141–2
Suprofen, 156

Tape closure of eyes, 164
Tear(s), 154–5
  evaporation rate, 72–3
Tear film interferometry in vivo, 5
Ten Ten, 85
Terrien's ectatic marginal
  dystrophy, 181
Tetracycline, 156, 178
Theodore's superior limbic
  keratoconjunctivitis, 182
Therapeutic uses of contact lenses,
  164–87
Thimerosal, 79, 82–3
  allergic conjunctivitis induced by,
    150
Thimerosal keratopathy, 128–32
  conjunctivitis, 130–2
  corneal epithelial dysplasia, 130
  erosive corneal epitheliopathy,
    129
  superior limbitis, 129–32

Three and nine o'clock infiltrates,
  114–5
Three and nine o'clock keratopathy,
  112–3
Three and nine o'clock staining,
  113, 114 (fig.)
Thygeson's superficial punctate
  keratitis, 165, 166, 182–3
Tight lens syndrome, 165, 182–3
Timolol, 171
Tinted soft lens, 167
Tissutex, 16
Tobramycin, collagen-shield
  delivery, 186
Topogometer, 24
Toric back surface lens, 61–3
Toric front surface lenses, 63–5
Toric hard corneal lens, 59
Toric hard corneal lens fitting,
  58–60
  prism ballast, 60
  toric back optic zone, 60
  truncation, 59–60
Toric soft corneal lens fitting, 60–1
Torisoft lens, 64–5
Total endothelial bedewing, 46
Trachoma, 169, 183
Transpore, 164

Trauma, 145
Trigeminal neuralgia, 176
Two o'clock in the morning
  syndrome (Lansche and Lee
  syndrome; overwear
  syndrome), 111–12

Ulcerative keratitis, 88, 89–90
Ultrazyme, 79

Vancomycin, 14
  collagen-shield delivery, 186
Ventilation, 7
Videokeratograph, 24, 25 (fig.), 26
  (fig.)
Vibrio cholerae, ultraviolet irradiation
  disinfection, 81

Weicon 38E bisoft, 218, 219 (fig.)
Wet filamentary keratitis, 183–4

Z-value, 79